The Neurological Side of Neuropsychology

The Neurological Side of Neuropsychology

Richard E. Cytowic, MD

A Bradford Book
The MIT Press
Cambridge, Massachusetts
London, England

Seventh printing, 1996

This book was set from text files provided by the author in Trump by Asco
Trade Typesetting Ltd., Hong Kong and was printed and bound in the
United States of America.

Library of Congress Cataloging-in-Publication Data

Cytowic, Richard E.
    The neurological side of neuropsychology / Richard E. Cytowic.
      p.   cm.
    "A Bradford book."
    Includes bibliographical references and index.
    ISBN 0-262-03231-7 (hc : alk. paper)
    1. Clinical neuropsychology.   I. Title.
    [DNLM: 1. Neuropsychology. 2. Brain—physiology. 3. Mental
Processes—physiology. 4. Brain—psychology. 5. Neuropsychological
Tests.   WL 103.5 C997   1995]
    RC341.C98   1995
    616.8—dc20
    DNLM/DLC
    for Library of Congress   92-1528
                                                                      CIP

To Bobby
in memoriam

Contents in Brief

Contents in Detail

Acknowledgements

I am grateful to many patients for their trust and the privilege of sharing intimate details of their person, mind, and spirit; and to colleagues in diverse disciplines for fruitful discussions regarding the biologic basis of mind.

The Neurological Side of Neuropsychology

1 What Is Neuropsychology?

The World Federation of Neurology officially dubbed the 1990s "The Decade of the Brain." Although I would have thought that every decade was one of the brain for professionals interested in the mind, what the Federation intimated by this label is humanity's ever-increasing understanding of mental life. Speaking as one of the world's 23,000 neurologists (surprisingly few, aren't there?), I recall that not too long ago only the most thoughtful, self-motivated, and philosophically-oriented practitioners pondered how mind emerges from brain. Today, that question challenges bright individuals from several disciplines. The public, too, is fascinated, judging by the number of television shows and popular books that promise to explain "how the brain works." Unhappily, we cannot yet fully meet that promise. Maybe we never can.

Through considerable effort, however, we have learned relatively more about the detailed workings of the brain in the past ten years than we have in the entire history of science. For example, we can now trace with superb precision the course of a visual stimulus from its earliest neural transformations in the retina through its every cerebral pathway, and thereby postulate how an image is built up at the cellular level (Zeki, 1993). We can similarly trace details for hearing and, to a lesser extent, touch and other sensations. For even longer, we have been able to describe in exquisite detail the brain mechanisms of movement.

But when we try to fashion an overall view that a newcomer might understand, we can nowhere find an anatomical spot, conceptual framework, or even a hypothetical process of integration to which we can point and say, "This is how we come to understand." We don't really know how physical events, about which we know so much, are experienced ultimately as mental ones. An understanding of how the mind's conscious and unconscious expressions are organized eludes us even as the sheer number of facts and hypotheses about its detailed workings threaten to overwhelm the working neuroscientist.

In addition to this avalanche of facts poised to overcome the newcomer, clear and descriptive texts are not readily avaiable that offer both a broad vista and an explanation of what students are seeing. Existing neuropsychological texts are either too test-oriented or organized strictly along behavioral lines. The unevenness of multi-authored books denies students a unified viewpoint, and they often delve into too much detail for medical residents, graduate students, or interested professionals from other fields who are trying to grasp the concept of neuropsychology for the first time.

As a practical primer, *The Neurological Side of Neuropsychology* introduces contemporary neurological ideas to the beginner. It combines behavioral neurology with clinical neuropsychology in an attempt to relate today's understanding of cellular anatomy, chemoarchitecture, and brain organization to clinical findings. This book is problem-oriented rather than actuarial in approach. For example, it presents a radically different view of brain organization and function than is typically understood by the average scientist. The hierarchical and mostly linear organization of what has long been regarded as the "standard model" has been replaced. The new model organizes the brain into multiplex, reciprocal, and distributed systems based on a host of new facts about anatomy and function. Although my bias is clearly biological, I believe that the reader will comprehend the methods, assumptions, and implications of neuropsychology as a multidisciplinary enterprise.

I answer this chapter's question, "What is neuropsychology?" by saying that it seeks to explain behavior in terms of brain function. Constrained by biology, it tries to provide structural, functional, and psychological concepts of behavior that are coherent. But it also hopes to discover "how we come to understand." This is a formidable task in that some people seriously doubt whether the brain is capable of understanding itself. These doubters believe our quest has the fate of a parabolic curve approaching a mathematical asymptote: It gets closer and closer but ultimately never reaches it. In another sense, neuropsychology is not so formidable because we can approach many complex phenomena by dissecting them and examining their parts (this method only works to a point, however). Exciting explorations are under way, for example, in probing the cellular basis of memory, in imaging and recording methods that permit brain mapping of cellular groups and their connections to be correlated with specific functions, and in understanding how oscillating electrical potentials in widely separated brain regions might assemble sense impressions into a single object.

Although neuropsychology is a dynamic field of inquiry, parts of it are relatively easy to understand, and the conceptualizations of both psychology and anatomy in these parts have remained stable for some time now. Don't think, however, that I will feed you only the easy stuff. That wouldn't be fair. What I will do is show you the forest rather than the trees by emphasizing method over facts because neuropsychology is, more than anything else, a *method*, a way of approaching a problem. It helps that the neurological side of neuropsychology emphasizes patients over abstractions. Facts out of context can be dry and dreary, whereas those gleaned in a human context can be fascinating, even seductive. For the newcomer, grasping the big picture is far more important than gathering details. It is the big picture that makes the multidisciplinary facets of neuropsychology coherent. For example, the older literature seems confusing and contrary until you understand how our conceptualizations of cognitive psychology and nervous tissue have changed over past decades. Without understanding the evolution of thought regarding the major issues, you may become lost trying to reconcile the disparate viewpoints that you will surely encounter. Only twenty years ago, interested persons could easily assimilate what was known about the brain as well as concepts of cognition. Received knowledge is not as well received as it used to be.

In seeing how conceptualizations have changed over time, the newcomer will also understand that so-called facts are not intransmutable but are subject to replacement or reïnterpretation. Therefore, throw your energy not into memorizing labile facts, but into learning how to acquire them and judge them critically.

BACKGROUND DISCIPLINES OF NEUROPSYCHOLOGY

The mind is a range of functions and experiences produced by the brain. Neuropsychology's interest in explaining human behavior in terms of brain function is relatively recent and comes from the convergence at the end of the nineteenth century of four fields: (1) neuroanatomy, (2) physiology, (3) biochemistry, and (4) psychology.

I will talk about how we conceptualize nervous tissue in chapter 3. For now, let me point out that its complexity was not appreciated until the appearance of the compound microscope. Well into the eighteenth century, the mind was thought to reside in the three cerebral ventricles and the nerves were considered hollow tubes that conveyed animating energy from the lungs to the body.

Although the silver impregnation stain invented by the Italian histologist Camillo Golgi (1843–1926) made it possible to see the entire span of individual neurons, "factual" observations of his day persuaded a majority of his colleagues to believe that nervous tissue was a continuous syncytial net (Golgi, 1873). In contrast, the Spanish histologist Santiago Ramón y Cajal championed the neuron theory (1901, 1933), and proved much later that the neuron was indeed the basic signaling unit of nervous tissue. Their rivalry over neuron versus network theory was still intense when Golgi and Ramón y Cajal shared the Nobel Prize in 1906.

It is striking to appreciate that nervous tissue is everywhere similar yet functionally different in various anatomical regions. Sensory receptors respond only to mechanical (touch, hearing), chemical (taste, smell), or electromagnetic (vision) flux. Regardless of the type of fiber or whether the process concerned is movement, sensation, or thought, neural signals per se are virtually identical. It is often said that a nerve fiber can either fire or not (a binary choice leading to claims that the brain is a computer), and can only alter the number of impulses per second if it does. (The fraction of neurons that selectively can secrete more than one transmitter have a slightly broader repertoire.) We will see that that preceding statement is not quite true, yet despite the evident sameness of nervous tissue, widely divergent functions are supported by *regional anatomy* (in which topology is the important factor) and *cellular anatomy* (in which connections with other cell groups are important). Augmenting these differences are the release of disparate neurotransmitters by different neurons and the fact that synapses can be either excitatory or inhibitory.

Neurophysiology showed the importance of electricity to animal physiology. An early example is Luigi Galvani's work with frogs in

1791. Much later, the discovery that drugs interact with specific cell-surface receptors formed the basis for understanding the role of synaptic chemistry in nerve transmission. Today we can trace the detailed anatomy of neurochemical pathways and their terminal projection fields. Where once we thought that the synapse was the whole story, we now know that peptides, hormones, and other molecules are carriers of information that—remarkably—does not even travel along nerve fibers (such signaling outside of the hardwired circuitry is called volume transmission). The dynamics between chemistry and behavior are becoming clearer.

The relationship between the mind and the brain is vast and old. Much of contemporary Western thought derives from Aristotle, and standard sources should satisfy any need for topical review (e.g., Lavine, 1984). The psychological part of neuropsychology has its strongest roots in philosophy and spans many centuries. However, the Descartian approach to behavior of systematically analyzing its component parts did not appear until the nineteenth century. Here, the work of Charles Darwin on the evolution of animal behavior and physical traits perhaps freed psychology from the penumbra of philosophy and religion, allowing it to become both an independent discipline as well as one that flourished by application of experimental method.

After it loosened itself from philosophy, the psychological part of neuropsychology developed along the lines of experimentation and clinical observation. William James (1842–1910), the American philosopher and psychologist, systematized much of what was then known in his *Principles of Psychology* (1890).[1] Early on, for example, experimental psychologists described the speed and limits of rudimentary sensory, motor, memory, and perceptual events. More recently, psychologist Saul Sternberg (1969) not only decomposed complex abilities into a string of simpler ones but also developed a method for characterizing those singular components. Psychologists have subsequently developed many sophisticated behavioral tasks to tease out the constituents of *seemingly unitary* cognitive skills.

Be mindful, however, that behavioral data alone can never explain mental operations. By honoring the concrete realities of the brain's biology, we can constrain any set of possible theories that might explain a given behavior. The fact that our historical understanding of what the brain is has been a moving target helps to clarify why evolution of and conflict among such theories even existed. The overlap of neuropsychology's four main disciplines further fueled the rivalry of ideas. All these factors can confuse the newcomer. For example, the French physiologist Pierre Flourens (1794–1867) observed how animal behavior was affected by removing various parts of the brain. His observations led to the view that behavior derived from the cortex as a whole, any part of which could support all mental functions. This *global concept* predicted that damage anywhere would affect all mental functions equally.

The concept of *cellular connectivity*, however, viewed the relationship between brain and behavior as just the opposite. British neurologist Hughlings Jackson (1835–1911) deduced from observations of focal epilepsy that specific motor and sensory functions were localized to discrete brain areas. His clinical insight was later supported by both Ramón y Cajal (1852–1934), who showed that neurons connected with a high degree of order and specificity, and Carl Wernicke (1848–1904), a German neurologist who showed that some behavior was determined by discrete pathways connecting specific brain regions.

In the next two chapters, I will say more about these two views and subsequent developments in our understanding of nervous tissue and the mind. Suffice it to say for now that both areas of conceptualization have undergone dramatic changes, yet each retains some aspect of earlier thought. It is sometimes hard for students to reconcile changing concepts. Our habit of polar thinking leads us to assume that one model must replace another. Yet each contains some truth, and one scheme is not necessarily mutually exclusive of another. The nineteenth-century hierarchical view was based on evolutionary theory and held that the brain develops in phylogeny by successive additions to existing structures. Regulation of the more "primitive" and caudal parts of the brain by the "higher" portions is explicit in this view. Dissolution of this hierarchy is supposedly revealed by focal brain disease in humans or by severing pathways in animals. This hierarchical view influenced brain research well into recent times but is now transcended by ideas about the *unit module* and the *distributed system*, concepts that see the brain as an assemblage of widely and reciprocally interconnected dynamic (and nonlinear) systems.

Therefore, I suggest that you think of neither neurology nor neuropsychology in hierarchical terms. Regarding neuropsychology's major disciplines, you might think instead of an equilateral triangle with behavior at any one vertex, neuroscience at another, and psychology at the third. This triangular arrangement represents the interplay among disciplines, with none paramount yet all interdependent.

The behavioral sciences, exemplified by cognitive psychology, linguistics, psychophysics, and anthropology, describe what the brain does. To be useful, however, such descriptions must relate to underlying neural mechanisms.

Neuroanatomy and neurophysiology, collectively called *neuroscience*, inform us about biological constraints. Neuroanatomy is the study of the brain's structure, whereas neurophysiology is the study of the dynamic properties of neurons. For example, it takes a millisecond for an impulse to cross a synapse and evidently longer for a series of such crossings. Psychology tells us that object recognition takes about one second (i.e., a thousand times as long). Therefore, any model that hopes to encompass both neural events and clinical behavior must include all necessary activity in a time span of just three orders of magnitude, or a thousand synaptic crossings. Additionally, advances in molecular biology and chemoarchitecture are opening up our understanding of the neurochemical foundations of brain function. Memory is one ability that is now yielding to multiple analytical levels of transmitters, synapses, and receptors.

Psychology deals mainly with mental function per se, typically by analyzing the effects of selective brain damage on behavior. You may substitute "cognitive science" for "psychology" if you believe that the mind is computational. I am skeptical about this possibility for reasons detailed in chapter 8. While neuropsychology and cognitive science share many features, even many of the same disciplines, they differ in one important respect: Cognitive science assumes that cognition is autonomous and can be studied in isolation from biological, cultural, and social contexts (or any context for that matter). It also relies heavily on computer science, especially artificial intelligence and neural networks (see, e.g., von Eckardt, 1993). In contrast to the minority of scientists who doubt that the mind is computational, most students of the brain do assume that human thinking is representational and speak of multiple representations, or "maps," of the world that we some-how assemble into subjective experience. These representations correspond to different operations at different levels of the brain.

Lastly, I should mention that an interdisciplinary interest in brain and mind sometimes causes unintentional problems, given that each discipline comes with its own grab-bag of assumptions and methodologies. For example, localization has long interested neurologists. Now, other scientists try increasingly to relate for-mally-defined cognitive operations to anatomy. Some of the tech-niques used in such attempts are imaging, the molecular biology of receptors, and the analysis of time-locked electrical and magnetic oscillations. The underlying assumptions of such disparate meth-ods, however, are often different. The necessary shift among con-ceptual frameworks that so often plagues the newcomer is the distinction between top-down and bottom-up approaches to any intellectual discipline.

Bottom-up approaches are usually easier to grasp. Students in a given science enter the field and are trained in its basic framework. As they work away and eventually approach the controversial frontiers, they may be struck by deep, baffling, conceptual prob-lems that they have come upon from the bottom up.[2]

A philosopher, on the other hand, confronts the same problem from the top down. A philosopher's education emphasizes broad questions throughout history, a methodology for science, and a theory of what theory is in general. All this gives the philosopher a particular approach to problems. Confronted with a quandary in biology, for example, someone with a philosophical background ponders with a frame of mind quite unlike that of a biologist who encounters the same problem from a grass-roots training. A broad education lets the philosopher comes down on it and see it in a different way. We are all looking into the same room through dif-ferent windows. What difficulties you might encounter in trying to understand neuropsychology depend in part on your own intel-lectual background.

DIFFERENT KINDS OF NEUROPSYCHOLOGISTS

Neuropsychologists occupy several camps, each having a some-what different interest. Professional jealousy and turf wars that have arisen from time to time can be understood in terms of how these distinctions came about. Knowing this can help when you read the older literature. The three camps of original neuropsychologists were physiological psychologists, neurologists, and clinical psychologists.

If you wanted to be a neuropsychologist before 1975, you simply called yourself one. A few universities offered some special courses and, if you were a psychologist, you could say that you knew something about neuropsychology when you finished your doctoral degree, but there was really no explicit training for either medical doctors or doctors of philosophy. Among the early American founders of neuropsychology, Ralph Reitan was a physiological psychologist, Arthur Benton was a clinical psychologist who became interested in brain function, and Norman Geschwind was a neurologist interested in the brain organization of behavior.

Each professional discipline possessed special skills, but each also had to supplement its knowledge if it hoped to explain behavior and cognition in terms of brain function. Physiological psychologists needed to acquire clinical skills in order to study brain-damaged patients, clinical psychologists needed to learn anatomy and physiology, and neurologists, despite their strong background in clinical diagnosis and the clinico-anatomical relationships between brain lesions and bodily dysfunction, were woefully ignorant of psychology. In 1973, the National Institute of Mental Health, sensing perhaps a shortage of knowledgeable individuals, began offering postdoctoral fellowships at the University of Houston for turning out certified neuropsychologists. Others soon followed suit.

Differences among the types of neuropsychologists split not so much along the line of medical versus doctoral training as they do between a "brain mechanism group" and a "neurotic-psychotic group." These two groups can be diametrically opposed in their search for a physical explanation of abnormal behavior. The brain mechanism group (those with physiological or medical backgrounds) tries to rule in brain damage, while the neurotic-psychotic group (usually psychiatrists and clinical psychologists) tries to rule it out.

It should not be surprising that the biases of different backgrounds lead to disparate results in treating the many neurological and general medical disorders that feature a change in mental status. Sbordone and Rudd (1986) showed that thirty percent of psychologists failed to recognize underlying neurological disorders. Geschwind (1975) showed that neurological causes of psychiatric disorder are far from rare and that misdiagnosis and inappropriate treatment of such patients are common. Mental symptoms or a change in personality usually are interpreted by family as "psychological" and explained away as anxiety or depression. Thus, Sbordone showed that when a relative brings a patient in for evaluation, psychologists are unduly influenced by the erroneous conclusions (interpretation) of the relative and are more inclined to recommend inappropriate psychotherapy for an underlying physical problem.

If there is a difference between MDs and PhDs, it seems to me that psychologists tend to emphasize standardized tests more than physicians do. A sharp neuropsychologist of whatever educational stripe should have a good idea of what is wrong with the patient in the first minutes of interaction. Physicians are likely to stop sooner and justify a clinical diagnosis, whereas psychologists are likely to spend more time demonstrating closure through testing. I discuss the important uses of formal neuropsychological testing in chapter 4.

Testing, of course, was a prime means for localization before the advent of computed tomographic (CT) scanning, which was invented in Britain in 1971 and introduced to the United States the following year. Previously, there was a huge emphasis on the neuroanatomical locus responsible for a patient's symptoms. Neuropsychology was the best tool for determining "where the hole was," to help direct neurosurgeons where to muck around, and to guide the differential diagnosis among stroke, tumor, subarachnoid hemorrhage and other conditions. (Yes, you read that sentence correctly—it was the *best* tool.)

Today, various scans tell us where the hole is and often what causes it, so we now look to neuropsychology to tell us how bad it is. We want a percentage impairment or suggestions for rehabilitation, if possible. Because we know where the lesion is (thanks to scanning) and understand the gross anatomy (thanks to earlier workers), we are now more interested in the mechanism of function at the cellular and cell-groups level than in localization per se.

Those who assume that neuropsychological analysis must be inferior to the capacity of computed tomography, magnetic resonance imaging (MRI), or some other technology to identify brain lesions might consider that as autopsy series once revealed brain lesions that went undetected in life, so also do modern techniques expose structural abnormalities that are clinically silent. Imaging is not the final word. It is also a fatal error to assume that function is strictly localized or that discrete lesions on scans are isolated. By this I mean a failure to consider the multiplex character of neural physiology, diaschisis, reciprocal interaction with anatomically remote areas, and even restoration of function.

Enthusiasm for a gold standard based on some technology is dashed by the reality that neuropsychology is often the dependent variable in determining whether a disease is present or not. Dementia is the obvious example. Furthermore, the behavioral sequelæ of cardiac arrest and heart-lung bypass, substrate deficiency, poisoning, and metabolic aberrations exist without any structural footprint at all. Technology has not made the practitioner's intelligence passé. Properly done, neuropsychological analysis remains a powerful tool.

LEARN BY HANDS-ON EXPERIENCE

It is difficult to imagine a time when human anatomy was not considered common property. Postmedieval medicine would be hard put to understand the human body more reliably than by direct observation—that is, by dissection. Up to the sixteenth century, ancient medical texts were believed to be more authoritative than any hands-on experience ever could be. Small wonder that Andreas Vesalius's *De humani corporis fabrica* (*Fabric of the Human Body*, 1543) was such an inflammatory publication. Blind faith in Galen had so long been the authority that the traditional dissection was performed by a seated professor reading from the book, a surgeon performing the dissection, and an assistant pointing out the details. Discrepancies with the text were either regarded as anomalies or not acknowledged at all.

The analogy is that you too must learn by direct observation—by dissecting your clinical interactions with patients. First, you must learn anatomy in detail. You cannot hope to understand neuropsychology without a good, three-dimensional grasp of anatomy. (Such understanding matures slowly, after years of experience.) If your institution offers brain cutting sessions, by all means go. Seize any opportunity to dissect a brain yourself. You will learn more from hands-on experience than from any amount of reading, and you cannot rely solely on texts or the opinions of others. What Vesalius did was to make science, specifically human anatomy, common property. You too must believe that human behavior is common property, yours for the taking through constant observation. Never decline the opportunity to examine patients. Engage them, analyze the interaction, and make the most of the gold mine in which you find yourself. No one would sail a boat solo without having first learned something about sailing, yet not examining patients is like reading about sailing while sitting on the shore, never taking to the water. Do not put off seeing patients because you don't feel "ready." Of course you will make mistakes—you're learning. Accuracy and efficiency come with repeated practice, as do the fun and intellectual satisfaction.

In the course of learning you must guard against sloppy thinking, faulty logic, self-delusion, incorrect leaps, judgemental bias, and seeing what you want to see. You will also encounter a wide range of practitioners and teachers, from those brilliant minds that make elegant formulations to plodding dolts devoid of any imagination or aptitude for sorting out facts. So, *en garde*!

Finally, you can expect to encounter laypersons fascinated by the brain, for whom no concept is too simple. In an old *New Yorker* cartoon poking fun at the popularization of split-brain research, a woman rebuffs a would-be seducer by saying, My right brain says Yes, but my left brain says No. This reminds me of the Parisian intelligentsia who flocked to Charcot's Tuesday evening public lectures, seeking a drought sufficiently shallow so that they might act fashionably knowledgeable about the then-new science of neurology. Beware of little knowledge.

NOTES

1. A blending of disciplines is seen in William James' own life. He studied philosophy and theology, received his MD from Harvard and, along the way, studied physics and physiology with Hermann von Helmholtz, pathology with Rudolph Virchow (inventor of cellular theory), and laboratory

science with Claude Bernard, the foremost experimentalist of nineteenth century medicine. He studied art as well and accompanied the naturalist Louis Agassiz to the Amazon.

2. Deep conceptual problems do not confront every science. Chemistry, for example, has none that I can think of, while evolutionary biology is full of them. Physics is plagued in two special areas: space-time, and quantum theory.

SUGGESTED READINGS

Goetz CG, tr. 1987 *Charcot, the Clinician: The Tuesday Lessons.* New York: Raven Press

Haymaker W, Schiller F, eds. 1970 *The Founders of Neurology,* 2d ed. Springfield, IL: Charles C Thomas

Wolpert L. 1993 *The Unnatural Nature of Science.* Cambridge: Harvard University Press

I   Conceptualizations

The traditional separation of philosophy, psychology, and neuroscience into distinct academic disciplines has led to several discrete approaches to the mind. Few areas of human inquiry remain static, yet neuropsychology is often taught without regard for its multipartite growth. The next two chapters review the evolution of fundamental concepts in neuropsychology. Chapter 2 deals with changing concepts of the mind, while chapter 3 addresses changing concepts of nervous tissue.

A concept is a general notion or idea, often in set form, that is taken into the mind. It originates in the mind as a design, idea, or a plan. Human minds interpret the physical facts of human brains and the clinical observations of human behavior, as they are given to our senses, to produce conceptualizations of what the mind and brain each are.

Although one intuitively supposes that the rules, observations, and facts that fill textbooks are "totally objective" (more on that assumption in chapter 8), I invite you to look at them for now as an *interpretation*, an attempt to explain, as Kant put it, "experience as we know we have it." Locke's philosophical musings tried to discover which properties of experience are "in the objects" and which are "in the mind," phrases which I hope heighten my point that conceptualizations are products of human minds and therefore dynamic entities that can never claim to be complete or ideally true. We will also come to see later how there is no escape from subjectivity, and that the notion of objectivity is a delusion.

SCIENCE IS COUNTERINTUITIVE

In the position of an armchair philosopher conducting a thought experiment, we can imagine how things "should" be and even extrapolate existing knowledge to predict future events. Invoking common sense to explain phenomenal things often make us scientifically wrong, however, whether we talk about behavior, celestial mechanics, or chemical reactions. This is because science is often counterintuitive (Wolpert, 1993), as experiment shows.

Experiment means to try, to put to the test. The point of scientific experimentation is to find out what *is*, not to guess what might be or to force matters to conform to our wishes. For centuries after Galen, anatomical observations that did not agree with his text were discarded as anomalies. Today, facts that fail to fit theory oblige that theory's revision.

The Royal Society of London took as its motto *Nullius in Verba*, best translated as "Take nobody's word for it, see for yourself."[1] Granted its charter in 1662 by Charles II, the Royal Society is the oldest and most venerated of English scientific societies. By insisting on exactness, it changed the dominant mode of scientific inquiry from *experience* to *experiment*. The Society judged that anecdotes of gentlemen naturalists often were random, frivolous, and even purposely misleading. Instead of transacting their findings in the language of "Wits or Scholars," the Society strove for "clear senses" and a "mathematical plainness." Experience was personal and never precisely repeatable, while experiment signified that some types of experience could not only be confirmed, but also coördinated and systematically added to the stock of knowledge. Measuring instruments, which were largely an outgrowth of clock making, especially helped transform singular experiences into repeatable experiments (Boorstin, 1983).

In learning neuropsychology, you must see for yourself by examining patients. Existing knowledge and theories can guide you, but you have to experience the operation of human behavior firsthand. You must also express yourself clearly and unambiguously so that others are not misled to wrong conclusions. You have at your disposal all sorts of measuring instruments, from paper and pencil (often still the best and almost always the place to start) to billion-dollar technology. The exquisite anatomical drawings in Vesalius's folio are visual summaries of multiple dissections and, as such, represent the collective experience that is common prop-

Constraining Cognitive Theories

Empirical facts of neuroscience must constrain any theory of cognition. Any psychological theory, no matter how self-contained or elegant, is useless unless we can reconcile it to the biological observations of neuroscience. We can determine through experiment how the brain is constructed and how external sense impressions are conveyed by the transduction apparatus of sensory receptors. Bear this in mind as we try to map a cognitive structure onto an anatomical one.

erty. By announcing not "This is what I saw" but "This is what was seen," these drawings allow anyone to replicate the experience of dissection. By analogy, you will prove to yourself that deficits, syndromes, and patterns of behavior do exist. *Nullius in Verba* is a good motto. Keeping a dose of doubt by your side is good, too.

SOME MODERN TERMS

You will hear some terms that denote different things to different speakers. The field itself that we are discussing is called *neuropsychology, behavioral neurology, behavioral neurobiology, neuropsychiatry, neuroimmunopsychiatry,* and other permutations of these root words. The dust has not yet settled, but we should take a stab at clarifying some of these labels.

Neuropsychology is an older term, now freely interchanged with *behavioral neurology.* I would prefer the term *cognitive neurology* to distinguish that discipline which seeks a neural explanation of behavior and cognition; unfortunately, it seems to foster the erroneous assumption of sharing a fondness for computation with *cognitive science.* Neuropsychology distinguishes itself from *clinical psychology* in that the latter is heuristic and claims no physical basis for its theories.

Cognitive psychology tries to describe, predict, and model thought. But how useful can such models be unless they match the physical facts of the brain? The neuropsychologist is more interested in those parts of cognitive psychology that suggest anatomical and functional relationships. The ideal case would be a theory that accepts "experience as we know we have it" as a given and then constructs how a mind "must be" in order to explain such experience. Theories of cognitive psychology can inform neuropsychology and vice versa.

Psychology is interested in brain pathology to the extent that philosophy of mind, introspection, and inferences from experiments on normal subjects can be confirmed or refuted by examples of disordered brain function. Similarly, neurologists have looked to psychological theories (behavioral, gestalt, and cognitive) to explain clinical findings. The theory of microgenesis, for example, believes that a psychology can be built up directly from a study of pathological symptoms (Brown, 1988; Hanlon, 1991). Microgenesis sees the aphasias, for example, as a window onto cognitive structure in believing that any theory capable of explaining the diversity of aphasic disorders will lead to a more general theory that accounts for disorders of action and perception, too. Implicit is the assumption that the principles underlying aphasic disorders are fundamentally the same as those of other cognitive domains.

Behavioral neurology encompasses developmental disorders of childhood, lateralizing disorders, rostral-caudal disorders, diffuse versus focal disorders, as well as more specific disorders of language, emotion, and the frontal lobes, to mention a few. It also encompasses the complex behavior of the declining brain as seen in dementia and other degenerative illnesses. *Adult neuropsychology* studies disturbances of established patterns of behavior, whereas *developmental neuropsychology* studies disturbed acquisition of cognitive functions regardless of the pathological origin. *Neurolinguistics* is considered a subdivision of neuropsychology dealing with disturbed verbal performance following cortical lesions.

Artificial intelligence (AI) concretizes the metaphor of the soul and believes that brains are simply "computers made of meat" (Marvin Minksy's phrase). Intelligent people believe that it is possible to make machines that think, feel, and even know they exist, machines that will be capable of satisfaction, doubt, and free will as soon as computational hardware and algorithms become good enough. Although computers perform operations speedily, can they, as Martin Gardner asks, "understand" what they are doing in a way that is superior to the "understanding" of an abacus?

METHODS FOR APPROACHING MIND AND BRAIN

Knowledge of normal and aberrant behavior comes from different approaches. Two classic ones are *hard wiring* and *black box*, methodologies frequently used by electronic engineers and that rely more on deductive rather than inductive logic. The classic Dejerine model of language, for example, is hard-wired in saying that language can be described by a network of three crucial perisylvian regions—Broca's area, the arcuate fasciculus, and Wernicke's area. The Chomskian school of modern linguistics supports a hard-wired structure common to all languages, arguing

Approaches to the Mind and Brain

Black box. Behavior is studied without any knowledge of the nervous system by applying different inputs and analyzing the outputs. Behavior can be predicted, but the brain itself is not studied. Cognitive architecture doesn't matter either.

Ablation. Abnormal behavior observed after a brain lesion reveals the function of the remaining tissue or the release of a previously inhibited function.

Electrical stimulation. Considered reversible ablation, ESB does not imitate any normal physiological state but disrupts ongoing activity.

Electrophysiology. Precise recording and quantitative analysis of single cells to well-chosen stimuli is possible. Correlations with EEG, evoked potentials and, in animals at least, oscillating potentials from specific brain regions have also been fruitful.

Pharmacology. Stimulation, blockade, or re-uptake blockade of neurotransmitters is correlated with behavior.

Introspection. Subjects observe their own behavior. Although such reports can be invaluable, they can also be actively misleading.

Human experimentation. Included are normal studies, case reports, and series of patients.

Conceptual analysis. We cast new hypotheses and test them with one or more of the methods available. It must be remembered that diagrams are sketches of hypotheses and not facts. Hypotheses are often cast in terms of metaphor. Do not confuse the symbol with the thing symbolized.

---

its uniqueness on grounds that its structure is different from that needed to describe elements in other cognitive domains (Chomsky, 1965, 1985). Although similar, hard-wired and black-box models are not identical. Extreme black-box modeling is represented by the behaviorists, who didn't care whether humans had a brain let alone a cognitive architecture.

Other classic methods include *ablation* and *electrical stimulation* of the brain (ESB). Magnetic stimulation is a more recently devised technique that is similar in principle to ESB (Devinsky et al., 1993). Most deliberate lesions are created in subhuman primates, although some have been created in humans during surgery. These methods assume that discrete structures or microstructures are related to certain functions or impairments. ESB is considered reversible, whereas ablation is not.

Ablation experiments also happen as so-called experiments of nature when lesions such as trauma or stroke occur in discrete brain areas that are exactly those the researcher wishes to study (Damasio & Damasio, 1989). The anatomical territory is often well-defined in vascular lesions and, therefore, volumes of reproducible data in stroke patients have been gathered. For example, the Aphasia Research Unit at the Boston VA Medical Center depended on this type of case to develop its theories of aphasia.

Higher functions have been studied with ESB during neurosurgery. In particular, the Canadian neurosurgeon Wilder Penfield espoused this approach (Penfield & Jasper, 1954). Others were later able to map areas in language-dominant cortex and subcortical regions correlated with naming, short-term verbal memory, and allied aspects of speech and language (Whitaker & Ojemann, 1977). ESB remains useful, and refinements of both technique and analysis have led to a reïnterpretation of Penfield's pioneering work.

Beginners commonly assume that an observed change in behavior is attributable solely to the tissue in the lesion. But acute lesions can also disturb remote function metabolically or physiologically, a term called *diaschisis*. A lesion may release other brain areas from facilitation or inhibition. It may disconnect areas from one another, disrupting spatially separate processes that require coördination. Because neuroanatomy is so compact, multiple functions, perhaps even contrasting ones, can course through a given region. Lesion analysis must be done with care. *Nonspecific effects* are always a possibility, which is why control lesions of similar size and type in a brain area other than the one under study are desirable. If such a control lesion has a different behavioral effect rather than no effect, then one has shown a *double dissociation*. Simply put, lesion A produces behavior X but not Y, while lesion B produces behavior Y but not X.

Acute lesions and the behavior associated with them are rarely static. Cerebral swelling, metabolic substrate availablity (oxygen, glucose, adequate blood flow to remove toxic metabolic wastes), and the capacity of the nervous system to reorganize itself slightly are all factors. Whole new atlases of neuroanatomy are being drawn based not on light-microscopical histology but on the distribution of neurotransmitters. New staining and tracing methods permit detailed mapping of cell bodies, projections, and connections. Better understanding of behavioral-chemical relationships has made *pharmacologic manipulation* another neuropsychological tool.

Many oddities in neuropsychology come to our attention by accident or with considerable coaxing of patients who feel embarrassed or ashamed by what they believe is "not real." Despite sometimes being dismissed as subjective and, therefore, vaguely unscientific, such *experiential reports* alone have occasionally changed our fundamental paradigms. The obvious example is dreaming during REM sleep. If no one had awakened sleepers during different electroencephalographic (EEG) phases and asked what was happening, the clinical meaning of this EEG stage would have remained undeciphered or been assumed to be meaningless. Verbal reports are often the neurologist's Rosetta stone. There are, of course, two sides to that stone. Experiential reports have advanced neuroscience; neuroscience should be able to help us better understand experience. However, patients' words must be interpreted with utmost caution: Blindsight research, for example, shows that verbal reports severely underestimate visual capacity, while research in split-brain patients shows that verbal reports can be actively misleading.

We often assume that *human experimentation* is increasingly difficult to do, largely for ethical reasons, but actually much can be unearthed from the study of normal individuals, from single cases that are studied in depth and over time, and from series of patients. Statistics can separate a real effect from a random event. Selective input into the nervous system (dichotic listening, tachistoscopic or contact lens half-field viewing) is one way of studying behavior in normals as well as in brain-damaged individuals.

There has been a particular renaissance of the case study method in Iowa City. A huge *case registry* of patients with specific symptoms or specific lesions is assembled there together with CT, MRI, or positron emission tomography (PET) scans and postmortem data when available. Such registries are tools for analyzing what psychological functions are impaired by specific brain lesions. Because of its size, a registry increases the chance of finding patients with damage in just the area researchers wish to study.

One's *conceptual analysis* embraces all the above considerations. Consciousness is associated with the way we observe things. There are levels of consciousness ranging from reflexive responses and automatic behavior, such as driving mindlessly to work, all the way up to observing oneself as an observer. Do not forget for a moment that every observer's interpretation includes personal bias, history, culture, and values that determine what is seen and not seen, what is relevant and irrelevant, and what is believable. Intentionally or otherwise, investigators always throw out data they deem irrelevant. Someone else with a different hypothesis or background may find this presumably irrelevant material crucially important. Different observers of the same events can arrive at alternative truths. The incompatible systems of Eastern and Western medicine, for example, show how different scientific communities invent incommensurable interpretations of identical physical phenomena. You should keep these facts in mind.

NOTE

1. Modern people often mistranslate the Latin *Nullius in verba* literally as "There is nothing in words," implying that talk is cheap and theories irrelevant. We misread the genitive singular *nullius* as the nominative *nullus*. We also fail, as no educated seventeenth-century person ever would have, to recognize the phrase as an allusion to a fuller statement from Horace's *Epistulæ*:

> *Nullius addictus iurare in verba magistri,*
> *quo me cumque rapit tempestas, deferor hospes.*
> (I am not bound to swear allegiance to the word of any master,
> Where the storm carries me, I put into port and make myself a home.)

The motto thus adjures freedom of thought and action, not the insignificance of words. Its meaning is that learned individuals would henceforth replace dogmatic philosophical musings with empirical facts and experiments that anyone could reproduce to determine for themselves what was true.

2 Concepts of Mind

What we think thinking is has been a moving target throughout history, and many books review the vast chronicle of both philosophy and psychology of mind. In this chapter, I restrict myself to exploring how a mental psychology heavily flavored with philosophy and religion evolved into a biologic one, and how mechanical concepts of mind have in turn led to the current view that cognition is the aggregate of autonomous, dissociable components. I will try to leave concepts of nervous tissue for chapter 3.

Modern science often uses René Descartes's method of detailed analysis that breaks down complex problems into smaller components. Such analysis is done when things are too complicated to be studied whole. What we lose in interaction among the parts we hopefully gain in accessibility to those parts. By showing how cognition breaks down we can put constraints on how it may be organized in the first place. In this spirit, we use preparations like *Aplysia* and *Limulus* in neurophysiology to study behavior; in psychology, fragments of real experience substitute as models of reality. While this approach does yield results, these kinds of compromises can also distort the very issue we are trying to understand.

MACHINE ANALOGIES OF BRAIN ACTIVITY

The idea that thinking is somehow a mechanical process is an old one. Ever since humans began thinking about the brain as the factory of the mind they have described it in terms of the latest technology. Aristotle did it. Descartes did it. We do it.

Like biting one's fingernails, this is a hard habit to break even though, despite their prevalence and surface appeal, one can hardly be impressed by machine analogies of neural activity. A long history of parallelism keeps neurological theory on par with current technology. In Mesmer's day, the paranoid was persecuted by malicious animal magnetism, his successors by galvanic shocks, the telegraph, radio, radar, and now extraterrestrial beacons. Impressed by the hydraulic figures in the Royal Gardens, Descartes developed a hydraulic theory to explain the brain. We next had brain theories based on telephone wiring, electrical fields, and waves. More recent analogies are grounded in computer science and quantum mechanics.

It is true that inanimate physical systems can manipulate symbols and thereby perform tasks previously done only by humans. This includes problem solving. Impressive as results may be, they are just restatements of the washing-machine analogy, namely, that any mechanization of a human task is hardly identical to it no matter how similar the outcomes may be. Still, what better incarnation of the Frankenstein myth could there be today than the supposed creation of mind?

The computer analogy is particularly poor, and the early artificial intelligentsia wildly overstated the promise of AI. Still, it is a sign of how deeply both faith in the machine metaphor and technology are rooted in our thinking that practitioners of AI, plus the *majority* of cognitive and behavioral scientists, take the separation of mind from brain as a given, believing mind to be an abstract program that can be instantiated on any machine capable of running it. They believe that "understanding" the mind is really a *technical* problem of reducing cognition to a series of formal logic statements and that the scope of human experience is, in fact, so reducible. The approach that sees the mind as software—some abstract, disembodied knowledge—is extremely attractive to people who think theoretically precisely because it liberates them from having to learn the biological complexities of neural tissue. This is not to say that the engineer's efforts at neural networks, the logician's computational theory of mind, or the mathematician's efforts at functional models may not help clarify what "thinking" is. Yet only a handful of biologically-oriented scientists successfully resist throwing themselves before the altar of computation.

The two essential reasons why the brain cannot be modeled faithfully by any computer are mechanical and moral. On the mechanical front, the distinction between software and hardware has become meaningless. Engineers of neural networks invent mathematical designs that can either be run as programs or translated directly into computer chips if need arises. This practice is then extrapolated to mind: Define the program, and running it on a machine will fall into place.

This confidence is overblown given our miserable failure at replicating far simpler biological parts. In 1970, for example, bioëngineers at Pennsylvania State University enthusiastically promised that an implantable, artificial heart pump would be developed in a few years and could be ready for routine surgery by 1975. After incalculable effort and currency, this goal remains elusive. Artificial kidneys or joints are likewise nowhere as sophisticated as the biologic counterparts they claim to replace, even though they are much simpler than the brain given that they lack the associated subjective state that is integral to mind itself.

Despite thirty-five years of AI, it seems unlikely that we can adequately model the brain, in any meaningful sense, when we have failed to model far simpler biological entities. But even this rebuttal is beside the point: The moral argument for why one cannot separate psychology from biology has to do with the roles of emotion and subjectivity in human life (Weizenbaum, 1976; Cytowic, 1993, Part II, cpt. 2, 3, 4).

More fruitful results are likely to come from studying the brain itself than by making physical analogies. Many of these poor mechanical analogies rest on the false supposition that a unique "sense datum" exists, one that faithfully measures some physical property of the environment and travels, unmodified and in isolation, from a peripheral sense receptor to higher brain levels. This of course is not what happens at all.

Real-World Understanding

Efforts to enable humans and machines to "communicate" have not succeeded as originally envisioned. This failure clearly illustrates the importance of a real-world understanding that lies outside of formal rules, especially formal rules of language. Possessing a character of standing outside itself, language has always appealed to individuals who think abstractly, and many rules for computational systems have roots in the formal rules of transformational grammar (Wasow, 1991; Chomsky, 1965, pp. 47–59).

We need to understand more about nonlinguistic knowledge, especially subjective experience and what philosophers call "qualia" (more on this later). Any scientific approach to mind must view mentation from the outside, from an objective third-person viewpoint. But there remain important aspects of mental life that are comprehensible only from a first-person perspective. Anthropologists, for example, have shown not only that culture can affect cognition, but that it is, in fact, a pervasive influence. This negates an earlier presumption that the mind was an abstract entity separable from both its "hardware" and any context.

If you believe, as cognitive scientists do, that reasoning denotes a problem solvable by applying some kind of logic, then the deep insights into symbolic representation that have arisen from anthropology's contrasting assumptions and presumptions may surprise you (D'Andrade, 1991). Because the *content* of propositions strongly affects how well individuals reason, for example, cultural anthropologists argue that it is implausible that people really do use formal systems in reasoning. They also find it ironic that initial emulations of human reasoning imitated either cognitive games such as chess or symbolic manipulation such as that found in formal logic and math. Neither represents a cognitive task that humans do either frequently or well. Mental puzzles and challenging sports are culturally-learned examples of how we enjoy entertaining ourselves with intellectual or physical ventures at which we are not very good.

Although many agree that we use representations (models) rather than logic to reason, anthropologists emphasize that our reasoning depends on cultural models that are more than just a self-contained information packet about the world. The assumptions of a cultural model are shared by members of the culture, and what makes a model a cultural one is how it is used, not how it is learned (whether, for example, its information is innate or acquired knowledge).

I raise such issues here in the hope that you will abjure too mechanical a viewpoint as we push forward to clinical issues. Neither intellectual nor conceptual boundaries are as sharply drawn as textbooks (including this one) manage to imply. Neuropsychology is really quite a soup: A system of mental concepts, empirical facts, theoretical constructs, suppositions, and a host of cultural, scientific, personal, and methodological biases. That it manages to bring any coherence to the vagaries of human behavior is really extraordinary.

HOW DOES MIND ARISE FROM MATTER?

Classical physics took for granted the separation of the world into mind (*res cognitans*) and matter (*res extensa*). Delbrück (1986) suggests that the lesson of contemporary quantum physics is to force us to view mind and matter as aspects of a single system. It is our evolutionary development that has come to regard the mind as an independent, nonmaterial entity. Though the mind-matter dichotomy may make it easier to categorize our experience (perceptions such as size, shape, time, space, and causality) he suggests it may be no more than a practical illusion.

The world as seen through the uncertainty principle, Delbrück continues, is remarkably similar to that of the infant who has not yet acquired the categories of adult cognition. "Since each of us made the transition from the infant's world, in which there is no clear distinction between subject and object ... it is not wholly incongruous that in our rational thought processes we should be able to reverse this process."

There is no pure objectivity or subjectivity. Quantum theory showed that matter is altered by perception (it is not purely "objective") while biology shows that mind is certainly a product of the material world (it is not purely "subjective"). Why then should one wait for science to produce a coherent explanation of mind when it has not yet produced a satisfactory explanation of matter and the end is not in sight?

Early twentieth-century quantum experiments led to the conclusion that physical phenomena are fundamentally shaped by our perception of them. Neils Bohr developed the idea of complementarity to resolve the particle and wave paradox, proposing that both are related aspects of a single reality that cannot be wholly observed from any perspective and that any experiment which demonstrates one aspect inevitably interferes with the other.

Though it may be a product of physical evolution, the human mind has actually become what most of us presume it to be: An entity that exists independently of the world it perceives. When we look in later chapters at what actually happens when we perceive, our common-sense presumptions about the nature of mind and reality quickly break down.

Investigating vision, for example, we find that our brains construct much of what we take to be "objective" visual data. Contrary to what most of us have been taught, color is not due to the wavelength of light reflecting off a surface, nor is it related to any obvious physical quality at a point on an object (Thompson et al., 1992; Cytowic, 1989, pp. 292–300; Land 1977). Another example is the detachment of shape. We have no difficulty recognizing a real tree from an artist's sketch of the same shape or a photograph of a tree, despite the enormously different images that each of these three examples casts on the retina. That we do not rely on "bits of data" from individual photoreceptors in constructing form is an obvious conclusion that can be logically developed into the premise that shape can detach from objects. This is an example of modularity.

This, of course, is Kant's idea that the mind receives information from the senses in a prestructured form (*Critique of Pure Reason*, 1781). He argued that we experience sensory impressions only after interpreting them in terms of *a priori* categories such as time, space, object, and causality, all of which reside innately in the mind. This idea has recirculated since Kant's time.

Many of the difficulties in the mind-body problem arise from our penchant to ask "what is" questions. We expect that we will one day really find out what mind is, despite the fact that we do not really know yet what matter is. Although we know a great deal about matter's physical structure, we are not sure whether so-called elementary particles are elementary in any relevant sense. Similarly, we know a great deal about the structure of mind but nothing about mind's essence. Just as Newton sought an ultimate explanation for mechanical phenomena, we too seek an ultimate explanation of what the mind is. Mind is a process, a phenomenon of life. Yet all we know about it is less than our collective knowledge of matter.

In suggesting a way out of this materialistic impasse, Sir Karl Popper (Popper & Eccles, 1977, chapter P1) extends the argument of Julien La Mettrie's classic book, *Man a Machine* (1747), in tracing the mechanical view of humans from robots all the way to present-day electrochemical machines. Both atomism and quantum physics grew out of a Newtonian clockwork universe and assumed that matter, in the sense of occupying space, was ultimate, something neither capable of nor in need of further explanation. Everything else could be explained in terms of matter. As knowledge progressed, however, it turned out that matter was not a substance, because it could be destroyed and be created. The conservation-of-mass law had to be discarded: Even the most stable particles can be destroyed by collision with their antiparticles as their energy is transformed into light. It turns out that matter is highly packed energy, something of a process, as it can be converted into other processes such as light, motion, and heat.

Sir Karl concludes that the outcome of modern physics dictates that we *give up the idea of a substance or essence, the idea of a "thing."* There simply is no self-identical entity persisting through time. There is no essence that is the persisting carrier or possessor of the properties or qualities of a thing. The universe, which includes human minds, appears to be not a collection of things but an interacting set of events or processes.

This is where we are today when pushed to the limit of the question, "What is mind?" Fortunately, just as Newtonian mechanics are good enough in many earthbound situations, we too retain some earlier ideas of what mind is because they are still useful. Let's now take a broad survey of two millennia's worth of changing concepts of mind-body.

HISTORICAL DEVELOPMENT OF MIND-BODY IDEAS

Because so much of contemporary Western thought derives from Pythagoras, Aristotle, and other Classic philosophers of antiquity, it is well to reflect on the *words* we use to describe modern ideas in neuropsychology. Students who are troubled by my inclusion in a "factual" textbook of anything smacking of religion or metaphysics are those most in need of expanding their capacity for subjectivity and the irrational, for appreciating the prominent roles that both play in the human psyche.

Furthermore, do not dismiss historical concepts of mind as merely academic and somehow irrelevant. It is all too easy to pat ourselves on the back and wonder how those who went before us could have been so stupid. We never suppose that today's great achievements might be derided as tomorrow's leaches. Students interested in only new ideas seriously handicap themselves.

A Modern Emphasis on Ancient Words

Psyche (Greek) = breath and, by extension, the mind, now meaning the mental life, both conscious and unconscious. Psyche is the animating principle in humans and other living creatures, the source of all vital activities, rational or irrational, the soul or spirit, in distinction from both its material vehicle, the body (*soma*), and the intellect (*nous*). Psyche is sometimes considered capable of persisting in a disembodied state after separation from the body at death. Psyche was extended by Plato to the *anima mundi*, conceived to animate the universe as the soul animates the individual organism.

Psychiatry = psyche + healing: The medical treatment of diseases of the mind, that branch of medicine dealing with disorders of the psyche. Reflect for a moment that most unhappy psychiatric patients are troubled by their feelings (affective disorders) or the content of their thinking (thought disorders).

Psychology = psyche + science: The science of the nature, functions, and phenomena of the human soul or mind. That branch of science that concerns mental operations, especially as evidenced in human behavior. Psychology is heuristic and does not consider any physical structure of mind, although it may describe and even correctly predict patterns of thought and behavior. Subgroups are *clinical psychology, physiological psychology,* and *experimental psychology.*

There is often much discomfort in America in relating psyche to concepts such as the soul, yet I cannot emphasize enough how deeply ideas of the mind are connected with spiritual ideas of the transcendent. This relationship with the vital force is rooted in our language. Most obviously, we use the root *pyche* (soul) in psychology; we do not call it nousology (*nous* = mind, intellect). Consider the following relations.

The ancient Greek *pneuma*, meaning "breath," and the modern Greek *pneumata*, meaning "inspiration, spirit, or ghosts," are all derived from *pneuma*, having to do with air. Greek and Roman physicians taught that air was drawn into the heart by the pulmonary veins and transformed into life-sustaining pneuma. Later, Galen (AD 119–200) taught the concept of pneuma that affected succeeding generations of physicians. Galen recognized both a psychic pneuma in the brain, *pneuma animale*, and a sustaining vital spirit, *pneuma zoötikon*, in the heart and arteries, which drew its nourishment, in part, from respiration (Quin, 1994).

In modern English *pneuma* introduces technical terms related to air and the lungs (pneumatic, pneumonia), but its link with the spirit has not been lost, because pneumatology refers to the study of spiritual beings. The Latin word for both "breath" and "wind," *spiritus*, reminds us of our link between respiration and spirituality. We talk about being inspired to great deeds and about expiring when we die. That pervasive ties exist between spirit and breath are especially apparent when we find different words for the same root that refer to both concepts. Take "animated" and "animal" in English, for example. For the former we can also say "spirited." Both "animated" and "animal" hail from *anima* (wind or breath), *animus* (soul), and the Greek cognate *animos*. While psyche now represents only soul and mind to us, it previously represented (in the *Iliad*) the breath of life, while *psycho* denoted "breath" and "blow" (Gravenstein et al., 1981).

It is therefore easy to see how old concepts that link breath, life, spirit, and mind have endured and been inflected by the cultural forces of successive generations until we can no longer feel the mythical ground from which these concepts arose. For centuries, humanity has sought to understand the vital force of life and the nature of its existence. This ancient quest is translated into *scientific terms* because we believe mysticism and metaphysics are not relevant to our lives today. These concepts have been sanitized, you might say, by a world view that emphasizes rationality and objectivity. So, in the guise of being objective, neuropsychology looks to the brain to understand what the human mind is and, by extension, to understand what it means to be human. Because Western thought insists that everything important will be discovered in the head, we stress the "meaning" of life. What does this emphasis cause us to miss?

Meaning Versus Experience

The list of eminent neuroscientists who have gone off looking for the seat of the soul is long. Oskar and Cécile Vogt, directors of the Kaiser Wilhelm Institute for Brain Research outside of Berlin, and Sir John Eccles, Nobel laureate physiologist, are but two sterling examples that humans still seek transcendence, something that customarily belongs in the realms of religion. Transcendence (literally, "to climb over or beyond") is that which exists *behind* everyday "experience as we know we have it" (Kant's words again). In describing the strange and fantastic fabric of the universe during the past twenty years, for example, theoretical physicists have sounded more and more like high priests of metaphysics rather than the cold, objective scientists everyone expected them to be. Today, it is neuroscientists who are on the threshold of becoming the high priests of transcendence in promising to explain us to ourselves.

This is problematic for beginners who want "just the facts" of neuropsychology. Unfortunately, humans feel as well as think. Since reason and emotion coëvolved, they are inseparable. Since some aspects of human experience just cannot be conveyed by facts, there is no escape from subjectivity. The totality of human understanding is more than a balance sheet of third-person observations.

This is precisely the point argued by the mythologist Joseph Campbell (1904–1987), whose exposure on public television turned him into a household word. Such holistic advocates criticize viewing the head as the supreme organ that directs all other energies of the body. The rational mind, they contend, is only one organ of the body and is often in conflict with other bodily energies, hence the self-conflict that we so often feel. Most people, Campbell contends, think that what they seek is the rational "meaning of life," but what they really are seeking is "the experience of being alive." This old debate dates back to antiquity: Aristotle (BC 384–322) chose the heart as the principal organ, Plato (BC 429–347) the head. In wrestling with this ancient dilemma, some contemporary scientists have concluded that humans possess "multiple minds" rather than just one (Gardner, 1983; Cytowic, 1993).

Neo-Wiganism: One Mind or Many?

Just looking at the two cerebral hemispheres naturally raises the question of whether we have a mind in each or only a single one in the whole brain. In 1844, Arthur Wigan published a formulation of this question in *The Duality of Mind*, which was based on the postmortem observation of someone he knew well in whom one cerebral hemisphere was totally absent! Wigan was sharp enough to conclude that a single hemisphere was sufficient to be a person. His astounding finding implied that the brain is not a single organ of two halves, but actually a closely apposed pair, just as the kidneys or lungs are paired organs. Wigan concluded that if one hemisphere was sufficient to have a mind then the usual two makes the possession of two minds inevitable. However synchronous they might usually be, there must be times when the two minds are discrepant. Wigan's observation suggested an anatomic and physiologic basis for that internal conflict so characteristic of humans (Wigan, 1844; Bogen, 1972).

Wigan's prescient speculation attracted little attention at the time. Today, psychophysical probing of normals and clinical evidence from split-brain patients both support Wigan's magnificent deduction that two hemispheres mean the possession of two minds. Our two minds differ in content, mode of organization, and possibly even in goals. Sectioning the cerebral commissures does not produce this duality of mind but merely makes it easier to demonstrate. More about the split brain appears in chapter 3.

Early Concepts of Mind

In the fifth century BC, Pythagoras regarded sensation and thought as different entities and believed, as did Plato, that an immortal soul resided in the brain. A century or so later Aristotle proposed a tripartite soul consisting of *memorativa* (which stores and reproduces recollections), the irrational *imaginativa*, and the rational *intellectus*. This triple concept was paralleled by the idea that the brain distilled the *spiritus animalus* into a carrier of the three faculties of thought, judgement, and memory. On evaporation, air inspired into the brain through the senses left its *quinta essentia*, Aristotle's fifth and purest element. Humanity has ever since debated the irreconcilable views of whether it has a Platonic immortal soul that temporarily resides in a mortal brain, or a finite Aristotelian soul that resides in the heart and perishes with it. Note how the soul, and not the brain, is considered prime.

The cerebral ventricles were discovered around AD 300, and were initially said to contain *imaginitiva, logistica*, and *memoria*. Now comes the first germ of modularity, the idea that mental faculties reside in different ventricles or "cells" of the brain. Localizing the soul's faculties in the brain's cavities appears to build on Galen's teaching of *pneuma*.

Religious and philosophical forces subsequently argued over the number of cells, and whether the soul's faculties resided in the solid brain tissue or in its fluid-filled ventricles. What gradually emerged after the twelfth century, however, was a cellular doctrine *not of brain function, but of mental function*. The soul (mental life) was explicitly separate from the physical body (brain). This era was dominated of course by the ecclesia, an early self-sustaining bureaucracy. Christianity infiltrated medieval communities not only with an ontological basis of the universe (God did it) but with the notion that only through the church could humanity be saved from eternal perdition.

The subject of finding the seat of the soul was alive among medical, theological, and philosophical savants well into the fifteenth century. In fact, it lives today in another form. The conflict between Greek and Christian philosophies—between reason on one hand and an unthinking faith that manipulated facts to fit doctrine on the other—eventually saw the end of religious scholasticism. Bruyn (1982) lists more than two dozen ancient schemes for compartmentalizing mental functions, and points out that there is no correspondence between the number of mental functions and the three physical ventricles. When a divine trinity corresponds with a Platonic tripartite soul, brain doctrine finds itself pictured in a tri-cellular fashion; when scholastic clerics deduced the existence of additional inner senses, more cells were simply invented to accommodate them (figure. 2.1).

A lack of correspondence between mental faculties and the three physical ventricles was irrelevant because what was actually being conceptualized was a *cellular division of thought*. It is remarkable that any useful ideas came out of this era given the clerical authorities' constraints: They were dealing with inconsistent medical data from Galen (AD 119–200) to Avicenna (AD 980–1037), were themselves incompetent in medicine and anatomy, and had to force Greek and Arabic pagan philosophy to fit Christian dogma.

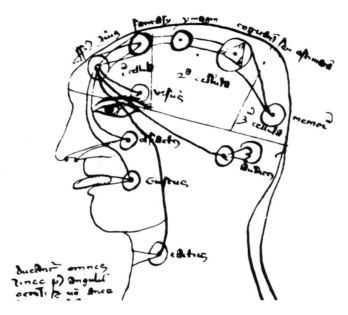

Figure 2.1
Bayærische Statsbibliothek, Munich, Codes Latin 527, folio 64ᵛ. A treatise on the anatomy of the head for physicians. This head contains three polygonal cells and five encircled faculties: *Sensus communis, fantasia, imaginativa, cogitativa sue estimativa,* and *memorativa.* From Bruyn, 1982, with permission.

The countless essays titled *"De Anima"* and *"De Spiritu"* reflect humanity's preöccupation with its own nature from Pythagorean times up to the present. It shows the split between soma and psyche, the conceptual discontinuity between what is taken as physical reality and what is taken as mental reality. Following Sir Karl Popper's suggestion that both matter and mind are processes rather than things, some suggest that we look at the brain as a spatially-organized grid of elements that process myriad energy transients. Its mathematical integral is a field property called "mind," something similar to the field force called "gravity" that emerges in the presence of sufficient mass. Ask yourself whether this modern idea is different from or similar to the ancient concepts of soul and mind.

Mind or Matter?

> Quantum physics suggests that mind and matter are two sides of the same coin. Rather than a split between psyche and soma, perhaps mind and matter do show duality's union just as light manifests itself, according to how we look, as either a wave or a particle. Descartes's conflict between *res cognitans* and *res extensa*, conceived as two totally separate worlds, was destroyed sequentially (1) by Kant, who showed the epistemological a priori elements of time and space, then (2) by Freud, who pointed to the workings of the unconscious mind (a conceptual contradiction to his contemporaries), and lastly (3) by Einstein, who showed that Kant's categories are relative rather than absolute.

Post-Renaissance Thought

The search for the seat of the soul was but the first step toward cerebral localization. The Greeks and medieval religious thinkers ascribed functions of the mind to the brain but did not localize them further beyond debating whether such functions were housed in the ventricles or in the brain tissue itself.

Since the earliest times, the contralateral representation of gross motor and sensory function was known as a consequence of open brain injuries. But absolutely no connection was made between these "lower" functions and the corresponding "higher" ones of volition and sensation. That is, the free will that initiates movement and the conscious perception of stimuli was simply not considered on the same level as these grosser abilities, and functions of the body were regarded as separate from functions of the mind. René Descartes (1596–1650) made this dualism of mind versus body explicit. Stated most simply, Descartes believed in the incommensurability of mind and body.

Descartes replaced Aristotle's three-part soul with a single, indivisible one as the agent of reason. Ever since, the West has held reason in extraordinary esteem, and not always with the best results. One has only to think of the silly excesses of the Age of Enlightenment in the eighteenth century. Descartes's views were entirely philosophical, not physiological. His philosophical premises required him to find a single location for a unitary soul as well as a single point for the conceptual convergence of the paired sense organs. The pineal gland, a single structure at the center of the brain, fit the bill. Its small size was irrelevant to his grand purpose, because what Descartes was localizing was not a physical relationship between structure and function, but a philosophical one between mind and body. Actually, Descartes was a bit like Galen in that his explanations of the body were unsupported by observations. Nevertheless, his approach to physiology ultimately did encourage observation and experimentation along mechanical lines.

The nineteenth century saw a progressive relaxation in the rigid separation between mind and body. Philosophically, Immanuel Kant (1724–1804) believed that all ideas were innate, and that the brain arranged sensation and supplied a priori concepts by which we understand experience. John Locke (1632–1704), however, argued earlier that ideas were not innate but *derived from experience*. Locke called the mind a *tabula rasa* that was written on by external sensation and "internal observations of our minds." Thus, external experience dictated the content of mind and implied a close physical relationship between the mind and the world.

We have since come to accept this view. In fact, a fundamental problem of any theory of mind is explaining how we move from a subjective, inner world of thoughts to an outer, objective world of things. A logical distinction between "thoughts" and "things" appears in most philosophies of the mind, and the more successful philosophies are based in experience. Such philosophies study our conscious experiences to arrive at the truth, and believe that all knowledge begins with experience. Holding such a view gives direction to the nature-versus-nurture debate. Read the box, "Genes or Environment?"

The Nineteenth Century and Localization

Comes now a famous dispute between Franz Josef Gall (1758–1828) and Pierre Flourens (1794–1867). Gall, a European anatomist and the founder of phrenology, believed that higher faculties could be localized to discrete areas of the cortex. Flourens, a French physiologist, held a contrary view that any part of an equipotential cortex could execute any mental function. Physiological evidence at first supported Flourens's equipotentiality, while later in the

Do Genes or the Environment Shape the Human Brain?

Modern philosophies of mind believe that all knowledge begins with experience. In the nature-versus-nurture debate, this premise assumes that nurture (the environment) largely shapes our minds. But any theory of mind or brain must address the paradox of how the small number of human genes can orchestrate the much large number of synapses. Mathematics suggests a direction.

Assume the null hypothesis that mind and behavior are genetically determined and that the environment plays a minimal role. Estimates for the number of human genes range from 2×10^5 to 1×10^6, whereas the number of synapses is estimated at 10^{14} to 10^{15}. Even if all the genes directed nothing but the structure of our brains, there is simply not enough genetic material to organize an entity with eight to ten orders of magnitude more elements.

Suddenly, the environment (nurture) seems to have the major burden in shaping our minds and brains. We could reduce this burden by rejecting the assumption that every synapse requires its own gene. We can further reduce it somewhat by knowing that the nervous system is organized not by single cells but by groups of neurons (columns, cortical modules). We can also consider *noncognitive external factors* such as nutrition (protein-calorie substrate, vitamins), hormones (thyroid, growth hormone), and biochemical factors (nerve growth proteins such as GAP-43). But these facts reduce the gap in our problem only by factors of 10^3 to 10^5.

This leaves two notions: (1) The brain's internal milieu may exert tropic organizing forces via physical and chemical factors, and (2) our actual experience does play a large part in shaping our brain after all. This refutes the null hypothesis.

So, we have come to believe that experience actually does change the brain physically (see chapter 3), but to understand how our experience structures the mind and leads to concepts of how the world is constructed, we must first look at how thought develops in infants as they interact with the world over time. To do so, we turn to the work of someone such as Jean Piaget.

century the localizationists got the upper hand. Flourens retained a lot of flavor from Descartes in defending the idea of an indivisible soul against Gall's separate "organs of the mind." Gall further believed in the psychological continuity between humans and animals in that the minds of each depended on neurological development. Elaborate development, he reasoned, begot elaborate functions.

Unlike Descartes, Gall rejected a central point where all nerves unite. Rather, he conceived that cortex was the expansion of lower and less complex nervous elements, thus foreshadowing the hierarchical view that partly persists today. Gall implied that the soul really had feet of clay in declaring boldly that all mental properties, intellectual as well as emotional, emerged from the brain. Because the separate faculties he proposed were each associated with a discrete organ of the brain, he reasoned that each faculty would mold the overlying cranium depending on its relative development. The science of phrenology analyzed the robustness of each mental faculty in a given individual via palpation of bumps on that individual's skull.

Phrenology excited huge popular interest. Scientific criticism exploded, however, after Gall's followers inflated his original twenty-seven faculties to more than fifty. Many were vaguely defined. Later in the century, the number of purported faculties eventually exceeded one hundred. Phrenology's disrepute unfortunately caused all subsequent schemes of localization to suffer. Nonetheless, Gall's idea of localization was both original and fundamentally correct.

The accident of Phineas Gage in 1848 provided fortuitous evidence for clinical localization of higher mental functions. Gage, a railway foreman in Vermont, was lobotomized when a hefty tamping iron was propelled through his left orbit, passed through both frontal lobes, and exited through the top of his skull (Damasio et al., 1994). After a brief collapse and convulsion, Gage was up and about. He had, however, a new personality. As his workmates said, he was "no longer Gage." His physician, Harlow (1868), wrote:

His health is good and I am inclined to say he has recovered.... The equilibrium or balance, so to speak, between his intellectual faculties and animal propensities, seems to have been destroyed. He is fitful, irreverent, indulging at times in the grossest profanity (which was not previously his custom), manifesting but little deference for his fellows, impatient of

restraint or advice when it conflicts with his desires, at times pertina-
ciously obstinate, yet capricious and vacillating, devising many plans for
future operation, which are no sooner arranged than they are abandoned.

Beyond the fact that someone could survive such an injury at
this time in medical history (Lord Lister, whose name we trivialize
with a mouthwash, had yet to invent antisepsis), Gage's injury was
astounding because it affected his "higher" mental functions, his
personality rather than gross sensation or the ability to move his
limbs. A small strip of the frontal lobe (the pre-central gyrus) had
already been associated with movement, but its greater bulk could
not be assigned any obvious function. For this reason the frontal
lobes were called "silent areas" for many years because damage to
them did not cause any obvious motor or sensory symptoms! This
is a prime example of circular reasoning. Today, the conceptual
poverty of simplistically dividing brain function into only movement and sensation is obvious.

In the twentieth century, a dispute between localizationists and
champions of globalism seems to have recurred. The similarity between the nineteenth- and twentieth-century disputants is superficial, however, because both twentieth-century parties believed
that mind emerged from brain. Nineteenth-century equipotentiality held that all parts of the brain were equal, whereas twentieth-
century holists believed that higher functions emerged from the
brain as a whole. Localizationists of both centuries asserted that
higher functions could be mapped to discrete brain regions.

The shift toward holism in the 1920s and 1930s was conceptual
rather than factually based, since available methods and materials
were quite similar to their nineteenth-century counterparts. Larger
cultural and historical factors possibly contributed to the rise of
holistic concepts given that one can find analogous shifts from localization to holism in most fields of twentieth-century thought.
In the biological and physical sciences, as in economics and politics, one finds a conceptual change from a reductionist viewpoint
to one favoring "organization." Historically, the conceptual shifts
that occurred in other areas of intellectual inquiry naturally could
have influenced those developing in brain theory.

Perhaps the most persuasive illustration of clinical localization
was Paul Broca's. A patient who for many years suffered from
right-sided paralysis could understand speech, but could say only

Biological Psychology—William James (1842–1910)

James received his MD from Harvard in June 1869 but remained a house-bound invalid for a year. This morbid state was relieved by reading Renouvier on free will, followed by James's decision that "my first act of free will shall be to believe in free will." With the resolution of his illness, James also abandoned all types of determinism, both the scientific kind, which his training had inculcated, and the metaphysical kind, which had been part of his theological upbringing.

In 1872, James was appointed instructor in physiology at Harvard, yet his interests were in psychology. Instead of the traditional, and deeply theological, mental philosophy, James developed and taught physiological psychology. He brought biology to mental science, defended free will, and championed psychophysics, the study of how physical processes affect mental ones. Through his efforts, psychology changed from a mental science into a laboratory one, and philosophy moved from dialectic to empirical metaphysical discovery. A contract for a textbook grew into the huge two-volume classic, *The Principles of Psychology* (1890).

James's work is dated only in the same way as that of Galileo and Darwin. His ideas are hugely original and transformative. His notion that the relations between things are as real, functional, and important as the things themselves radically did away with the empirical belief in a hidden metaphysical ground, such as the mythical turtle that supports the world. He championed the search for truth by direct experience instead of through philosophical arguments that defended already-decided beliefs.

For example, in researching the psychology of religion, James went directly to religious experience. In *The Varieties of Religious Experience* (1902), James's description of transcendent experiences is classic and unambiguous. "The subject says that it defies expression, that no adequate report of its content can be given in words. It follows from this that its 'qualities' must be directly experienced, it cannot be imparted or transferred to others." We will recall his description of the transcendent in dealing with some clinical aspects of human subjectivity, especially knowledge without awareness (subception) and split-brain patients.

one word. At postmortem, Broca found a large lesion involving the left second and third frontal convolutions, a place that became known as Broca's area. Strong evidence for left-hemispheric dominance of language first appeared in Broca's series of eight patients (1865).

In his *Symptom Complex of Aphasia* (1874), the German neurologist Carl Wernicke drew on earlier work showing that the posterior parts of the hemispheres were sensory while their anterior parts appeared to be motor. Wernicke noted that posterior temporal lesions produced an aphasia marked by lost comprehension and fluent, but meaningless, utterances. He proposed that the posterior temporal region, which receives auditory input, contained sound images while Broca's area contained the patterns for speech movement. He guessed correctly that a white-matter commissure (the arcuate fasciculus) connected these two cortical regions, and that a lesion of this tract would disconnect the receptive area from the motor one (figure 2.2). Wernicke's proposal introduced a language model that considered both clinical and anatomical facts. It predicted different forms of disturbed language based on the site of lesions, and accounted for motor, conduction, and sensory aphasia with poor repetition. Elaboration of Wernicke's ideas predicted additional types of language disorders that were soon confirmed. These were summarized by Jules Dejerine in 1914. The success of association models unfortunately encouraged the interpretation of observations in light of prior theoretical deductions, causing the hypothetical centers and pathways to multiply until association models started collapsing under their own weight.

Support for cerebral localization continued to accumulate. German physiologists Gustav Fritsch and Eduard Hitzig (1870) elicited specific movements by electrically stimulating the cortex of dogs. These movements were lost if that area of the cortex was removed. British neurologist John Hughlings Jackson (1835–1911) studied paralysis and focal epileptic seizures, correlating the clinical picture with postmortem pathology. Not only did Jackson localize brain function to anatomical areas, but made explicit the reduction that mental life was "nothing but" the combined motor responses to sensory stimuli.

But of what substance can the organ of mind be composed, unless of processes representing movements and impressions; and how can the con-

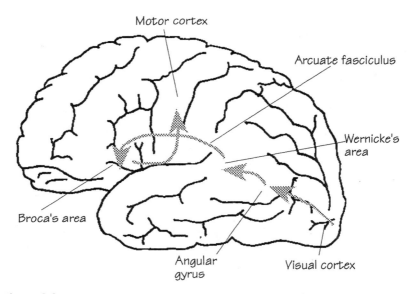

Figure 2.2
The Wernicke model of language is characteristic of approaches that "associate" one "center" with another. To speak a written word, its visual impression must first be transferred to the angular gyrus, which associates the visual form of the word with its corresponding auditory pattern in Wernicke's area. A representation of the word then travels by the arcuate fasciculus to Broca's area, evoking its pattern for the articulation that is finally executed by the lip-tongue-larynx-etc. segment of the motor cortex.

Association diagrams usually feature cell clusters, interconnected by short U-fibers, that are associated by long tracts, such as the arcuate fasciculus shown here. Association theories demand a direct correspondence between associationist psychology and physical anatomy, sometimes leading to a confusion of symptoms with function. Adapted from Geschwind, 1979.

volutions differ from the inferior centers, except as parts representing more intricate co-ordinations of impression and movements in time and space than they do?... Surely the conclusion is irresistible that mental symptoms of disease of the hemisphere are fundamentally like hemiplegia, chorea, and convulsions. They must all be due to lack, or the disorderly development of, the sensory-motor processes (Jackson, 1870).

The German neuroanatomists Paul Fleschig (1847–1929) and Korbinian Brodmann (1868–1918) finally provided anatomical footing for the concept of localization. Fleschig partitioned the cortex into motor and sensory areas according to its pattern of myelination, whereas Brodmann (1909) studied the cytoarchitectonics (i.e., the architectural arrangement of neurons in different regions) of both gray and white matter, carving up the brain into the fifty-two parcels that we now refer to as Brodmann areas (figure 2.3). (Parenthetically, careful counting shows areas 12 to 16 to be apparently missing, while areas 43 and higher are rarely pictured. See Markowitsch, 1993; Gorman & Unützer, 1993.)

Psychology marched in step with anatomy as anatomy increasingly divvied up the brain: Ideas were also conceived of as discrete units (atoms) that might be mapped to specific structures. Darwin's theory of evolution allowed psychology to bid good-bye to the long-accepted gulf between animal and human behavior. In fact, animal behavior (usually that of rats) was now extrapolated to humans. Behaviorism emerged from such extrapolations and, by perpetuating the idea of thoughts-as-atoms (in this case, discrete stimulus-response units), it continued to support the concept of localization (see figure 2.4). Later on, Gestalt psychology seriously challenged this atomistic view.

Ideas of localization as well as reduction were evident in other areas of science. Viennese pathologist Rudolph Virchow, for example, introduced his "cellular theory" in 1858 by showing that all bodily tissues, from skin to viscera, were composed of microscopic subunits that he called "cells." After the Spanish histologist Ramón y Cajal discredited the idea that the brain was an amorphous network and proved instead that neurons were discrete cells, a marvelous parallelism grew between physical brain cells and their connections, on one hand, and atomistic ideas and their psychological associations, on the other. This idea of quanta also appeared in other fields such as physics (particle theory and quantum mechanics) and chemistry (atomic theory and optical isomers).

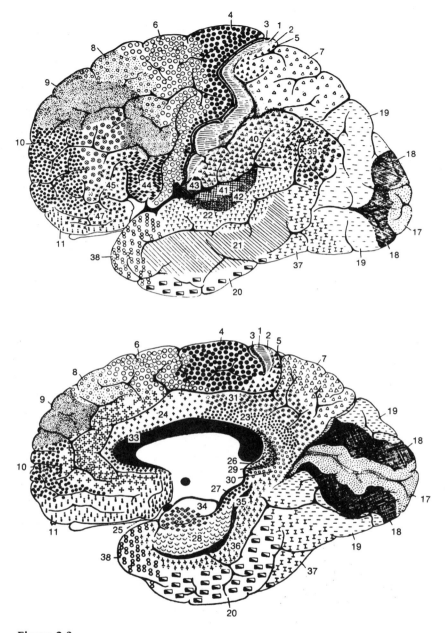

Figure 2.3
Brodmann's map of the human cortex appeared in 1908 and divided the cortex into some fifty regions based on cytoarchitecture. Correspondence between architectural regions and gross function is satisfactory, but not precise. The postcentral gyrus, for example, corresponds to Brodmann areas 3, 1, and 2, and is somatotopically organized as shown in figure 2.4 (*top*). From Brodal (1969), with permission.

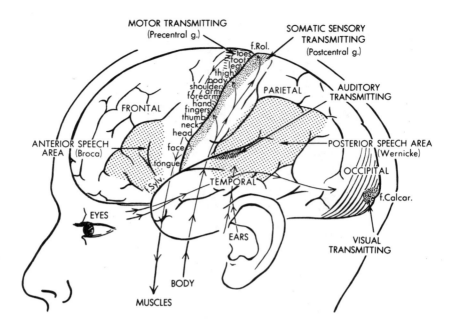

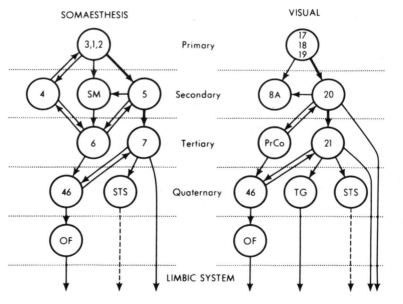

Figure 2.4

(*Top*) A "standard" view of the primary cortical areas for motor and sensory functions, as well as speech. A somatotopic map is shown over the precentral motor strip; an analogous one exists along the postcentral sensory strip. (*Bottom*) Schematic cascade of connections for somasthetic and visual systems. The numbers refer to Brodmann areas, the letters to standard cortical areas. Note the hierarchical progression from "primary" centers to association areas. From Popper & Eccles (1977) with permission.

Perhaps one measure of the confidence that philosophy, psychology, and neuroscience all had in localization was the exponential growth of psychosurgery. In 1936 the Portuguese psychiatrist Egas Moniz began destroying the frontal lobes of psychiatric patients. This technical attempt at assuaging deranged minds was popular throughout the late nineteenth and early twentieth centuries. While Moniz later invented the invaluable tool of cerebral angiography, by which the cerebral arteries were made visible to X rays, it was for inventing the lobotomy operation that this physician was awarded the Nobel Prize in 1946.

Aside from their easy access through the eye sockets or directly through the frontal bone, the frontal lobes were chosen for surgical destruction because they were believed to house personality, emotion, and memory. The reason for this assumption is twofold. The lobes are silent to experimentation, being without obvious motor or sensory signs following stimulation or ablation. That the frontal lobes are largest in humans and higher apes "obviously" reflects their importance to higher intelligence. Perhaps as a holdover from phrenology, people with bulging foreheads were also regarded as especially bright.

WHAT WE THINK OF MIND TODAY

Trying to understand what the mind is has historically been a search for the seat of the soul. A separate historical issue has been whether the relationship between mind and brain is a one-to-one correspondence, a dualist interaction, or whether they are entirely incommensurable. A third issue concerns the nature of nervous tissue itself, a concept that has gone from the idea of hollow tubes conveying pneuma to one of "centers" that are associated with one another and whose output somehow manifests itself in the physical world.

To understand contemporary concepts you should know four things: (1) a standard hierarchical map of primary and association cortices, (2) a topographic map of neural connections, (3) the distributed system, and (4) limbic anatomy. These concepts are complimentary rather than mutually exclusive depending on the purpose for which you use them. The standard map, for example, is good enough for the bedside and for first approximations, but inadequate for proposing mechanisms.

Korbinian Brodmann's famous map of the human cortex appeared in 1909. Brodmann showed that the anatomical organization of the cortex is similar in all mammals. His use of cellular arrangements (cytoarchitecture) to classify cortical types as well as his nomenclature of the six horizontal layers were instrumental in clarifying the hopeless confusion that existed before Brodmann entered this field. At the time, however, his work was so strongly opposed that the medical faculty at Berlin refused to admit him. Politics, jealousy, and narrow-mindedness always impede real progress.

The next step was understanding the cellular origins of nervous-system components in vertebrates. Anatomy did not mature as a science until embryology showed how structures developed and attained their adult configuration. The American anatomist George Coghill (1872–1941) laid to rest behaviorist assumptions that the reflex constituted the quantum of behavior. Studying salamanders from first motility to their final adult form, Coghill correlated developing morphology to the exact sequence of behavioral patterns. He gave the first account of relationships between the progressive differentiation of bodily structures and the role of a given structure in overt behavior.

Broad-minded and synthetic scientists were able to assimilate structure, function, and clinical experience. It is hard to select a few individuals from among the many persons whose names are now eponyms for anatomic structures or household words in modern neuroscience. Interested students should consult *The Founders of Neurology* (Haymaker & Schiller, 1970) not only for biographical sketches of these pioneers, but also for historical vignettes of the trying circumstances in which they worked. It is not romantic exaggeration to say that people working with high-technology probes today often cannot match their superior specimens with ideas as well as men and women of the nineteenth century could.

The mere coöccurrence of aberrant behavior and a disordered brain is not sufficient to prove cause and effect. But we do believe today that both normal cognition and diseased minds obey natural laws that we can discover. This approach tends to do away with metaphysical speculations about the relationship between body and mind. Much of the philosophical and psychological discussion in the twentieth century contains the explicit assumption that the character of both mind and brain is understood and that the driving issue is simply understanding the link between the two. This, of course, is hardly true.

The expectation of linear process is deeply embedded in our thinking despite ample evidence for the abundance of parallel, recursive, and other non-linear events. This is true whether we consider history, technology, or the various schemes that propose to explain how we get from thinking to movement, or from sensation to thinking. We are still much taken with the idea of a linear, sequential psychology. Although we think that "cascade" or "information flow" concepts of cognition are modern concepts, they are nothing more than a rehash of the medieval cells that were arranged in a line. The generic flow from transduction of physical energy flux to internal mental representations is often depicted as follows:

Sense organs → Sensation → Perception → Cognition → Memory

Each mental stage is mapped onto a physical one and a "togetherness of function" is assumed in such a scheme. The components of vision, for example, that psychology had named only two decades ago (shape, color, stereopsis, location in space, etc.) were conceived to be together at the retina, together at the geniculate, together at the striate cortex, the association cortex, and so on down the line. The sequential cells of medieval times have simply been replaced by a succession of cortical tissue. In only two generations, the anatomical ground of cognition just scattered itself, first more and more finely over the cortex, and then into the microscopic realm.

We now believe that several concepts can be simultaneously valid and that, for instance, many functionally distinct cortical fields process information in parallel as well as through more or less traditional hierarchy. Traditional motor and sensory maps were static; now, we appreciate that each individual's experience (learning, environment) influences that individual's cortical maps. Four important themes of neuroscience today are (1) multiplex information flow, (2) physical plasticity during both development and adult life, (3) the richness and complexity of cortical pharmacology, and (4) the search for cerebral circuits.

One of the most challenging questions within the framework of modularity is how information processed in separate areas is assembled into a seamless experience. The nature of the questions we pose today also differs from those of earlier times. We ask not so much, "Where is a cognitive function or a symptom localized?" but, "How does a lesion (or selective input, or stimulation) modify the function of the brain so that a definite symptom appears?"

The astute student will see that the progression of ideas I have presented remains linked to a one-to-one mapping between psychology and anatomy. What has changed over the millennia is simply the fineness of the map, from the tricellular one of Aristotle to the microscopic ones of today. In the past quarter century, we have seen proposals for both *one-to-many mapping*, in which a given psychological function has multiple neuronal representations, or a *many-to-one mapping* in which several psychological functions are mapped onto the same neuronal substrate. Both these ideas have matured in recent years, and both seem to be correct.

The one-to-many anatomical mapping implies multiple maps of cognitive function that differ in their representational style. In vision, for example, the task of knowing "what" we are seeing (shape recognition) is processed in one anatomic region; the task of knowing "where" that shape is located (spatial recognition) is processed elsewhere; color is processed yet somewhere else; and so forth. There are almost two dozen anatomically distinct regions that are now identified with vision. The psychological many-to-one mapping is characteristic of the distributed system that we will discuss in chapter 3. This shows how multiple functions can be mapped through a single anatomic region. We have given up the idea that the deeper we dig and the more finely we divide, the closer we will come to the elusive link between mind and brain. Rather, we now seek multilevel theories, understanding somehow that mind and brain are more than the sum of their parts.

SUGGESTED READINGS

Churchland PM. 1990 *Matter and Consciousness*. Cambridge: MIT Press

Finger S. 1993 *Origins of Neuroscience: A History of Exploration into Brain Function*. New York: Oxford University Press

Gardner H. 1987 *The Mind's New Science: A History of the Cognitive Revolution.* New York: Basic Books

Hundert EM. 1989 *Philosophy, Psychiatry, and Neuroscience: Three Approaches to the Mind. A Synthetic Analysis of the Varieties of Human Experience.* Oxford: Oxford University Press

La Mettrie JO. 1748 *Man a Machine.* Reprinted, 1991, La Salle, IL: Open Court

Lavine TZ. 1984 *From Socrates to Sartre: The Philosophic Quest.* New York: Bantam Books

Schrödinger E. 1944 *What is Life?* Reprinted 1967, New York: Cambridge University Press

Searle JR. 1992 *The Rediscovery of the Mind.* Cambridge: MIT Press

Young RM. 1990 *Mind, Brain and Adaptation in the Nineteenth Century.* New York: Oxford University Press

3 Concepts of Neural Tissue

Permit me a bit of hyperbole in starting this chapter with an explanation of "how the brain works." Anyone with a modicum of knowledge in neuroscience would normally huff at such presumption, given that we cannot explain how the brain ultimately produces thought and behavior despite our detailed knowledge of its inner workings. This deluge of substantive neural knowledge has perhaps already exceeded the ability of any one individual to comprehend it all. It is precisely for this reason that students from other fields must have a synopsis (Greek *syn* [together] + *opsis* [view] = "to see altogether") to keep them from becoming hopelessly lost.

This big picture is necessarily stripped of the many qualifications and nuances with which those who come to neuroanatomy from the bottom up are familiar. I have also chosen to present not one view of the big picture but two, starting with the "standard," or hierarchical, concept of neural tissue. This is the view with which most scientists and knowledgeable laypersons are familiar. Unfortunately, while a number of its concepts are no longer tenable to those working intimately in the field, they are still widely believed by those who are not. This is largely a matter of dissemination rather than contention. Because neuroscientists are in the middle of changing our minds about the nature of neural tissue, I do consider compendiums of both the standard hierarchical view and the current "multiplex" one necessary. You may consider both as first approximations of how the brain works. We will discuss nuances in due course.

THE STANDARD HIERARCHICAL MODEL

Typical surveys found in popular books and television programs, what one might call *Neurology 101*, explain how the brain works in terms of how we conceived of its organization several decades ago. The three prime concepts of this standard model are (1) that information flow is *linear*, (2) that physical and mental functions can be *localized* to discrete parts of the cortex, and (3) that a *hierarchy* exists in which the cortex dominates everything else.

Although the standard model is no longer very standard, I will continue to use the terms "standard" and "hierarchical" to refer to this dated concept of nervous tissue that conceives of a linear flow of nervous impulses (information, if you like). It casts perception as a one-way street, traveling from the outside world inward, our sense organs transducing the energy flux and dispatching a linear stream of neural impulses from one relay to ever more complex ones, so that the process is metaphorically like a conveyor belt running through stations in a factory, until a perception rolls off the end as the *finished product*.

Both sense impressions coming in and motor commands going out of the brain are conceived metaphorically in this way: The sense organs transform the flux of electromagnetic energy (vision), mechanical energy (hearing and touch), or chemical energy (taste and smell) into nervous impulses. These impulses then travel to various relays in the brainstem and thalamus and from there to progressively more complex stations of the cortex where different aspects of the external stimulus are sequentially extracted from the stream. These aspects are somehow assembled at the end of the line into a conscious experience so that we understand what it is in the external world that triggered our sensory transduction in the first place.

Localization of function is the second major tenet of the standard model. For example, the occipital lobe is concerned with vision, the parietal lobe with touch, and the temporal lobe with hearing. The division of the brain into "lobes" was done so long ago as to retain no current validity, though the names of the four different lobes are still used as a general point of physical reference, as the top of figure 2.4 shows. (As late as 1844, according to Wigan, the brain's lobes numbered only three.) This century's several schemes for dividing the brain into some fifty discrete units are based either on its microscopic patterns of cellular arrangement (the technical term is *cyto-architecture*) or on patterns of myelination (*myelo-architecture*). Those who mapped the brain's architecture at the turn of the century were surprised to discover that the discrete areas they had found by looking through their microscopes did not at all follow the natural boundaries of the brain's bumps and fissures.

The word *cortex*, meaning "rind" or "bark," refers to the bumpy surface of the brain. Of all brain parts, the surface cortex is the largest and has the most complicated architecture. It also is the youngest component in terms of evolution. For these reasons, together with the fact that human cortex is said to be more developed than that of other mammals, the standard model pointed to it as the essential entity that distinguishes us from other creatures. In our efforts to understand the brain, however, we have often emphasized the cortex to the near-exclusion of everything below it. Perhaps one practical reason for its emphasis historically is that it *was* the surface and so could be easily approached experimentally.

In 1949, the American neurologist Paul MacLean originated the triune brain model, an embodiment of what was known as the *accretion hypothesis* at its height. This view, long popular but now much modified, held that newer structures were added on to those of the reptilian brain and were accompanied by correspondingly new mental skills and behaviors. MacLean's conceptual refinement of three-brains-in-one proposed that human brains contain three neural systems, each of different evolutionary age and each governing a separate category of behavior. The oldest "reptilian" brain, represented by brainstem and basal ganglia, deals with self-preservation. The middle "paleo-mammalian" brain is our inheritance from the mammallike reptiles and is concerned with preservation of the species (e.g., sex, procreation, and socialization), plus supposedly unique mammalian behaviors such as nursing, maternal and paternal care, audiovocal communication, and play. The components of the paleo-mammalian brain are collectively called the *limbic system*, which in humans deals mostly with emotion. The evolutionarily youngest "neo-mammalian" brain is embodied in the huge expanse of cortex that is seen as a chief executor. MacLean originally questioned the role of paleo-cerebral structures in behavior and was most interested in showing that *subcortical structures were vital for the expression of species-typical behavior.* The triune brain's apparent agreement with the

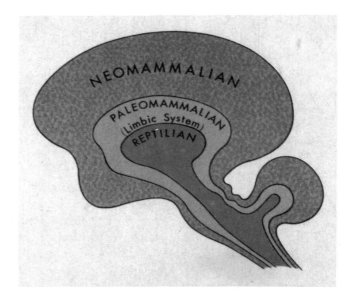

Figure 3.1
The triune brain represents the *accretion hypothesis* of brain evolution
and conceives of three-brains-in-one, each segment relating to particular
categories of behavior and reflecting a distinctive inheritance from earlier
life forms. From MacLean (1967), with permission.

standard model's concept of hierarchy and cortical dominance is
evident from figure 3.1, even though its originator did not intend
to perpetuate those ideas.

In 1902, the British neurologist Lord Sherrington had shown that
the brain's central fissure separates a *precentral* motor area in front
of it, whereas in 1909 the American surgeon Harvey Cushing
showed that a *postcentral* sensory area lies behind it. A central
fissure dividing a motor brain in front from a sensory brain in back
exists in all placental mammals. In 1952, Woolsey showed by
electrical mapping that the organization of the sensory area behind
the central fissure is a mirror image of the motor area in front of it.
The existence of two spatially separate areas, each with its own
function, became a fundamental concept of neuroscience. Later,
detailed electrical mapping of the cortex during surgery held out
the hope that we might establish a point-to-point correspondence
between brain tissue and function, both physical and mental.

Within the sensory half of the brain, the *primary sensory areas* were determined for vision, hearing, and touch. Those for taste and smell were debated for a long time, but the point is that all sensation was believed to have a cortical representation. The primary area for a given sense was its first cortical relay station, and damaging it caused total loss of function—such as blindness, deafness, and tactile anesthesia. *Secondary association areas* were soon found for each sense. These additional maps were conceived of as relays further along on the conveyor belt of perception that received more highly processed information. Damage to these secondary areas caused a distortion of a given sense rather than its total loss. An example is the failure of recognition called *agnosia* (meaning "not knowing"). In visual agnosia, for example, one can see and describe an object but neither recognize it nor understand its use. Agnosia can occur in any sense. At the end of the line was the *tertiary association cortex* in the parietal lobe. This was where sight, sound, and touch converged and where associations between and among the senses was assumed to occur. Though each sense had its own primary and secondary association areas, there was but a single tertiary area, where the highest, most abstract levels of association were believed to take place.

You will notice that smell and taste do not fit this model because their cortical representations are removed from the tertiary association area. Another function that received scant attention was emotion, a human trait known to be served in great part by structures beneath the cortex. If earlier scientists considered emotion at all, they conceived of it as a detour branching off the linear stream of neural flow. Even then, emotional calculations were thought of as secondary to those that took place in the cortex itself.

These three ideas (linearity, localization, and hierarchy) melded to inspire the further assumption that *the cortex is the seat of reason and the mind, the seat of those things that make us human.* The accident of Phineas Gage in 1848 is the classic example of this idea (see chapter 2, p. 41). The assumptions of the standard model are still in the minds of the general public as well as the average scientist. Perhaps they persist in part because the standard model is easy to grasp and useful to a point—just as Newton's mechanics are still useful even though everyone has known for decades that Einstein's relativity is a more accurate description of the universe.

A historical parallel might be the Renaissance astronomers who kept piling epicycle on epicycle to explain the retrogression of Mars's orbit until their scheme of planetary reaches was a patchwork that no longer held together. Kepler's conceptual shift of planetary orbits from circular to elliptical explained all observed facts much better and without the need for piling on special exceptions. The standard model of brain organization has similarly collapsed: It could no longer bear the weight of having to explain the avalanche of observations made in the recent past. We now know that as a model its generalities are true, whereas its specific predictions are sometimes erroneous.

Lastly, neuroscientists have just lately come to acknowledge how important emotion is in our mental life. In believing reason to be the superior and dominant force that guides our thinking and behavior, we simultaneously hold the dichotomous view that emotion must be primitive and disruptive, an interference to clear logical thinking. People who think of their brains at all usually imagine a computer in their heads, a reasoning machine that runs things. This is consistent with the hierarchical model of brain organization. However, like the carnival barker who pretended to be the Wizard of Oz, hiding behind the curtain while shouting, "Pay no attention to the man behind the curtain," placing reason and the neocortex foremost really overstates the case because emotion and the mentation that is not normally accessible to self-awareness are often what's behind the curtain pulling the levers.

THE NEW MULTIPLEX MODEL

The contemporary concept of neural tissue puts the role of the cortex not at the top but more in the middle of multiplex, parallel, and recursive pathways. "Highest," when used to describe cortex, is a meaningless attribute. Cortex is just one of several types of brain tissue. (Besides, there are several kinds of cortex, as we will see in an upcoming section.) Intense but recent interest in consciousness and emotion, after decades of disinterest, has led neuroscientists to reëvaluate the role of the limbic system (sometimes called the *emotional brain*).

Paul MacLean's triune brain captured popular attention over the last forty years for several reasons, one being that it is easy to understand. Like Gall's phrenology, the idea of three-brains-in-one was appropriated by others for purposes that MacLean never proposed. It is best taken today as a useful metaphor rather than a faithful model of brain organization. The triune brain did help to show that specific categories of behavior could be assigned to different types of brain tissue, each of which had a distinctive evolutionary history. It was enormously helpful in showing that tissue *below the cortex* was not just inert filler that could be neglected but that subcortical tissue was essential to behaviors that could not be dismissed as merely "instinctual" (e.g., reproduction, feeding, and fight-or-flight situations). In general terms, the behaviors in question include grooming, routines, rituals, hoarding, protection of territory, deception, courtship, submission, aggression, socialization, imitation, and other human proclivities (MacLean, 1990, pages 228–244).

MacLean coined the term *limbic system* in 1952 because of the extensive relation of entities below the cortex to the limbic lobe of the brain. Broca first defined the limbic lobe in 1878 in structural terms, as the inside rim (*limbus*) of the hemispheres where they meet the brainstem. MacLean's experimental work showed that one part of the limbic system was concerned with preservation of the species (being the substrate for behaviors related to sex, procreation, and socialization), while a second part was involved with self preservation (feeding, fear, and fighting). He identified a third segment as controlling suckling, maternal and paternal care, audiovocal communication, and play—behaviors supposedly unique to mammals.

Because he pictured the neomammalian brain (the neocortex) as enfolding everything else, MacLean's illustration of the triune concept inadvertently led people still to cede the cortex prime importance. The elevated role in human behavior that MacLean assigned to subcortical tissue (as represented by the reptilian and paleomammalian complexes) was undermined by his drawing. People came away with the hierarchical notion that the cortex was still boss.

Whether a neural structure is visible on the surface or tucked out of sight has no bearing on hierarchy or whether it is controlling or controlled. Function is what matters. As the contemporary model clarifies, the complexity of anatomic connections between cortex and subcortical entities are reciprocal and thus interdependent.

The contemporary model has three main points: First, neural propagation is not strictly linear but is also parallel and multiplex, including transfer of information that does not even travel along nerves; thus, the idea of strict hierarchy makes no sense. Second, we no longer speak of localization as a one-to-one mapping, but of the *distributed system*, a many-to-one mapping in which a given chunk of brain tissue subserves many functions and yet, conversely, by which a given function is not strictly localized but is distributed over more than one spot. Third, although the cortex contains mental representations (our models of reality) and analyzes what exists outside of ourselves, it is the limbic brain that determines the salience of that information. An emotional evaluation, more than a reasoned one, guides our behavior.

Nonlinear Information Flow

Information is transferred through the nervous system in more ways than most people realize. Multiple communication channels exist in addition to what we typically know of as nerves, synapses, and the hard-wired circuitry familiar from classic neuroanatomy. This abundance of alternate routes is denoted by the word *multiplex*.

The multiplex ways of transmitting information in the brain is not hierarchical, as would be the case if the flow were straightforwardly linear, but involves parallel, recursive, feedforward, and feedback connections. There also exists a wide assortment of molecules, such as hormones and peptides, that likewise act as information messengers. More than fifty are known and more are being discovered annually, not just in the brain but throughout the body. Information can therefore be transmitted throughout the body not only by neurons and axons (the traditional long wiring system of the brain) but through the extracellular fluid that surrounds the entire system itself. This method of communication is called *volume transmission* (Agnati, Bjelke & Fuxe, 1992; Fuxe & Agnati, 1991).

Think of electrical transmission along nerves as a train traveling down a track; volume transmission is the train leaving the track. The idea that molecular messengers communicate information over short or long distances, and at rates that can be very fast (up to 120 meters per second in axon fluid) or slow (e.g., the diffusion of peptides in cerebrospinal fluid), has opened up our understanding that the human brain has systems, which are much more complex than we had ever supposed, communicating at different ranges, different velocities, and different methods. A few examples should convey the fecundity to which volume transmission leads.

One protease found in the brain (PN-1) acts with thrombin, normally known as a blood-clotting agent, to regulate neurite outgrowth and neuronal connectivity. Another protease (PN-2) helps maintain cerebral blood flow. A family of five muscarinic receptors is now implicated in various neurological diseases. Perhaps the best-known information regarding volume transmission concerns the role that nitric oxide, a highly toxic, soluble gas, plays in the brain (Barinaga, 1994).

Long term potentiation (LTP) is a well-known process by which synapses linking active neurons appear to grow stronger through use. How LTP worked remained unknown for twenty years. It now seems that a nitric oxide molecule serves as a diffusible signal that spreads LTP to the synapses of nearby neurons. Nitric oxide is also implicated in neural degenerations such as Alzheimer's disease. Other gases, such as carbon monoxide, serve as physiological neural messengers too (Verma et al., 1993). The spread of LTP to only active synapses may be one way that experience sculpts clusters of neurons in the embryonic brain so that they will respond only to similar stimuli. Such a process could lead to the ocular dominance columns that exist in mature brains, for example.

Just as four base pairs can code all genetic information, so too sixty to seventy peptides can act as intercellular messengers in a variety of life forms (Brown, 1993). Nervous and immune systems share many specific, cell-surface recognition molecules that are highly conserved, meaning that they appear across all life forms. These receptors for neuropeptide-mediated intercellular communication are not uniquely human but seem to be hard-wired in even the simplest of creatures. Unicellular organisms (e.g., *Tetrahymena*) synthesize such complex peptides as endorphins and insulin, and even tumor cells (e.g., oat cell carcinoma) can secrete several neuropeptides in addition to bearing receptors that enable chemotaxis toward neuropeptides.

The classic one-to-one synapse turns out to be valid for acetylcholine but not for most other transmitters. Furthermore, neuropeptide receptors are not confined to the brain, but operate all over the body in transferring information. Action characteristically occurs at a distance, a substance and its receptors being physically far apart. The action of a given peptide also varies according to its location. Cholecystokinin (CCK), for example, is known as a satiety peptide. In the gut it affects intestinal motility, whereas in the spleen CCK receptors are present on macrophages. Furthermore, about five percent of monocytes have CCK receptors, meaning that subtypes exist that function in this case to make the monocyte move someplace else by chemotaxis. Another example of variable function is angiotensin: In the brain it influences thirst, while in the kidney it conserves water.

It is most noteworthy that peptide receptors are associated with *sensory* pathways, not motor ones. They therefore act like *filters*. One resulting speculation is that each peptide may be associated with a specific emotional state. Another speculation is that emotion exists in two realms, the physical one and the mental one.

One reason that current approaches to artificial intelligence have failed is that they try to imitate logic and are largely modeled on the circuitry of the cortex. Aside from the fact that humans are hardly ever logical (Cherniak, 1986), AI does not accommodate the biologic brain's many different ways of transferring information.

If you are wondering whether the stuff conveyed by volume transmission has anything to do with cognition, the answer is "yes." The two systems are integrated via reciprocal neurochemical links. Lymphatic tissue, for example, has sophisticated innervation (Felton & Felton, 1991). In humans, the integration of the hard-wired and volume-transmitted systems is most easily seen in the "neuro-immune-endocrine network," wherein synergistically acting transmitters and peptides regulate endocrine and immune activity as well as chemical feedback to hard-wired portions of the nervous system (Cotman et al., 1987; Husband, 1992). Additionally, immune functions are coupled with sleep and similar biological rhythms.

Both the nervous and immune systems have a remarkable capacity to receive and react to specific events in both internal and external milieus. Neither system is autonomous; complex homeostatic relationships integrate behavioral, neural, endocrine, and immune processes. It is such integration, rather than just an expanded cortex, that made it possible for human brains to develop from more primitive and highly deterministic organisms (Ommaya, 1994). To successfully reproduce the flexibility that this kind of integration affords, AI would have to incorporate some kind of regulating system to organize the different means of information transfer.

In the human brain, it is the limbic system that performs this regulation, a fact confirmed only in the last decade or so (Armstrong, 1990, 1991). You might wonder why it has taken until now to figure out something that seems rather fundamental. It is because only recently have anatomic techniques emerged that permit neurotransmitter molecules to be tagged with special dyes that can be seen microscopically. One can now follow the journey of neurotransmitters through both nerve fibers and the extracellular spaces in which volume transmission takes place. Classic anatomy at first allowed us to map the brain's general circuits, but having accurate knowledge now of the *direction* of flow as well as the precise origins and targets of various transmitters has forced us to make revisions. It turns out that every major division of the nervous system, from the frontal lobes to the spinal cord, contains some physical limbic structure related to emotion. In the neocortex are the prefrontal lobes; in the mesocortex, the cingulate gyrus; in the archicortex, the hippocampal formation; in the basal ganglia, the amygdala; in the diencephalon, the dorsal thalamus and hypothalamus; in the midbrain, the central gray matter; in the pons and medulla, the nuclei of the integrated autonomic relays; and in the spinal cord, the cell column nuclei. In other words, the limbic system forms an *emotional core* of the human nervous system.

Function Is Not Strictly Localized

The idea that circuits rather than "control centers" support the expression of emotion was first suggested in 1937 by the American anatomist James Papez (1883–1958). Major entities of what we now call the limbic system were hooked together into the Papez circuit, through which cognitive, visceral, and motor aspects of emotion were manifest. The implication for the neurologist's habit of localization was profound: Emotion was no longer localized in a discrete control center but was spread out over pathways. Of course, the pathways must be somewhere, and so some localization is involved. However, it is qualitatively a much more diffuse localization than that imagined by the standard model.

Over the next forty years, this approach caused a fundamental and permanent change in how many people working closely in the field conceived of information traveling through the brain. The linear idea of discrete workstations along a conveyor belt yielded to the concept of multiple mapping (modularity) in which a brain with multiplex communication channels can transform information in several locations at once.

Multiple mapping is possible by linking one input to several outputs. As soon as nervous impulses from the sense organs synapse in their respective primary sensory cortices, they simultaneously branch out to *multiple* areas of association cortex for further transformation, each area being concerned with a *different* facet of the experience. In vision, for example, each of some *two dozen* areas handles a different aspect of seeing (Van Essen et al., 1992; Zeki, 1993). The job of analyzing whatever it takes to yield the experience of color goes in one direction. The many things that constitute shape and lead to the recognition of an object, or the space where that object is located, are handled somewhere else. The neat image that the geometry of foveation casts on our retinas is shattered as the world is multiply mapped in our brains, a different map in each of several areas per sense. In addition, collateral branches to both cortical and subcortical entities form recursive feedback and feedforward circuits that contribute to a massively parallel "digital" transformation of the original analog image.

The ability of a discrete brain area to process several *uniquely different maps* of the world arises from the complicated pattern of its inputs and internal connections in each architectural region, and the linking of this calculation to *several* outputs. This is what we call a distributed system, which means that the many aspects of complex functions (e.g., vision, audition, memory, or emotion) subserved by a particular circuit are not rigidly located in any one of its segments but rather *in the dominant process* occurring at any given time in the circuit itself. (Recall Sir Karl Popper's formulation, on page 31, that both mind and matter are an interacting set of *processes*.) The number of distinct regions transmitting to and receiving from other cortical areas varies from ten to thirty. The exponential level of complexity is apparent and far beyond that inherent in the conveyor-belt progression of the old view.

It seems that the globalists and the localizationists of the nineteenth century were both right, but in a way that neither could appreciate at the time. Any complex ability depends not on a single lump of brain but on an array of underlying processes, each of which confers but a single facet to the ability. Simpler processes are localized, whereas complex abilities are distributed (Farah, 1994).

LEARNING ANATOMIC DETAILS

Having glimpsed the big picture, which I grant is still changing, let us now turn to some anatomic details on which our concept of nervous tissue is based. At the end of this chapter, we will discuss some advanced considerations that revisit the two views of the big picture that I have just presented.

Just as with clinical experience, your experience with neuroanatomy must also be of the hands-on kind. Otherwise, you will merely be talking about abstractions that may not have much to do with human minds. Many individuals professing an interest in neuropsychology have never held a human brain, let alone dissected one. This circumstance is absurd. Although behavior does not reduce even to microscopic anatomy, the physical reality of neuropsychology is nevertheless grounded in the brain, not transcendent box diagrams.

You should own an atlas of the nervous system showing gross structure, cell bodies (Nissl stains), and tracts (myelin stains). I recommend Nieuwenhuys, Voogd and van Huijzen's *The Human Central Nervous System* (1988). You must be able to visualize gross brain dissections in horizontal, coronal, and sagittal planes with corresponding radiographic and magnetic planar images. Familiarity with microscopic sections will develop as your knowledge grows. I suspect that knowledge of such biological circuits will ul-timately be more fruitful than knowing comparable circuits of the theoretical kind.

Group study is a time-honored way to learn functional anatomy. Beyond your ability to diagnose lesions and formulate mecha-nisms, you will use your expert understanding of three-dimen-sional anatomy to interpret the CT, MRI, and PET scans of your own patients. Even though scans come with an "official" inter-pretation, neuropsychologists should arrive at better-informed conclusions regarding patients, especially their own, who have be-havioral problems.

Three General Arrangements of Neurons

The principles of neuronal function are remarkably similar in ani-mals as far apart as the snail and the human. The human brain re-sembles the brains of "lower" animals much more than it differs from them (Sarnat & Netsky, 1981). It contains roughly 10^{11} (100 billion) neurons and 10^{14} synapses (100 trillion), give or take a fac-tor of ten. A typical neuron has a cell body 5 to 100 μm in diameter from which emanate one major axon and a number of dendrites. The axon usually branches extensively near its end and may give off branches near its beginning. Generally, the dendrites and cell body receive incoming impulses: The cell body averages these sig-nals, and the axon distributes the result to a new set of neurons. Circuitry is not serial but richly cross-linked. Elements operate at low speeds of thousandths of a second. Neuron processes are in-tertwined in a dense thicket with adjacent branches separated by fluid films only 0.2 μm thick. Virtually all the space is filled with cells and their various processes.

Comparing the above magnitudes, you will note that the average number of synapses per neuron is only 1,000, an amount eight orders of magnitude less than the total number of neurons. Even if each of a given neuron's 1,000 synapses were with a different neu-ron, it could still connect to only a small fraction of all neurons (roughly 1 in 10 million to 1 in 100 million). As a network, the brain is vastly underconnected despite popular notions otherwise. Furthermore, most of a given neuron's synapses exist within a surrounding area of just 1 to 2 mm. Thus, the energy transformations that concern any individual neuron, or group of neurons, are predominantly local. We will return to this fact shortly.

Many scientists have pondered how to arrange this galaxy of nerve cells. The Russian-born physician Paul Yakovlev (1894–1983), who later worked in America, organized the brain according to three types of neuronal arrangements that can be found in all vertebrate brains and the operational representations of which, in humans, he derived empirically (Yakovlev, 1948, 1970). His is a very broad view of neural organization and therefore quite helpful to those just learning their way around the forest of neuropsychology. The three arrangements of neurons are reticular, nuclear, and laminar. As a first approximation, different behaviors can be associated with each type.

The three types of neuronal arrangement are shown in the coronal brain slice of figure 3.2. The reticular system (from the Latin *rete*, meaning "net") is an aggregation of loosely arranged cells having an expansive vertical distribution within the central core of the brainstem. The dendrites of these cells are arranged in bundles that form a net-like pattern. The reticular formation continues caudally as the intermediate substance of the spinal cord, while rostrally it projects to the intralaminar thalamic nuclei. The reticular formation is concerned with consciousness and arousal (so-called state functions, as opposed to channel functions that are conveyed by more self-contained sensory or motor pathways) and the internal homeostatic milieu.

Nuclei are clumps of neurons, just as galaxies are aggregates of individual stars. Nuclei range in size from a grain of sand, containing perhaps a few thousand neurons, up to the size of an almond that would contain a few 10 million cells. Examples of nuclear aggregates are the thalamic nuclei, medial geniculate body, red nucleus, and substantia nigra. Nuclear aggregates are either the cells of origin of a single entity or a sensory ganglion of second-order or third-order neurons.

A laminar arrangement of neuron groups permits more complex interactions such as feedforward, feedback, facilitation, recurrent inhibition, and defacilitation. Structural complexity increases through the five types of laminar tissue in the cortex. The corticoid tissue of the amygdala and the four-layered hippocampus, for example, are simpler than the six layers of the neocortex (figure 3.3).

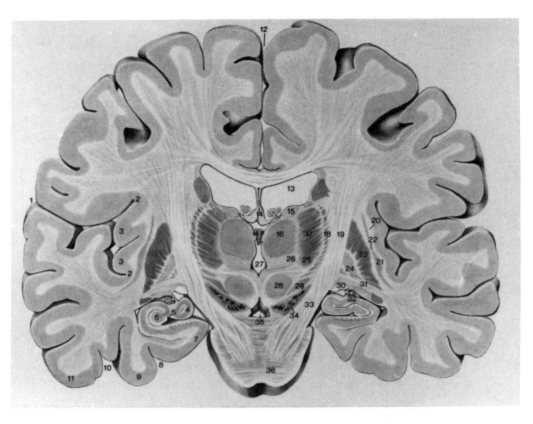

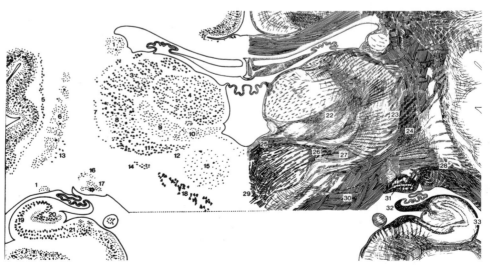

Figure 3.2
Gross anatomy (*top*), cell bodies (*bottom left*), and myelin tracts (*bottom right*) in a section cutting through the thalamus, cerebral peduncle, and the pons shows that most nuclear aggregates are centrally placed. Simple laminar arrangements occur in the colliculi and amygdala; four layers exist in hippocampus, six layers in neocortex. Lamination (layering) is best seen with a cellular stain. The reticular system is visible only microscopically. From Nieuwenhuys et al. (1988), with permission.

Ways to Arrange the Cerebrum

Reticular, nuclear, and laminar arrangements each are associated with specific behavior (movements of the body within the body, movements on the body, and movements outside the body, respectively).

State versus channel functions highlight general behavior and distinguish those functions more dependent on chemical or hormonal activation from those subserved by more self-contained pathways.

The cortical column, orthogonal to the surface, is the basic unit of the cortex.

The distributed system, a complex of reciprocally interconnected dynamic systems, allows us to conceive of multiple mapping of psychological functions.

Patterns of neural connection in cortex can be reduced to five types: limbic, paralimbic, heteromodal homotypical, unimodal homotypical, and idiotypical.

Subcortical versus cortical categorization of behavior emphasizes that cortex is not necessary for many types of behavior or sensory discrimination.

Lateralization and hemispheric specialization remind us that brain function segregates in utero, probably under hormonal influence. Cognitive ability is unevenly distributed in the general population.

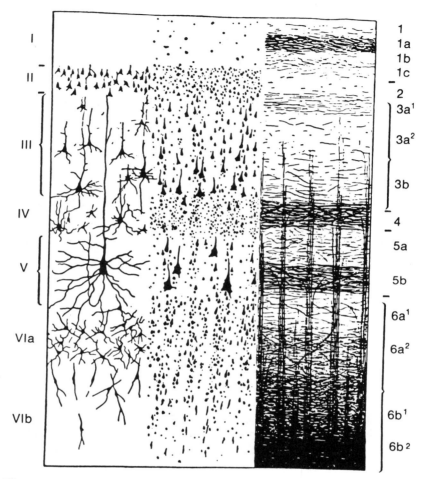

Figure 3.3
Vertical chains and horizontal lamination in the cortex. (*Left*) A Golgi stain, which shows branches. (*Center*) A Nissl stain, which shows cell bodies. (*Right*) A myelin stain, which shows pathways of axonal projections. From Popper & Eccles (1977), with permission.

In his classic 1948 paper, Yakovlev reduced behavior to movement (which it fundamentally is) and conceived "three spheres of motility" comprising (1) movements in the internal milieu, which he called *visceration*, (2) the physical expression of internal states (*emotion*), and (3) manipulation of the external world (*effectuation*). Yakovlev drew a correspondence between neuronal arrangements and behavior as follows: (1) The reticular arrangement yields movements of the body *within* the body (the essence of autonomic and visceral action); (2) the nuclear arrangement yields movements of the body *upon* the body (axial and postural action of the extrapyramidal system); and (3) the laminar arrangement yields movements of the body *outside* the body (the pyramidal action of effectuation). Yakovlev's scheme is beautifully concise and remains generally valid.

Three corresponding clinical examples of Yakovlev's organizational scheme are (1) hemiplegia caused by a stroke in the *laminar* cortex, impairing operation on the external world; (2) Parkinson's disease caused primarily by degeneration of the substantia nigra *nucleus*, which impairs movements of the body upon itself, especially postural and axial adjustments; and (3) destruction of the pontine *reticular* activating system causing coma or sleep-wake disturbance.

Phyletic Development

There exists a basic blueprint from which all vertebrate brains are built. Phyletic development compares the elaboration of fundamental neural components across species. This very traditional view, peppered with evolutionary theory, says that as we ascend the phylogenetic scale we find an increasing separation and elaboration of neural building blocks. This is how discrete faculties supposedly emerge out of a less specialized brain during evolution.

This is how, for example, lateralization and multiple specialization emerge in human brains, which reputedly rest at the top of the phyletic scale. Of course, some features of complex organisms, such as lateralization (asymmetry), are present in simpler forms such as fish and even plants. What matters to phyletic theory is the degree of a feature's development and its relevance to cognition in a given species. At its simplest, there is a conceptual parallel

Table 3.1
Phyletic Development

Species	Developmental Feature
Humans	Separation of projection areas, marked lateralization
Primates	Developed association cortices
Mammals	Separation of motor and sensory areas, multiple specialization
Marsupials	Overlap of primordial zones

between the complexity of neural development and its correspondingly sophisticated mental expression the "higher" we travel on the evolutionary scale (table 3.1).

The behavior of simple organisms has little or no plasticity. The brains of simple creatures tend to react immediately to the stimuli in their environment with a limited, invariant repertoire. They are unthinking brains that, partly because of their small size but mostly because of their hard wiring, have little room for flexible responses or for assembling information from several senses. For example, the hydra or sea anemone (phylum Cnidaria, class Anthozoa) has a mostly reticular nervous system. Neuroëpithelial cells located on the body surface make direct contact with underlying muscle cells. By poking the animal, as any marine aquarist knows, *stimulating one cell stimulates all of them*, and the anemone recoils and closes up.

This simple reflex arc between sensor and effector has been replaced in higher organisms by a series of interneurons poised between the sensor and effector cells. More advanced animals such as the crown jellyfish (Ctenophora) or tube worm (Phoronida) retain throughout their bodies the reticular nerve net, which stimulates undulating contractions that guide food into the mouth. Additionally, however, isolated conduction in a separate ring of neurons around the rim of the creature's umbrella causes the synchronous contraction of the marginal lappets by which the jellyfish swims and the tube worm withdraws into its tube. You now find *conduction of a nervous impulse over a long distance without stimulating all the neighboring or intervening cells* (that is, it does not stimulate the reticulum). This separation of a wide-band reticular system from a narrow-band conducting system in the ring represents a major advance in neural architecture. An analogy could be drawn with the separate human pathways serving channel and state functions. It is in the great proliferation of these intercalated neurons (*interneurons*) that central nervous systems of higher organisms find a corresponding plasticity of behavior.

The American Nobel laureate Roger Sperry performed a famous experiment in which he caused a visual displacement in a newt by surgically rotating its eyeball. The relatively inflexible wiring between the creature's retina and its higher visual brain kept it from ever finding food targets or behaviorally adapting to its new visual orientation. Humans (and subhuman primates) can experience similar, though reversible, visual displacements by wearing prisms that reverse the up-down and left-right orientations. These more flexible brains with their cloud of uncommitted interneurons can adapt within fifteen minutes of donning such spectacles so that the subject can operate fully in the new visual environment. (I have ridden a bicycle in traffic while wearing such prisms and can assure you that it is indeed an exciting experience.)

As we ascend the phylogenetic scale, the gradual elaboration of interneurons that eventually gives rise to association areas is considered a later stage of the process by which the primary motor and sensory areas first became individuated out of a less specialized brain, such as that of sea anemones and jellyfish: That is, cytoarchitectonic differentiation increases as associative activities become separated from receptive and motive ones. Patterns of cellular organization and connection become more distinct, and the topographic relationships among individual types of organization are highly ordered and regular. Such constant relationships allow us to derive principles about neural organization and its relation to specialized behavior.

Even though the evolutionary trend seems to be for increasing separation of function, dividing lines are not perfectly sharp. In many species, including humans, we can stick an electrode into what is supposed to be a visual neuron and discover that it also responds to sound or touch. In addition to such multimodal cells, unit recording also shows modality-specific ones amidst cells responding to a different modality. Rather than all or nothing, it is a question of degree that a cell responds robustly to a specific

modality and not very much to other kinds of input. Figures 2.4
(*top*) and 3.4 are standard illustrations of motor and sensory maps
along the central fissure. On the macroscopic scale, however,
electrical stimulation studies have proven that the boundaries of
functional regions (e.g., language) are not as sharp as conventional
diagrams usually suggest (Ojemann & Whitaker, 1978; Penfield &
Jasper, 1954).

Cortical Columns

Our conceptualization of nervous tissue has changed radically over
a short time from an amorphous reticulum to an arrangement of
intrinsic power modules raging a battle of excitation and inhibition. In addition to the six major layers of horizontal lamination
that Brodmann clarified in 1908, Lorente de Nó (1943) discovered
that neurons were also arranged in vertical chains throughout
the depth of the cortex (see figure 3.3).

Investigations by the American physiologists Vernon Mountcastle (1957) and David Hubel and Thorsten Wiesel (1972) showed
that neurons in tiny columns orthogonal to the cortical surface re-
sponded similarly to highly specific afferent inputs. These sharply-
defined columns for feature detection have an average cross-section
of 0.1 mm². Szentágothai (Szentágothai & Arbib, 1975) elucidated
the structural basis for what has become called the *modular*
organization of these neuronal columns. In both structure and
function, the column of specific cell types was conceived as the
basic unit in all cortical areas. The basic circuit of the columnar
module is (1) afferent fiber input, (2) complex interactions within
the module, and (3) output through the axons of the pyramidal
cells. There are major functional differences between connections
in laminæ I and II, and connections in laminæ III, IV, and V (figures
3.5, 3.6).

Cortical layers are numbered from the surface inward and are
arranged as follows: Layer I contains mostly horizontally directed
dendrites from other layers and other areas; it has few cells. Cells
in layers II and III project to deeper cortical layers as well as horizontally outside the cortical column. In turn, these cells in layers
II and III receive input from the deeper layers and adjacent cortical
columns. *Layer IV receives the direct projection from thalamic*

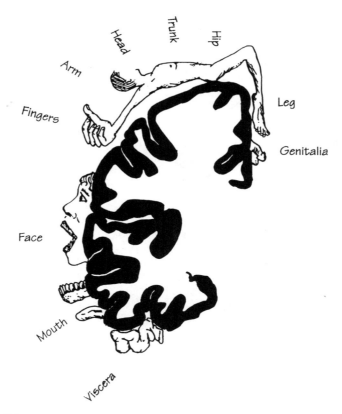

Figure 3.4
Electrical mapping during surgery produced motor and sensory homunculi, an orderly projection of the body surface onto the brain surface. Note the greater amount of area given to the face and hand compared to the trunk. Compare to figure 2.4 (*top*). (Adapted from Penfield & Rasmussen, 1950.)

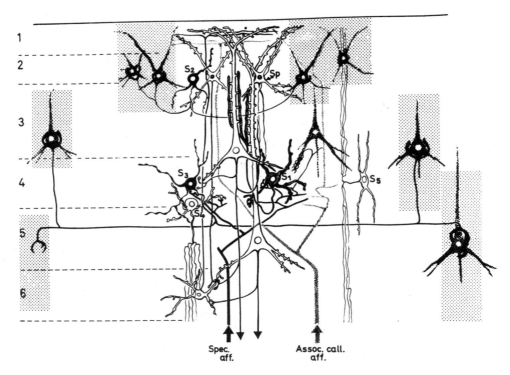

Figure 3.5
Neuronal components of a cortical column. Two pyramidal cells are in layers III and V. The specific afferent (spec. aff.) pictured excites a stellate interneuron S_1 (crosshatched), whose axon makes a cartridge-type synapse on the apical dendrites. The specific afferent also excites a basket-type stellate interneuron, S_3, that inhibits the pyramidal cells in adjacent columns. Interneurons S_6, in layer VI, and S_5, in layer IV, help spread excitation through the whole depth of the cortex. Sp, stellate pyramidal cells; S_2, short-axon inhibitory cells in layer II. The afferents formed by association and callosal fibers are shown ascending in layer I where they branch. From Popper & Eccles (1977), with permission.

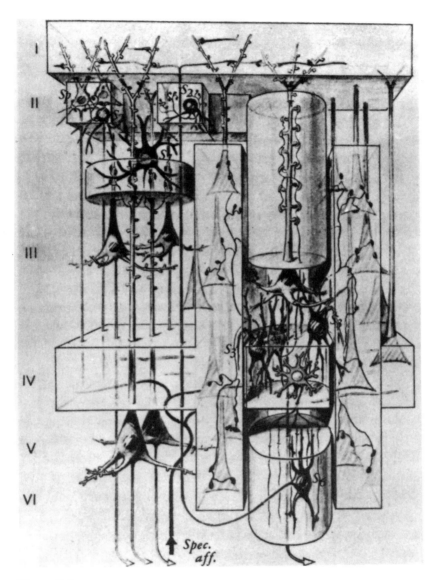

Figure 3.6
Three-dimensional sketch of a cortical column and its connections. From Popper & Eccles (1977), with permission.

nuclei. Not surprisingly, therefore, this layer is best developed in primary sensory cortex and least so in motor cortex. The giant pyramidal cells of layer V provide the main exit from the cortical column; they often give off recurrent axons that engage in feedforward or feedback operations. Layer VI contains spindle cells whose dendrites travel only in the lower three layers.

To summarize, the modular concept is of well-defined groups of cells (approximately ten thousand) with a unitary existence as a result of their mutual connections. They build up power within themselves and inhibit the cells of nearby columns. There are two levels of performance: A powerful one in laminæ III, IV, and V, involving specific afferents and pyramidal output, and a finer grain of influence in laminæ I and II that is exerted mainly by association and callosal afferent fibers. The delimitation of internal power and inhibitory surround is what defines a module. Each column tries to overcome its neighbor by building up its own power through its vertical connections and by projecting horizontal inhibition onto neighboring columns (Szentágothai, 1974).

It is not easy for the beginner to reconcile changing concepts of nervous tissue. Over a half century, the concept of an amorphous network yielded to that of hierarchy in which commands from supposedly higher centers were carried out by less complex brain systems. Cytoarchitectonics became increasingly complex as it more finely divided the cortex on the basis of number or type of cell, packing density, or degree and temporal sequence of its connecting fibers' myelination. At present, we think of the cortical column as the brain's basic *functional module.* Beyond the fundamental unit of the cortical column is the distributed system that sees the brain as a collection of widely and reciprocally interconnected dynamic systems (Mountcastle, 1979).

The Distributed System

A highly repetitive structure is characteristic of cortex. Though an expert eye (with the help of a microscope) can distinguish one region from another, the sameness of cortex suggests that it repeats the same task over and over. This repetition is in space rather than time, however, given evidence that different regions of cortex perform roughly the same transformation on their given inputs.

The distributed system develops this idea that there is nothing unique about the structure of one region versus another. Rather, it is the pattern of connections among entities, any one of which can belong to several distributed systems and onto which multiple variables can be mapped, that constitutes the distributed system. You will likely need to read the following section several times, because the distributed system is not easy to understand. However, *the idea of multiple mapping is its essence.*

The classic reticular, nuclear, and laminar divisions (such as the reticular formation, dorsal horn, basal ganglia, and neocortex) are referred to as *entities* that, as such, are composed of local circuits that are similar within any given entity (Szentágothai, 1974). Modules are grouped into entities (e.g., nuclei or regions of laminated cortex) (1) because of their specific external connections, (2) owing to the way they interact within a module, or (3) by cloning a particular function over a topographic region. The function of modules is everywhere the same, with nothing inherently motor about the motor cortex or sensual about sensory cortices.

Phylogenetically, the neocortex of primates achieved its enormous size *with hardly any change in its vertical organization,* one feature that led to the vertical minicolumn being regarded as the basic structural unit in this part of the cerebrum. This 30 x 25–μm cylinder of cells, perpendicular to the brain surface, forms as neurons migrate from the germinal zone of the neural tube along the radial glial cells to their destined locations in the cortex.

Different species of mammals all have an invariant 110 cells in each minicolumn of different neocortical areas, except for the striate cortex where the fixed number is 260. The number of pyramidal and stellate cells, the two main classes of neurons, is a constant 2:1 ratio in such diverse cytoarchitectonic and functional areas as motor, somatic, and visual areas of different mammals (Gatter et al., 1980). Mountcastle (1979) considered it unlikely that wholly new cell types unique to other brains, including more primitive ones, have appeared at any particular stage of mammalian evolution.

Just as atoms form molecules, several hundred structural minicolumns join to form the larger and fundamental functional unit of the cortical column, onto which *several* variables can be mapped. The human neocortex contains approximately 1 million of these larger columns, each of which is a complex processing and distributing unit that links a number of inputs to several outputs. The number of other regions transmitting to and receiving from a traditionally defined cortical area varies from ten to thirty. The cells of origin of different output pathways are sharply separated by cortical layer.

Note how several features from the hierarchical and cytoarchitectonic models of brain organization can be subsumed under the newer concept of a distributed system: (1) There exist distinct cortical areas that are homologous over a series of mammals, (2) each distinct architectural region has a unique function (in the conventional sense), and (3) each neocortical area that has a distinct architecture and function also has a unique set of extrinsic connections (that is, it has its own pattern of thalamic, cortico-cortical interhemispheric, and long descending connections). *These three variables of cytoarchitecture, extrinsic connections, and function define a cortical area.*

One great advantage of the distributed system is that several variables can be simultaneously mapped onto it while preserving the area's topology. Many variables can be mapped through a single area while preserving orderly relationships among (1) sets on the input side, (2) those within the area, and (3) those in the target. Thus, a number of distributed systems can be mapped through a given area of cortex, allowing an integration of their functions with other properties of the area that are determined by some different input to it. In this way, for example, selective processing (feature extraction) is possible via intercolumnar pathways that diverge to different outputs.

Neither the laminar nor the columnar organization of the cortex precludes other systems (e.g., nuclear, reticular) from operating throughout the cortex in different ways. This is seen particularly in systems that subserve state rather than channel functions (see below, pages 120–121). The noradrenergic system arising from the locus coeruleus of the pons, for example, reaches every cortical region and all cortical layers. Immunohistochemistry reveals a fine web of noradrenergic fibers at 30 to 40-μm intervals, indicating that any single cell of the locus coeruleus sustains an immense and divergent axonal field. Catecholamine-containing neurons are phylogenetically old and relatively few in number, and their

The Distributed System

> A cortical area is defined by its cytoarchitecture, its extrinsic connections, and its function.
>
> Distinct cortical areas can be homologized over a series of mammals.
>
> Every neocortical area that has a distinct cytoarchitecture also has a unique function in the conventional sense.
>
> Every distinct neocortical area also his its unique set of extrinsic connections (thalamic, corticocortical interhemispheric, and long descending).
>
> Several variables can be simultaneously mapped through an area while still preserving an area's topology.
>
> The distributed system does not preclude the operation of other systems, such as those serving state functions.

terminals are found both with and without synaptic connections, implying both transmitter and modulatory functions. The noradrenergic system is, in fact, capable of directly modulating the entire neocortex (Gold & Zornetzer, 1983).

The functions of various distributed systems were elucidated through three discoveries (Mountcastle, 1979). First it was determined that a distributed system's major entities are built by iterating identical multicellular units joined together by complex intermodular connections. Hundreds of structural minicolumns are packed together to form the functional unit of the cortical column. Second, extrinsic connections between large entities of the brain are far more numerous, selective, and specific than previously was supposed. Third, the many modules of a large entity do not each contain all the connections known for that entity. Instead, a large entity is split into subsets of modules, each linked by a particular pattern of connections to similarly segregated subsets of other large entities. The linked sets of modules of the several entities thus define the distributed system.

In contrast with older models of brain organization, the number of distributed systems in the brain is perhaps several orders of magnitude larger than previously thought. By definition and empiric observation, distributed systems are both reëntrant pathways and links to input and output channels of the entire nervous system. *Major entities are, moreover, nodes of more than one distributed system*, contributing to each system, as Mountcastle explained it, "a property determined for the entity by those connections common to all of its modular subsets and by the particular quality of their intrinsic processing. Even a single module of such an entity may be a member of several (though not many) distributed systems." The distributed system allows us to conceive of multiple maps of a given psychological function.

Topography: Patterns of Neural Connection

In trying to correlate the structure of nervous tissue (not just the neocortex!) with behavior, one looks for patterns. Compared to the sameness and repetitive structure of the modules that comprise distributed systems, *topologic organization stresses a region's common characteristics*. Topology bears the same relationship to topography as does geology to geography. It means a science of place, a qualitative geometry. Your study of this section of the text should be fortified with standard anatomic references, as necessary depending on your individual familiarity with cerebral anatomy.

The topologic approach divides the cortical mantle into just five common types that display a progression in structural complexity and differentiation. Figure 3.7 shows this topological schema on the left and, on the right, these same topologic regions superimposed on the conventional Brodmann areas. As the figure graphically depicts, the functional topologic zones widely overlap conventional architectonic divisions. The five topological types of nervous tissue are listed in table 3.2 and are shown schematically in figure 3.8, where their relationship to extrapersonal space and the internal milieu also are indicated.

With reference to table 3.2 and figure 3.8, we can see that brain tissue becomes more differentiated as we proceed from limbic tissue on the one hand to the primary motor and sensory areas of idiotypic cortex on the other. Note that the simplest structures have an in-between architecture that is partly nuclear and partly laminar. These are the *corticoid* tissues of the septum, the substantia innominata, and the amygdaloid complex. A substantial part of the amygdala has a nuclear architecture, though its location

Table 3.2
The Five Topographic Divisions of Cortex

1. Limbic areas	
Corticoid	Septum, substantia innominata, amygdala complex
Allocortical	Hippocampal formation (archicortex)
	Piriform (olfactory) complex (paleocortex)
2. Paralimbic areas (mesocortex)	
Temporal pole	
Caudal orbitofrontal cortex	
Insula	
Parahippocampal gyrus	Ento-, pro-, and peri-rhinal areas
	Pre- and para-subicular areas
Cingulum	Retrosplenial, cingulate, and parolfactory gyri
3. Modality-specific (unimodal) homotypical association isocortex	
4. High-order (heteromodal) homotypical association isocortex	
5. Idiotypic cotex	
Primary motor cortex	
Primary sensory cortices	

on the hemispheric vesicle actually makes it part of the cortical mantle.

Nomenclature proposed more than a century ago is still used next to more modern terms. Not much can be done to alleviate the resulting confusion other than to learn the terms, which roughly reflect the evolutionary age equivalence of laminated tissues as well as their increasing differentiation into granular and more distinctly laminated forms. The piriform complex is called *paleo*cortex ("old"), and the hippocampal formation *archi*cortex ("first," or "beginning"), and both are examples of *allo*cortex ("other"). The entire paralimbic region is called *meso*cortex ("middle"), whereas homotypic and idiotypic cortex are known collectively as *neo*cortex ("new"). Although all of these tissues are laminated, and thus technically are cortex, each is distinguished by a different level of organization. The word cortex used without a prefix commonly means the *neo*cortex.

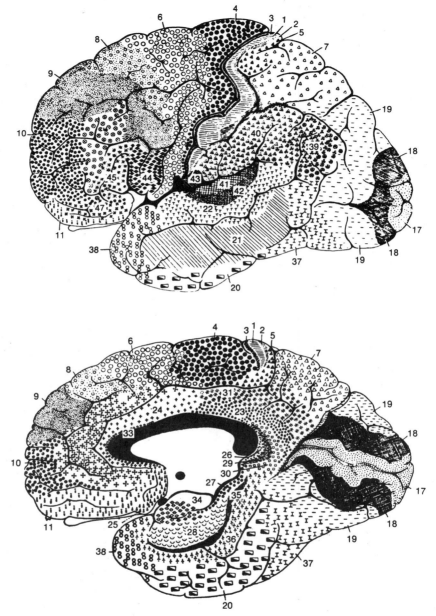

Figure 3.7
(*Left*) Brodmann's cytoarchitectonic map of the left hemisphere in lateral (*top*) and medial (*bottom*) views. Compare with the topographic organization shown at right. From Brodal (1969), with permission. (*Right*) Distribution of topological and functional zones in relation to Brodmann's map. Boundaries are not precise. Adapted from Mesulam (1985a), with permission.

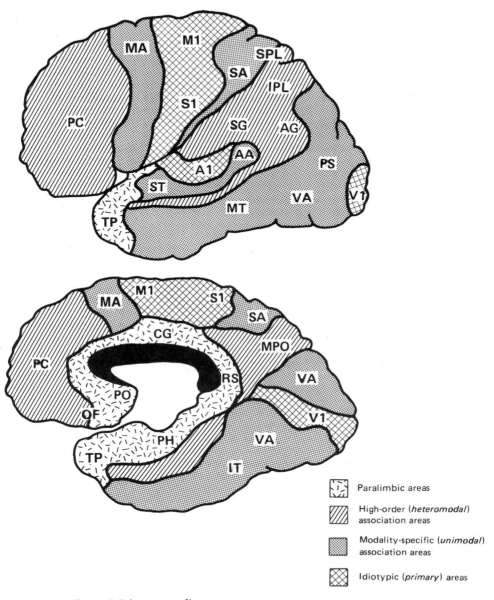

Figure 3.7 (continued)

Paralimbic areas

High-order (*heteromodal*)
association areas

Modality-specific (*unimodal*)
association areas

Idiotypic (*primary*) areas

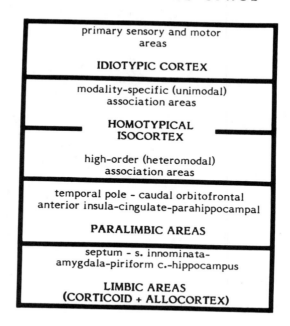

Figure 3.8
Schematic organization of the five topologic types of nervous tissue. See text for further details. From Mesulam (1985a), with permission.

Simply memorizing these names leaves you with mere abstractions, a poor substitute for the direct experience of viewing the histology of different types of cortex. You can see for yourself (*nullius in verba*) the gradual changes in complexity and differentiation. Both the horizontal lamination and the vertical chains appear more striking in newborn or fetal tissue, should you be fortunate enough to have access to any.

Homotypical association isocortex is either modality-specific (unimodal) or high-order (heteromodal). Analogous older terms would be *secondary association cortex* and *tertiary association cortex*, respectively. Heteromodal cortex actually is closer in structure to paralimbic cortex because it is less granular and its layers are less differentiated. Such classification on anatomic grounds makes the highly granular and striated idiotypic cortex of the primary motor and sensory areas the most advanced of cortices. This view is opposite that implied by older concepts that traced neural impulses linearly from thalamus to primary cortex, thence to secondary association cortex, and then to tertiary association cortex. Today we view primary (idiotypic) motor and sensory cortex as the most differentiated and the most advanced.

Three features define unimodal isocortex: (1) neurons in this area respond only to a single sensory modality, (2) input is by primary isotypic or other unimodal regions in the same modality, and (3) damage causes modality-specific deficits.

Heteromodal cortex is identified by three contrasting characteristics: (1) neurons respond to more than one modality, (2) inputs are from unimodal areas in more than one modality, from other heteromodal areas, or both, and (3) damage yields behavioral deficits that are not modality specific. Some neurons in heteromodal cortex are themselves multimodal, but the region is mostly a mixture of neurons that prefer different modalities.

Idiotypic cortex contains the well-known motor and sensory areas: The primary visual area in the calcarine cortex of the occipital pole, the primary auditory cortex (Heschl's gyri) in superior temporal cortex, the postcentral primary somatosensory cortex, and the precentral primary motor cortex.

Figure 3.8 schematically represents the five cortical types in relation to extrapersonal space and the internal milieu. You can deduce quickly from this schematic, together with figure 3.7, that the physical arrangement of cortical types is highly ordered. For example, paralimbic cortex is always surrounded by isocortex on one side and allocortex on the other; primary sensory cortex is always separated from heteromodal association areas by unimodal isocortex.

Figures 3.8 and 3.7 should also help you to observe that paralimbic and limbic areas have the closest relationship to the hypothalamus, which essentially is the cerebral ganglion for homeostasis. It is involved in temperature and metabolic control, autonomic outflow, sexual arousal, hormonal release, circadian rhythms, and immune regulation. It should be no surprise that limbic tissue is involved in four closely related behaviors: (1)

memory and learning, (2) modulation of drive, (3) emotion, and (4) higher control of hormonal balance and autonomic tone. The primary motor and sensory areas are more closely related to the external world. Sensory input has its first cortical relay in idiotypic cortex, whereas the motor cortex is the upper motor neuron outflow path that leads to manipulation of the outside world (what Yakovlev called *effectuation*). The heteromodal association and paralimbic areas occupy an intermediate position and permit the further elaboration of sensory processing and the integration of this processing with drive, emotion, and other aspects of mental content.

The five cortical zones also have horizontal and vertical connections with one another, although the pattern is not at all homogeneous. The vertical connections of a given zone are strongest with the immediately adjacent zone. For example, though all areas receive some hypothalamic projections, the most intense projections connect limbic entities. Similarly, unimodal cortex may receive input from other association areas in the same modality, but there is essentially no connection among areas belonging to different modalities. Instead, all modalities converge downstream in the limbic system.

Multiplex Communication
Figure 3.9 attempts to summarize this section on patterns of neuronal connections. Obviously, no illustration can successfully convey the rich *multiplexing* of the brain that I discussed earlier. Schemes organizing the brain into cortical versus subcortical, gray matter versus white matter, left hemisphere versus right hemisphere, and so forth are merely conceptual divisions that make comprehension a little easier for us. Though the brain is multiply specialized and regional differences in structure and related function do exist, all its parts are constantly active.

SUBCORTICAL ENTITIES

Scientists and laypersons alike tend to overemphasize the neocortex for reasons already noted. It is counterintuitive to learn how much sophisticated behavior is possible without any cortex at all. For example, cortex is unnecessary for many kinds of auditory, visual, and somesthetic discrimination (e.g., Weiskrantz, 1986; Diamond & Neff, 1957). MacLean showed that cortex is unnecessary for the expression of many complex behaviors that are usually called *innate*, and Konrad Lorenz showed that birds, which have virtually no cortex, exhibit sophisticated behaviors such as imprinting, parenting, and socialization. Monkeys in whom large stretches of cortex have been removed can hardly be distinguished from their cagemates (MacLean, 1990). This suggests that rather than being an obligate component of any meaningful behavior, cortex provides only a finer grain of discrimination to other brain areas that might be the final effectors of behavior.

It is also counterintuitive to learn that "decisions" can be made at the lowest human brainstem level. The gustofacial reflex, for example, is a well-differentiated motor reaction of the facial muscles to taste stimuli (Steiner, 1973). Controlled by neural structures of the brainstem, this reflex is a rigidly fixed behavior. Ethologists such as Peiper (1951) and Lorenz (1965) call the gustofacial response an innate behavior, an inherited motor coördination. Characteristic of such innate behaviors is its rigidly fixed expression, resistance to exhaustion by repetition, and homologous distribution among lower and higher mammals.

In the gustofacial reflex, different tastes produce fixed facial expressions (sweet = smile, bitter = disgust with tongue protrusion, sour = pursing of the lips). The gustofacial reflex is universal, evoking identical responses across individuals. The neural apparatus of gustation is well developed and functions long before birth. The adult form of the human taste bud is clearly visible in histologic preparations of the human embryo in the fifth gestational month. The reflex is even present in anencephalic monsters, babies who are born without any cerebrum but only a brainstem and diencephalon.

The striking point of the gustofacial reflex is the ability of the human brain's pontomedullary region, one of the lowest levels of the brainstem, to discriminate between sensory signals and to "decide" that some events are welcomed by the organism while others must be rejected as harmful or noxious. People often are inclined to believe that discrimination between good and bad is a cognitive function based on life experience, conditioning, learning, and an emotional attitude. This is simply not always true.

E
x
t
e
r
n
a
l

R
e
a
l
m

Outside World
Not Self

Sense Receptors
Mechanical, chemical, or
electromagnetic transducers

Local Architecture & Centripetal Tracts
(e.g., retina, cochlea)

*Most cortical areas feedback
to nuclei*

Nuclear Relays
One or more (e.g., thalamus)

*Primary (idiotypic) Sensory Cortices
First cortical relay, each sense projecting
to multiple & different association areas

Above connections, more linear;
those below, multi-directional

*Sense-Specific (unimodal)
Association Cortices
Highly concerned with external world

*Multi-Sensory (heteromodal)
Association Cortices

Bridges between external
realities and internal urges ******

Para-Limbic Areas
(portions of temporal and frontal lobes)
Behavioral relevance now more important
than the physical aspects of a stimulus

All areas
project to
striatum

Limbic Areas
Memory, learning, modulation of drive,
emotional coloring of experience, higher
control of hormonal & autonomic tone

Concept of linearity
increasingly disappears

I
n
t
e
r
n
a
l

M
i
l
i
e
u

Hypothalamus
Head ganglion of Internal Milieu
Immune regulation, circadian rhythms,
sexuality, temperature, metabolism,
electrolyte balance, drives and instincts
for species- and self-preservation

Internal Milieu
Sense of Self

Subcortical tissue does more that just hold up the surface. To confuse cortex with the whole brain is a bad case of synecdoche. The human neocortex constitutes only a fraction of the brain's bulk. Although gyral folding confers on it a large surface area, cortex averages only 1 to 2–mm thickness compared to a thickness up to a hundred times that for the whole brain.

I discuss the clinical correlations of subcortical lesions in chapter 6.

The Limbic System

The limbic system is complex in its evolution and in its connections. Do not fret if you feel confused initially. You must study it first-hand and via a standard brain atlas before its details become coherent. The Nieuwenhuys atlas that I recommended uses twenty-four separate illustrations to convey the limbic system's pertinent anatomic features, and forty-three pages of text to detail

Figure 3.9
Conception of linear and parallel sensory processing in unique zones of different neural tissues. This is a complex and recursive pathway from the outside world to an internal sense of self. Processing can be thought of as mostly *linear* in early stages, whereas *parallel processing* of multiple maps starts roughly at the dark horizontal line, mostly through vertical intercortical connections with other zones and horizontal *intra*cortical connections within the same zone. There are no interconnections among primary sensory or sense-specific association cortices belonging to *different* senses. Yet in the multisensory, paralimbic, and limbic zones, there are strong horizontal connections with other components in the *same* zone. Hence, early on there is an emphasis on rich linking that combines the neural transformations of many structures. The limbic system is what gives *salience* to any event.

*The idiotypic, unimodal, and heteromodal cortices are all kinds of neocortex.

**Multisensory heteromodal and paralimbic types of cortex perform two kinds of neural transformation: (1) further parallel elaboration of multiple sensory maps and (2) integration of the result with drive, emotion, and mental content. Earlier cortical types are fairly homogeneous transformers of a single sense; later types of cortex have heterogeneous input-output relations, and no uniform type of behavior can be ascribed to them. Sense specificity gives way to intermodal associations. Even the distinction between what is motor and what is sensory is lost now.

its connections. What I present here is a broad overview. Clinical correlations of important structures such as the septal nuclei, pyriform cortex, amygdala, and hippocampal formation are addressed in chapter 6.

Recall that Paul Broca (1878) used the term *limbic lobe* to designate the tissue of the inside rim (*limbus*) of the hemispheres where they meet the brainstem. Grossly, this includes the cingulate and hippocampal gyri, the tissue connecting them, and the various gyri that surround the olfactory tracts. This is what is usually shown in midline sagittal brain sections, although the three-dimensional span of the limbic system is too great to be seen in any one section alone.

Broca emphasized the common presence of a limbic lobe in all mammalian brains. Because natural selection has likely made existing animals considerably different from their long-extinct ancestors, it is most surprising to find uniformity in the connections among limbic structures in all vertebrates presently living. Two independent evolutionary trends in higher mammalian brains are an expansion of the neocortical surface and the development of limbic structures. A given species tends to be high in only one dimension, however. Monkeys, for example, show substantial neocortical development but little limbic enlargement; rabbits have the opposite trend of robust limbic elaboration but poor neocortical sophistication. Humans are unique in being substantially advanced in both limbic and neocortical dimensions.

Portions of the diencephalon, telencephalon, and mesencephalon are so structurally and functionally related that we consider them an autonomous functional unit called the *limbic system* (figures 3.10, 3.11). There is nuanced argument among bottom-uppers regarding exactly what entities constitute the limbic system, although its widest boundaries include the following:

- The hypothalamus
- Limbic cortex (corticoid and allocortical)
- Paralimbic cortex
- Limbic striatum (olfactory tubercle, nucleus accumbens), parts of globus pallidus, ventral tegmentum, and habenula
- Limbic and paralimbic thalamic nuclei

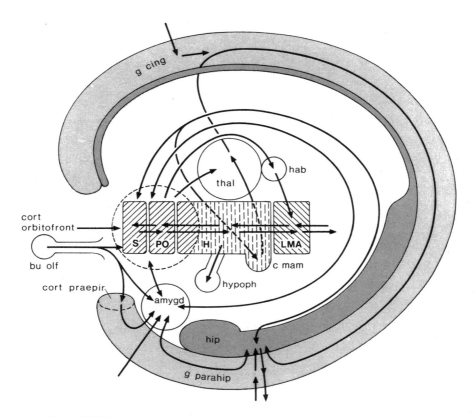

Figure 3.10
A schematic of the limbic system showing its central units and surrounding limbic rings. g cing, cingulate gyrus; hip, hippocampus; amygd, amygdala; LMA, limbic midbrain area; H, hypothalamus; hypoph, hypophysis
(pituitary); PO, preoptic region; S, septum; thal, thalamus; hab, habenula;
bu olf, olfactory bulb; cort orbitofront, orbital frontal cortex; cort praepir,
prepiriform cortex; g parahip, parahippocampal gyrus. From R. Nieuwenhuys, (1985), with permission.

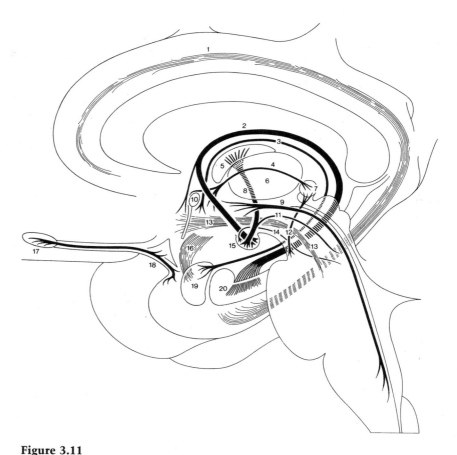

Figure 3.11
Subcortical components and major pathways of the limbic system: 1,
cingulum; 2, fornix; 3, stria terminalis; 4, stria medullaris; 5, anterior thalamus; 6, medial thalamus; 7, habenular nuclei, 8, mammillothalamic
tract; 9, dorsal longitudinal fasciculus; 10, anterior commissure; 11, mam-
millotegmental tract; 12, habenulointerpeduncular tract; 13, medial
telencephalic fasciculus; 14, mammillary peduncle; 15, mammillary body;
16, ansa peduncularis; 17, olfactory bulb; 18, lateral olfactory stria; 19,
amygdala; 20, hippocampus.

Note first that each of these structures is more concerned with drive, emotion, homeostasis, autonomic control, and memory than with straightforward perception or action. What feeds into the limbic system is a highly processed and highly abstract transformation of neural signals from both internal and external environments. Partly because of this, *the context of any stimulus strongly modulates the specific behavioral response (or lack of response) to it.*

Lower mammals and vertebrates, by contrast, appear insensitive to context. Turkeys, for example, will attack anything in the nest that does not peep like a chick. A bird made deaf will kill even its own offspring. One of Konrad Lorenz's best-known experiments showed that male sticklebacks, which have red underbellies, attack any floating object with a red undersurface whether it looks like another fish or not. We call such context-insensitive behaviors *instinctual.*

In humans, the situation is much different. Here, the paralimbic regions interpose themselves between external stimuli and the urge to act, they direct drive toward appropriate targets, and they add emotional coloring to thought and perception. The cingulum appears to direct motivation to the appropriate location in space. All these make it difficult to answer simply, "What does the limbic brain do?" Examining the preceding list of entities should help you deduce that sensual, motor, autonomic, and mental manifestations are all possible expressions of neural firing in the limbic brain. Still, what is fundamentally distinct about expressions of the limbic brain is a *qualitative alteration* of perception, of well-coördinated motor actions, or of consciousness itself. Why is this so?

The two major inputs to paralimbic and limbic cortices are (1) heteromodal association cortex and (2) the most distal synapses of modality-specific association cortices. Here is a convergence of highly abstracted qualities of the external world where, as the flow of figure 3.8 tried to convey, the *relevance of a stimulus* is more important than are its physical properties. Limbic dysfunction can severely disrupt the synergy among experience, thought, behavior, and emotion. Clinically, this causes the emotional coloration of mental life to be both unpredictable and incongruous. Feelings of unreality, distortion of perception, time dilatation, the feeling of a presence or familiarity (*déjà vu*), memory flashbacks, out-of-body experiences, synesthesia, and a sense of certitude (the "this is it" feeling) are some of the experiential correlates of limbic brain that I discuss in later chapters.

There are few places in the brain where it is possible to bring signals together from functionally different and geographically independent areas. As I pointed out in the beginning of this chapter, the brain as a network is vastly underconnected. Perhaps the most important togetherness that connects every sense as well as the internal milieu happens in those limbic entities that are housed in the anterior temporal lobe. Information can be fed both stepwise and by direct long relays into the temporal lobe, where they converge on the entorhinal cortex, which is the primary gateway to the hippocampus lying immediately underneath.

Through its outputs to the entorhinal cortex and fornix, the hippocampus can respond back to virtually every entity that originally fed into it. Fragments of information that were processed in geographically separate parts of the brain come together as signals in a singular structure that knows about the internal milieu as well as the fundamental drives of the organism as a biological entity. It can also respond back to the different types of cortex that fed into the circuit and further act on autonomic structures that govern the internal milieu. Limbic entities constitute a fundamental device for bringing information together in the context of how the organism is and what it wants to be.

The Papez Circuit

Paul Yakovlev, James Papez, and Paul MacLean are three neurologist-neuroanatomists who proposed classic formulations of behavior and who each happened to divide brain and behavior into three categories. We reviewed earlier Yakovlev's divisions of reticular, nuclear, and laminar tissue together with their corresponding "three spheres of motility." Visceration, emotion, and effectuation corresponded, respectively, to autonomic movements "within the body," the extrapyramidal movements of the body "upon the body," and the pyramidal movements of the body "outside the body."

Yoking the words "extrapyramidal" and "emotion," as I just did, may confuse top-downers, most of whom know the term *extrapyramidal* in the context of Parkinson's disease. They tend to equate the extrapyramidal system solely with postural and locomotor movement. While emotion is *experienced* as an internal sensation, it also is *expressed* by outward action. Consider the common circumstance of stroke patients who have what is called a *central facial weakness* whereby they cannot voluntarily move the lower half of their face on the side opposite the stroke. When commanded to smile, only the unaffected side of the face moves upward. Should the patient be amused or surprised, however, the face instantly assumes a symmetrical smile because a different pathway is involved in movements that are emotionally incited. Voluntary movements use the pyramidal motor system, whereas emotionally-triggered ones use extrapyramidal paths (see, e.g., Cascino et al., 1993). Often, this fundamental distinction regarding the *context* of motor acts is forgotten.

James Papez first proposed the idea that midline structures were the anatomic substrate of emotion, a then-novel notion that sealed the physician's lasting fame (Papez, 1937; MacLean, 1978). Papez noted that the word "emotion" implies both a way of acting and a way of feeling. Since emotional actions were known already to depend on the integrating power of the hypothalamus, Papez argued that emotional feelings require the participation of cortex.

He convincingly showed that sensory afferents split at the thalamic level into three paths, each carrying "a stream of impulses of special importance." The route conveying afferents through the dorsal thalamus and internal capsule to the striatum represents the "stream of movement." The conduit from the thalamus through the internal capsule to the lateral neocortex of the hemispheres is the "stream of thought." The third set, with one branch from the ventral thalamus to the hypothalamus and a second branch via the mammillary body and anterior thalamic nuclei to the cingulate gyrus, represented the "stream of feeling."

The hippocampo-mammillo-thalamo-cingulate-hippocampal circuit is the classic *Papez circuit* (figure 3.12). Papez took pains to point out connections whereby all sensation could project to the cingulum through the mammillary bodies. In his often-quoted words, "It is proposed that the hypothalamus, the anterior thalamic nuclei, the gyrus cinguli, the hippocampus and their interconnections constitute a harmonious mechanism which may elaborate the functions of central emotion as well as participate in emotional expression" (Papez, 1937, page 743).

Papez's Three Thalamic "Streams"

Stream of movement
    Dorsal thalamus → internal capsule → striatum

Stream of thought
    Thalamus → internal capsule → lateral neocortex

Stream of feeling
    Ventral thalamus → hypothalamus
    Mammillary body → anterior thalamic nucleus → cingulate gyrus

---

The bottom of figure 3.12 shows that new knowledge has forced an expansion of the original Papez circuit: (1) the hippocampal formation influences distant regions by acting on the subiculum, (2) the cingulate cortex receives multiple thalamic inputs, and (3) the nucleus accumbens is an important target in the basal ganglia for both cingulum and hippocampus, the two major cortical components of the Papez circuit. This link with the basal ganglia offers a new route for *expressing* behavior that is also consistent with Yakovlev's correlation of nuclear structures with gestural movements.

The hypothalamus participates in both the hard-wired and volume-transmitted transfer of information. A good deal of its input arises from either direct physical or chemical stimulation (e.g., light, temperature, circulating steroid hormones, and the concentration of glucose, salt, and other substances in the blood). Likewise, its outputs are both conventional (synapses) and *neuroendocrine*. Some hypothalamic hormones modulate the secondary release of pituitary hormones, while others directly affect distant targets. An example of the latter is oxytocin, a participant in orgasm (in both genders), parturition, and lactation. These three experiences obviously have both physical and mental components. In general, hypothalamic function is another good example of the fundamental role that volume transmission plays in neural regulation, as well as the inseparable interplay between cognitive and visceral forces.

The Primacy of Emotion
The limbic system and the neocortex perform different functions. The neocortex processes information that has too many fine de-

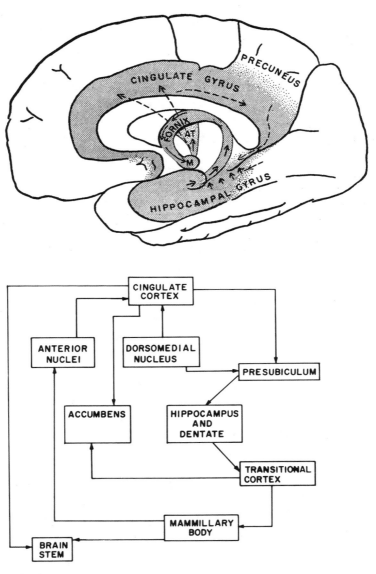

Figure 3.12
(*Top*) The original Papez circuit loops continuously from hippocampus, to mammillary bodies (via the fornix), to anterior thalamic nuclei, to cingulum, and thence to other cortical areas where they recurse to the hippocampus. From MacLean (1949), with permission. (*Bottom*) An expanded Papez circuit incorporates new knowledge. See text for further details. From Isaacson (1982), with permission.

tails to be handled by simpler, more direct, and often evolutionarily earlier systems. The complexity of multiple mapping is one reason we have historically believed that the role of the cortex is to analyze the external world and house our models (representations) of reality. It is the limbic brain, however, that decides questions of salience and relevance and so determines how we act on the information we have.

Let me suggest that it is an emotional calculus, more than a logical one, that animates us. This is a counterintuitive proposition given that, for centuries, emotion has been looked down on as primitive and reason esteemed as the superior development. Some possible physical reasons for this belief are found by surveying the general development of mammalian brains as well as the earlier notions of hierarchy that fostered the truism that a massively expanding neocortex overwhelmed and suppressed earlier neural systems.

Additionally, we know that environmental and cultural changes do not directly affect the direction of evolution. In other words, acquired traits such as knowing how to speak German or having a broken nose are not passed through genes to your offspring. What environmental changes do create are different niches for adaptation, and these niches are filled up by the natural selection of organisms with favorable genetic mutations. Before the development of big-brained human beings, change occurred through the force of evolution acting slowly over eons. Once brains develop any kind of organizing system for memory, however, with its ability to influence present and future actions, we immediately leap beyond the slow gene-by-gene mutation that physical evolution allows (Purves, 1994). This is because cultural change accumulates rapidly and can be passed on to others not genetically but through cultural transmission (which, for example, happens as you read this book).

This is an oft-cited advantage of having big, well-developed brains. It also provides one explanation for why humans have achieved so much in terms of culture and technology compared to other vertebrates. Our large frontal lobes are especially credited for this. Because the neocortex appears to have developed far out of proportion to subcortical tissue, we usually point to the cortex when we say, "This is what distinguishes us from less advanced species." The flip side of this assumption, however, is precisely why emotions usually are regarded as primitive.

The common assumption that the developed cortex makes humans unique implies that human limbic structures are no different from those of other mammals. If true, then human emotions are comparatively primitive. However, exhaustive anatomic studies such as those mentioned earlier show that the limbic system was not left behind by evolution. Because limbic and cortical circuits coëvolved, reason and emotion burgeoned in tandem.

The general blueprint that all vertebrate brains would follow started to emerge in the reptilian line. It was with the appearance of early mammals, though, that the limbic system underwent major changes. It is now a constant feature in all mammals and is not seen *in its developed form* in submammalian species. Its robustness in humans makes the human emotional system more powerful than that of other mammals. Additionally, the transformation of impulses that constitute emotional information seems to be qualitatively different from the processing of other information. Compared to the Draconian restrictions of behaviorism only a few decades ago, when any interest in emotion, consciousness, or other so-called subjective states was taboo, today's scientists are unearthing more and more evidence that emotion plays a greater role in our mental life than hitherto suspected.

I mentioned that limbic pathways did not wane as the neocortex developed. Although the relative volume of limbic structures is less in mammals with robust neocortical development, the number of axons in limbic fiber tracts is actually greater both in absolute number and relative to other fiber systems in the brain. In humans, there are five times the number of fibers in the fornix as in the optic tracts, which alone are customarily cited to carry 85% of sensory afferents into the brain (Isaacson, 1982). Our earlier discussion of multiplex communication suggested that the neocortex is not the highest rung on a hierarchical ladder of evolution but a detour interposed between brainstem nuclei and limbic entities. The neocortex provides analytic space, as suggested by its structure, and contains our model of reality. However, it is the limbic brain that is primarily involved in determining what we do with the analysis that the neocortex has carried out. The limbic brain's role in determining salience is what gives it such behavioral clout.

There is no doubt that the neocortex and limbic system are reciprocally connected, and that one system influences the other. As earlier hierarchical notions actually assumed, the real question is, "Does the influence of one outweigh the other?" The fate of the spiny anteater from Australia can shed some light on this hoary question.

The Australian anteater echidna is a prosimian on a very low branch of the mammalian family tree. Its tremendously developed frontal cortex is far larger than that of primates, our much closer genetic relatives. If we had frontal lobes as massive as the spiny anteater's per unit volume of brain we would have to carry our heads in front of us in an extra-large wheelbarrow. This contradiction of a simple animal with a proportionately huge frontal cortex suggests a dead-end evolutionary strategy. Having more analytical space for more computations, representations, or transformations may not make an efficient brain or even one that is especially smart.

The Australian anteater also appears not to dream, illustrating a general rule that for every gain there usually is an accompanying loss elsewhere. It is as if the anteater paid for its massive frontal lobes of cortex by forfeiting limbic function. The evidence is this. All other mammals dream, and when we do we emit an EEG signal in REM sleep called the *theta rhythm*. This rhythm is particularly prominent in the hippocampus of the limbic system. The anteater has no theta rhythm and presumably does not dream. When any sensory signal comes into the human cortex, the hippocampal theta rhythm becomes active only if the stimulus is evaluated as relevant and we attend to it. I used the word *salience* to describe a prime limbic function. The word means to "leap up" or "stick out," which is exactly what relevant stimuli do to grab our attention. That the hippocampus and the limbic system are a gateway, or valve, to perception is a crucial point to which I shall return later in this chapter.

By looking at the direction of flow and the scope of connections with their latest methods, authorities in neuroanatomy have confirmed that the hippocampus is a point where everything converges. All sensory inputs, external and visceral, must pass through the emotional limbic brain before being redistributed to the cortex for analysis, after which they return to the limbic system for a determination of whether the highly transformed, multisensory input is salient. If so, we will likely act; if not, we will ignore it just as we ignore most of the irrelevant energy flux that constantly bombards us.

It turns out that the brain's largest and latest development, the neocortex, receives more inputs from the limbic system than the limbic system receives from the neocortex. Compared to earlier hierarchical assumptions, the functional significance of these connections turned out to be the reverse of what we had long assumed. Obviously, there is a reciprocal relationship between the cortex and the limbic system, each modulating the other and each ultimately influencing our mental life. However, the volume and nature of recursive feedback suggests that the limbic influence may be greater than the neocortical one.

Emotion exerts a constant tone. An impressive example of its force is seen in epilepsy. Persons with epilepsy are always afraid of seizures and attempt to control all excitement because they know that emotional stress can trigger seizures. Nonetheless, patients have seizures because they have an underlying medical problem, and there is only so much that self-will can do. Their failure to stop all seizures nonetheless leads to self-recrimination, frustration, depression, social withdrawal, decreased gratification, more frustration, and soon more seizures. They are in a no-win situation because an underlying emotional state constantly acts on the whole system.

Specially dedicated seizure units at research institutions vividly highlight this relationship. Persons who have thirty to forty seizures daily come into a ward that is devoted entirely to understanding epilepsy. They are taken off all medication and kept in a room where injury is unlikely. Data on exactly what kind of seizures they have is collected by constant video monitoring and EEG recording. Remarkably, these patients' seizures often stop for weeks because they are in a place where they believe they will be better. They experience such a tremendous relief of stress from being in the hands of perceived healers that, with simple faith, their condition is better for a while. Of course, this change in environment cannot cure the underlying problem, but it does demonstrate the tremendous impact that emotions have in daily life.

Two further clinical examples illustrate how emotion rather than reason appears to be primary. The first concerns epilepsy originating in limbic structures of the temporal lobe. These structures have a low threshold for seizures that do not spread outside of the limbic brain. Temporal lobe epilepsy (TLE) can produce involuntary actions (called *automatisms*) that seem purposeful to an uninformed observer but of which the patient is unaware and has no recollection. TLE also can cause compulsive thinking, florid psychosis, and episodes in which one cannot distinguish between dreaming and reality. The overlap between the behavior of TLE and that of psychiatric disorders is striking: Fifty percent of those with temporal lobe seizures show psychiatric symptoms compared to only ten percent in all other types of epilepsy. Thus, the emotional brain seems physiologically able to overwhelm the rationality of the cortex.

The second example concerns patients in coma. In the sequence of their recovery, coma patients first manifest automatisms, then voluntary movement and speech that is childlike and emotionally childish. If recovery continues, their behavior becomes what we would describe as more rational and adultlike. The pattern of recovery from all comas shows that intellect cannot be reclaimed unless emotion recovers first.

We can conclude that emotions play an important and inadequately understood role in our behavior, perhaps a role even greater than that customarily assigned to reason.

The Triune Brain, Revisited
In the decades since its introduction, the triune brain concept has been challenged, revised, and largely relinquished. Notwithstanding critics who preferred that MacLean not attempt to yoke "big" behaviors to any specific anatomy, the model nonetheless has value for reasons I gave earlier. Because this topic's literature is unwieldy for beginners, I recommend MacLean's 1990 book on the triune brain's role in *paleo*cerebral functions as a good summary. MacLean's classic 1949 paper on the limbic system is clearly influenced by Papez and makes neural and behavioral distinctions from three types of anatomic systems found in mammalian brains

(MacLean, 1949, 1990). The usefulness of his triune brain lies in its description of behavior in terms of the actions and interactions of relatively self-contained anatomical entities.

The three-brains-in-one (see figure 3.1) are (1) a protoreptilian brain, or R-complex, (2) a paleomammalian brain, and (3) a neomammalian one. The R-complex, conceived as a fundamental core of the nervous system, consists of the upper spinal cord, midbrain, diencephalon, and basal ganglia. The paleomammalian division is essentially the limbic system, whereas the neomammalian brain is the neocortical expansion so prominent in primates. What MacLean believes to be the R-complex in living mammals derives from early mammallike reptiles, called *therapsids*, that disappeared in the Triassic period. Skeletal remains and other evidence of these reptiles' existence is found on all continents. Modern mammals may have developed from these mammallike reptiles.

The Reptilian Brain   The protoreptilian brain is responsible for stereotyped behaviors based on what MacLean calls "ancestral learning and ancestral memories." These species-typical behaviors are involved in establishing home territory, finding food and shelter, breeding, social dominance, aggression, and ritual displays. MacLean considers the reptilian brain nature's tentative first step toward self-awareness, particularly of the internal milieu (i.e., the emotions). It is a "visceral brain" (again, one of MacLean's terms) in the sense of dealing with strong, inward feelings that often are ignoble.

The formation of significant memories requires the elaboration of one's internal state. The hippocampus is an especially good place to combine internal information from the septal area and external information from sensory systems that project to nearby transitional cortices. A number of experts agree that the limbic system is a strong modulator of the R-complex; exactly how this is achieved is a current topic of inquiry.

In contrast to the R-complex, MacLean calls the neocortex the "mother of invention and father of abstract thought." Compared to the internal signals that project to limbic cortex, the neocortex provides fine-grained analysis of the external world and has a predilection for dividing things into smaller and smaller units. The neocortex affords "a vast neural screen for the portrayal of symbolic language and the associated functions of reading, writing, and arithmetic.''

The Paleomammalian Brain   Compared to the R-complex, the paleomammalian limbic system is an advance in neural tissue. Its transformations are better at helping an organism cope with the unpredictable vagaries of the environment and for integrating one's internal and external worlds. Parts of the limbic system concern primal issues of food and sex, others are concerned with emotions and feelings, and still others combine information from the internal and external worlds.

 The hippocampus can be thought of as an entity that suppresses the action of the R-complex when the unexpected happens. Life becomes uncertain when old patterns of responding fail to pay off (the price of inflexibility). This suppression prevents an organism both from responding in its old ways and from overreacting in general. The paleomammalian brain can be viewed as an entity that aims to reduce influences of the past, the stored memories of the protoreptilian brain.

Finally, each limbic structure, including the hypothalamus, is actually a complex set of subsystems in terms of anatomical relationships with other regions and in terms of overall behavior. Isaacson (1982), for example, adjures us to talk about limbic *systems*, not a single limbic system.

Lateralization and Hemispheric Specialization

Cerebral lateralization refers to the capacity of each hemisphere to govern particular skills. Anatomic and chemical differences between the hemispheres underlie the brain's capacity for multiple specialization. Endocrine, immune, and genetic factors affect the brain's development, its structure, and its lateralization—which means the final distribution and robustness of different talents between the two sides. The blueprint for the preordained parcellation of mental talents often gets rewritten in intrauterine life as the fetal environment exerts forces that alter the properties of individual brains. Critical periods exist for the development of nervous structures during which they are particularly susceptible to external influences.

In the adult, the primary role of circulating steroid sex hormones is to activate sexual responses. In the fetus, however, sex hormones direct the differentiation of sensitive body tissues. The brain is one of these steroid-sensitive tissues. Chemicals such as nerve growth factor or cortisol, for example, can influence a neuron's fate, guiding it to become either a sympathetic neuron or an adrenal secretory cell. Either male or female genotype is compatible with a physical brain of either phenotype; the phenotype is determined by circulating sex hormones in utero.

Sexual differences in neural structures (called *sexual dimorphism*) and sexual differences in behavior are somewhat advanced topics (for example, McWhirter et al., [1990] discuss the biology of sexual orientation, while Halpern [1991] reviews gender differences in cognition). In *The Sexual Brain*, LeVay (1993) gives a broad but succinct biological overview of the hereditary and environmental factors involved in sexual differentiation—somatic, neural, cognitive, and behavioral. Among the topics he reviews are sexual behavior (e.g., reproductive, courtship, maternal and paternal care), sexual feelings, gender identity, sexual orientation (gay, bisexual, straight), and differences between men and women that fall outside the sphere of sex itself. In particular, LeVay reviews evidence that sexual behaviors typical of men and women depend on distinct and specialized hypothalamic nuclei that are subject to sexual polymorphism. The influence of hormones on both sexual and nonsexual behavior generally is referred to as *behavioral endocrinology* (see e.g., Becker et al., 1992).

Lateralization is a central theme in biology and medicine, not something esoteric. Advantageous and disadvantageous consequences of cerebral dominance include the elevated rate of left-handedness in certain highly skilled occupations and its association with childhood learning disorders, immune disease, allergies, migraine, and twinning. For example, architects and the mathematically gifted tend to have superior right-hemisphere skills but are much more likely to be left-handed and afflicted with elevated rates of allergies and autoimmune diseases (Tønnessen et al., 1993; Dellatolas et al., 1990). These observations suggest that some of the processes that lead to lateralization also affect the development of the immune system and are in turn affected by it. The issues of lateralization are not yet settled, but it appears that processes which disturb cerebral lateralization frequently have widespread effects on other bodily systems. Hormone concentrations, especially of testosterone, also influence the development of various nuclear structures in the hypothalamus and limbic system, including sexually dimorphic structures.

Standard Brain Development

Neurons do not form in the cerebral hemispheres. They are generated midline in the neural tube and then migrate from the germinal center of the fetal brain to their future positions in the periphery. After furious DNA replication, cells move toward the lumen of the neural tube and proliferate in what is called the *ventricular germinal zone*. The differentiation of neurons begins at the sixth week of life. Cells migrate outward only after completing their last division and follow strict spatial and temporal gradients. Cells destined to populate separate architectonic zones have different origins and are produced in an ordered sequence of sizes, large ones migrating first. Phylogenetically older parts of the brain, such as the limbic system, appear earlier in development.

The brain forms inside out, with later-migrating cells passing through the inner layers that have already formed in order to reach the cortical mantle. The ventricular zone becomes thinner as cells continue to migrate out of it, and the primitive cerebrum becomes increasingly layered. The deeper layers contain more mature cells that migrated first; the more superficial layers harbor later-migrating and more immature cells. Migrating neurons are constantly in motion and may pass back and forth several times through their eventual resting place (figures 3.13, 3.14). Only after neurogenesis is finished does specification of cortical areas occur (Walsh & Cepko, 1992).

Starting in the sixteenth week of life, neurons develop dendrites and axons and then compete for synaptic contacts. Neural migration, assembly, and synaptic connection are influenced by a variety of factors that together account for the uniqueness of every individual brain. The intrauterine environment is especially influential. Neuronal migration and assembly may be modified by circulating sex hormones as well as prenatal and perinatal stressors (e.g., prolonged labor, anoxias, Rh incompatibility, breech births, multiple births, prematurity). In every species studied, neurons are

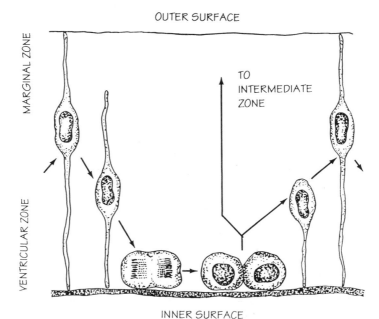

Figure 3.13
Developing neurons are in constant motion. During DNA replication, embryo nerve-cell nuclei migrate to the center of the neural tube (the ventricular zone), detach their peripheral process from the tube's outermost layer, and then round up. After cell division, the daughter cells either extend a new process, migrate back to the middle of the germinal epithelium, and divide again, or they move out of the epithelium altogether toward the intermediate zone in the wall of the brain.

formed in huge excess only to die in utero and during the first years of postnatal life when they fail in the competition to form connections with other neurons. This process is called *physiologic necrosis.*

The cell death of physiologic necrosis reduces the number of superfluous neurons produced in fetal life and is perhaps the most crucial factor in helping to match the number of neurons to available synaptic sites. That neural circuits can reroute themselves even across the midline is remarkable testimony to the developing nervous system's flexibility in that it can alter the availability and location of synaptic sites. A variety of intrauterine influences, as

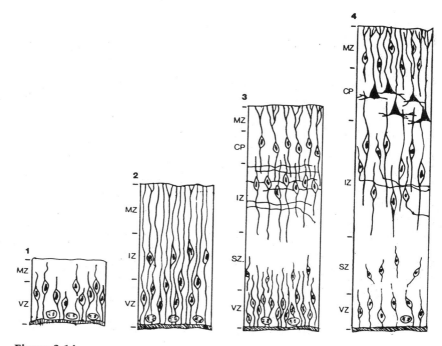

Figure 3.14

Progressive thickening of the developing brain wall. At stage 1, the ventricular zone (VZ) contains cell bodies and the marginal zone (MZ) contains only extended cell processes. As cells stop dividing (2), they migrate outward to form the intermediate zone (IZ). In the forebrain (3), cells that pass through this zone gather into the cortical plate (CP), from which the six layers of the neocortex develop. At the end of neurogenesis (4), the original ventricular zone becomes the ependymal lining of the ventricles, and the relatively cell-free subventricular zone (SZ) becomes the white matter through which fibers enter and leave the cortex.

noted, can cause anomalous segregation of standard mental skills and the emergence of special talents.

The right hemisphere begins its development before the left. We can speculate a reason for its precocious development based on its specializations, which include the analysis of external space and the orientation of the body within it. The right hemisphere plays a major role in emotion, including its subjective experience, external expression, and the interpretation of emotion expressed by others. It also helps shift the focus of attention from oneself to external stimuli and exerts control over important autonomic functions. This further suggests that the right hemisphere plays a special role in behaviors essential for survival. Thus, its early development relative to the left hemisphere seems advantageous.

Men and women normally differ on average in their patterns of abilities. As a group, women have superior verbal skills, whereas men are better at spatial perception. Normally, the male brain matures later than the female brain and the left hemisphere matures later than the right. *Anything that delays the development of the left hemisphere will cause a nonstandard pattern of cerebral lateralization.* It is such delays of left-hemispheric cellular migration, synaptic target formation, and maturation of connections that produce left-handedness, so-called learning disabilities, and weakening of typical left-hemispheric skills while prompting the emergence of superior right-hemispheric talents (see the box, "Left-handedness and Anomalous Dominance"). Though there is little doubt that sexual differences in cognition exist, they are not as robust as introductory texts often suggest (Halpern, 1991).

Conditions such as Turner's syndrome have been fruitfully used to separate the role of sex hormones from that of genetically-determined sex-linked characteristics in cognition. Turner females (XO karyotypes) are hypogonadal and therefore unable to produce estrogen. They do show selective impairments on mental tasks such as spatial rotation and right-left discrimination (Johnson et al., 1993). The question now remains whether such cognitive deficits are due solely to congenital factors or whether the absence of circulating sex hormones engenders a maturational difference.

Men have a higher frequency of left-handedness, a physical trait that is associated with mental ones. Stuttering and dyslexia, for example, are markedly higher among strong left-handed men than

The Standard Pattern of Cerebral Dominance

> The standard pattern of cerebral dominance is for strong left-hemispheric asymmetry for language and handedness.
>
> The right hemisphere normally matures before the left.
>
> Female brains normally mature sooner than male brains.
>
> As a group, women may have superior verbal skills whereas men, as a group, may have better spatial perception and an increased frequency of non-right-handedness.

Left-Handedness and Anomalous Dominance

> Frank left-handers constitute only one readily identified group with an anomalous (nonstandard) pattern of dominance. The basic pattern of the brain is one of strong left-hemispheric asymmetry for language and handedness. Influences that delay left-hemispheric growth therefore tend to reduce the typical brain asymmetry: As a result, many individuals experiencing delays in left-hemispheric growth will have *random handedness*. Frank left-handers, therefore, constitute only about thirty percent of the population with anomalous dominance. Although there are other reasons why left-handedness is not present in the majority of individuals in whom left-hemispheric growth has been delayed, it is the main reason, and left-handedness can usually be taken as a sign of anomalous dominance.

among strong right-handers (Smith et al., 1989). Histologic examination of dyslexic brains has uncovered abnormal cellular architecture in the left parietal lobe, the left temporal speech region, and even in the right hemisphere. A delay in cellular migration appears to disrupt normal cytoarchitecture.

Because the influences that produce delays in the left hemisphere lead to expanded growth of other regions, this phenomenon may also be a mechanism of giftedness that could account for the elevated level of non-right-handers among male architects and other men with talent for spatial relationships, including athletes, sculptors, engineers, and mathematicians. Instances of disjunctive neuronal migration may thus be not only a pathology of defect but also a so-called pathology of superiority, which explains both the presence of extremely high talents in many persons with autism, dyslexia, and stuttering and the common occurrence of superior right-hemisphere talents in dyslexics and their families.

The Pathology of Superiority   Because the developing brain can reorganize its connections, minor malformations caused by delays in cellular migration also can give rise to superior talents. Though we habitually think that a deviation from a prescribed pattern always results in abnormality, a superior outcome is not unusual, for reasons already cited. For example, a large proportion of those scoring among the top 1 in 10,000 individuals on the Scholastic Aptitude Test (SAT) are left-handed (Benbow, 1988). Such superior outcome may or may not be a trade-off with deficits in other areas.

When the growth of a hemisphere segment is stunted, other regions will then be larger than they normally would have been and superior talents may emerge. The spatial grasp of architects or musical affinity are common examples. Clinical instances of persons with remarkable artistic talents in the face of limited linguistic capabilities are even more illustrative (Galaburda & Kemper, 1979; Gordon, 1983; Sano, 1918). In fact, Geschwind and Galaburda (1987) have speculated that "the mechanisms that delay left hemisphere growth have been selected in the course of evolution because they often produce individuals of elevated talent." They suggest that the high talents created through this mechanism may also explain the high occurrence of childhood dyslexia. Dyslexia can, of course, often be overcome by effort and good teaching so that only the superior talents remain evident. The fact that whole families can exhibit special talents without obvious disabilities further suggests that disabling impairment may actually occur in just a fraction of those in whom left-hemisphere development is slowed compared to the general population.

The evolutionary advantage conferred by many talented individuals presumably outweighs the disadvantage of a linguistic learning disability that appears in a small number of individuals and that would be irrelevant anyway in nonliterate societies. Such a pressure on cortical development may well be advantageous to the population as a whole, inasmuch as it leads to diverse patterns of lateralization and corresponding patterns of talent. Even when growth is excessively retarded, high talents may emerge as a result of compensatory enlargement in brain regions whose growth is not impeded. The Geschwind-Galaburda model of cerebral lateralization is not without its critics, however, who argue their case in volume 26, issue number 2 of *Brain and Cognition* (1994).

Hemispheric Specialization

Although humans appear to have an axis of external symmetry, our internal organization, including that of our brains, is asymmetrical. Most creatures, and even some single-celled organisms, have an asymmetrical nervous system. The development of cerebral dominance and the differing specialization of each hemisphere perhaps contributed to human survival and the ability to adapt to almost any ecological niche.

Some people think, wrongly, that duplication of neural function is advantageous because it ensures a "spare part" in case of damage. The cat, for example, recovers from hemiplegia particularly well, a fact that may comfort pet owners though this capacity means nothing to felines in their natural habitats, where a brief disability portends likely death. Asymmetrical organization means that each side of the brain can control different functions. Overall capacity can theoretically double. Cerebral dominance packs more talents in each brain and in the species as a whole, so that some individuals will survive any catastrophe affecting the mass population. The further influence by the hormonal environment of the fetus produces even greater diversity than would genetic selection alone.

Asymmetries of the temporal planum, sylvian fissure, corpus callosum, and occipital lobe can easily be seen with the naked eye and measured with rulers (Geschwind & Galaburda, 1987). There are cytoarchitectonic asymmetries too, particularly in language areas, just as there are chemical and pharmacological asymmetries throughout the brain. This means that drugs may act asymmetrically (LSD being a famous instance) or that asymmetrical symptoms may emerge during illnesses, such as depression, in which there are large changes in certain classes of neurotransmitters that themselves are asymmetrically distributed. Finally, the well-known asymmetries of the peripheral nervous system, especially the autonomic innervation of the grossly asymmetrical thoracic and abdominal viscera, imply corresponding differences in visceral outflow from the two sides of the brainstem and hypothalamus.

There is no single dichotomy that describes the organization of the hemispheres. Verbal-nonverbal, analytic-intuitive, nor sequential-gestalt will not do. The left hemisphere has been variously characterized as linguistic, voluntary, linear, logical, and sequential, while the right has been described as spatial, automatic, synthetic, appositional, or holistic. During the first twenty years of split-brain testing, a cottage industry developed around the easy techniques of dichotic listening and tachistoscopic viewing. Predictably, a good number of experiments were ill-conceived and their claims regarding hemispheric specialization ill-founded (Efron, 1990; Christman, 1994). Bottom-uppers appreciate that these naïve shorthand characterizations miss important nuances of hemispheric specialization.

Language was the first function for which hemispheric specialization was widely recognized. Paul Broca's patient, who for many years suffered from right-sided paralysis and aphasia, could understand speech but could say only one word, "tan." At postmortem, there was a large lesion, the different parts of which Broca dated by techniques in common use at the time. He determined that the lesion in the frontal lobe was coincident with the patient's aphasia. The left second and third frontal convolutions became known as *Broca's area*. A left-hemisphere dominance for language was first demonstrated in Broca's series of eight patients (1865). The left hemisphere is specialized for linguistic tasks and for numerical calculation. Its superior skill for fine motor control is manifested in the right hand's dexterity (Latin *dexter*, meaning "right"; also French *droit*, meaning "right," as in *adroitness*).

Regardless of whether one is right-handed, left-handed, or of mixed dominance (a term favored over *ambidextrous* or *ambilateral*), language resides in the left hemisphere of most individuals (table 3.3).

Four general abilities relatively dependent on the right hemisphere are (1) non-linguistic perception, especially that involving spatial configurations, (2) spatial distribution of attention, (3) expression of emotion, and (4) the nonlinguistic aspects of communication (e.g., the melodiousness or *prosody* of speech, facial expression,

Table 3.3
The Speech Hemisphere and Handedness

Handedness	Speech Hemisphere (percent)		
	Left	Right	Mixed
Left	60	20	16
Right	90	10	0
Mixed dominance	60	10	30

gesture, emphasis, intonational pitch, attitude, comprehension of situational context, and cues regarding the interpersonal dynamics of a conversation). Hemispheric specialization is not always the black-and-white situation suggested by introductory texts and popular writings. Although the right hemisphere is more involved in recognizing faces, for example, the left hemisphere also plays a role (prosopagnosia requires bilateral lesions).

The right hemisphere's talent for visuospatial perception and manipulation have received the most attention, even though its skill at complex perceptual tasks extends to hearing and touch. Even memory is handled differently by the brain's two sides. For example, patients with right-hemisphere lesions have more difficulty than controls in tactile shape recognition or tactile assessment of object orientation; in recognizing variations in melody and rhythm; and in visually identifying objects when viewed from unusual perspectives. They can recall details but often forget the overall configuration (*gestalt*) of individual elements and their relationship to one another. Left-hemisphere lesions often cause the reverse pattern of forgetting the details but retaining the general layout.

Techniques such as dichotic listening and tachistoscopic viewing demonstrate the presence of these asymmetries in healthy individuals by selectively filtering input to only one hemisphere. Such work shows a left-hemisphere advantage for words and numbers, and a right-hemisphere advantage for pitch and melody. (The situation is different in professional musicians, however, implying a shift in talents that is a topic for advanced discussion.) The right hemisphere is also superior at depth perception, locating objects in space, identifying geometric shapes, and assessing spatial orientation by touch. Technologies such as regional cerebral blood flow measurement (rCBF), PET, and single photon emission computed tomography (SPECT) can take a "snapshot" of cerebral metabolism during certain tasks that can suggest metabolic grounds for asymmetry of a given function.

Emotional asymmetries bear special comment. It is a common clinical observation that patients with left-hemisphere lesions may respond to their illness in an extremely negative manner, whereas patients with similar lesions on the right may act inappropriately indifferent or even euphoric. These differences in comportment are evident too when a hemisphere is anesthetized briefly by the injection of sodium amytal into one carotid artery. Called the Wada test, this usually is done to evaluate aspects of memory or to determine in which hemisphere language resides in a particular individual. Anesthetizing the left hemisphere makes patients dysphoric, whereas anesthetizing the right makes them euphoric. Precisely because emotional expression can be dissociated from emotional feeling, utmost care is needed in interpreting overt behavior. Emotion is discussed in detail in chapter 8, but let me state generally here that the right hemisphere appears to be dominant in all aspects of emotional expression and experience.

The Cerebral Commissures

The cerebral commissures are discussed in chapter 7. Like the special abilities of the right hemisphere, the function of the commissures has been learned only in the last twenty years even though patients with agenesis of the commissures have been known for a century, and surgical cutting of the commissures as a treatment for epilepsy has a long history.

The problem with signs and symptoms of callosal lesions is that the standard neurological exam so often fails to disclose any abnormality in patients who have them. Casual conversation also fails to suggest that anything is amiss. Yet logic says that severing the commissures is an extreme thing to do to someone's brain. After all, more fibers cross back and forth between the two sides than enter from the outside via the senses.

Channel and State Functions

I referred earlier to multiplexing and diverse kinds of communication systems present in the brain. It is the self-contained tracts of the long wiring system of axons and synapses, operating on a narrow band, that carry what are called *channel-dependent* functions.

The anatomic substrate of channel-dependent functions usually has a point-to-point correspondence, or *topographic arrangement*. For example, the projection of retinal neurons to the geniculate nucleus, the striate cortex, and beyond maintains at each stage a retinotopic arrangement. The orderly point-to-point correspondence of cochlear hair cells projecting to the transverse auditory gyri is tonotopic; the lemniscal system is somatotopic: The disruption of pathways at different points in a channeled function produces clinical syndromes that often are so characteristic.

In contrast, there exist seven groups of nuclei that sustain huge terminal fields in either cortex or thalamus (see the box, "State Functions"). Each one of these small cell groups can modulate rapidly the state of the brain as a whole. Arousal, vigilance, and even some aspects of mood and memory are referred to as *state-dependent* functions. These broad-band pathways can affect the efficiency of channel functions without affecting the content of those channels.

Distinguishing between channel and state functions is sometimes useful in clinical assessment, whether at the bedside or during formal testing. Obviously, one cannot attribute a failure of performance to a specific lesion until one is certain that more fundamental state functions, such as attention and concentration, are intact. For example, it is impossible to test memory and other aspects of the mental status in someone who is disoriented. Sadly, clinicians attempt this all the time.

The distinction between state and channel functions, of course, also concerns the psychology of nothing, a fascinating topic that I can refer to here only briefly (Hearst, 1991). Absence, deletion, and nonoccurrence can be physical as well as psychological, though we are far more likely to note an event's occurrence than either prevailing conditions or something that does not occur. Yet human judgement often requires consideration of events that fail to occur. Because we are biased to accentuate the positive and because we give little weight to disconfirming instances, we often draw overly strong conclusions regarding causality.

When the Gestalt psychologist Kurt Koffka wondered why we "normally see things and not the holes between them," he was pondering why we associate things with one another rather than the spatial or temporal emptiness that envelops them. To most people, this is an odd thought. Artists, however, seem to be an exception in being attuned to the meaningful and æsthetic functions of gaps, pauses, open spaces, and intervals. Cultural differences figure widely too: Where the Western mind sees nothing, the Japanese mind considers both the interval—or *ma*—between elements and the elements themselves. The box, "A Feeling for Quiet" gives additional examples for you to ponder.

Chemoarchitecture

The term *chemoarchitecture* connotes chemical neuroanatomy and refers to the physical distribution of various neurotransmitters. At the moment, twenty-eight different neuronal populations, each of which contains a different transmitter, are generally recognized. These include acetylcholine, the various monoamines, the amino acid transmitters, and eighteen peptides. More such chemical systems are being discovered and characterized every year.

State Functions and Wide-Field Projections

Cholinergic neurons in the septum (Ch1–Ch4) project to the entire cortex, with overlaps.

Hypothalamic neurons project widely to cortex.

Serotoninergic neurons in the brainstem raphé project diffusely to the entire cortex.

Noradrenergic neurons in the locus coeruleus project to the entire cortex.

Cholinergic neurons in the pontomesencephalic reticular formation project to the entire thalamus and, less robustly, to the entire cortex.

Dopaminergic neurons in substantia nigra and ventral tegmentum project to the striatum, limbic, paralimbic, and heteromodal association areas.

Intralaminar thalamic nuclei project diffusely to the cortex.

A Feeling for Quiet

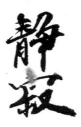

In English, *quiet* is defined by passivity, a negative absence. In contrast, Japanese has five words that describe the æsthetic quality of a full, voluptuous quiet.

The "loneliness" of *sabi* is the beauty of the solitary, the isolation by space, circumstance, or history, the wear of time or uniqueness of an object. *Sabi* is the ancient, lone pine on a mountain whose branches are molded by the wind.

Wabi denotes beauty in the "poverty" of the simple, the wonder in the commonplace, the poignancy discovered in the obvious. *Wabi* is the amazing quality of things just as they are.

Shibui is the "bitterness" of strong green tea. The beauty of *shibui* is an absolute simplicity that reduces something to its essentials and nothing more.

Aware is the beauty of fragility, a sensitivity to everything's transient nature. The "pity" of *aware* implies the ultimate submission of everything to a vast fate.

Yugen means both "hidden" and "obscure," the beauty of the unrevealed, the reality behind appearances: The snowy heron hiding in the bright moon, the vague object at the bottom of a clear pool. *Yugen* is unfathomable depth.

The top Japanese character above represents the word *quiet*, the bottom one *solitude*. In combination, the two mean "tranquility."

As a student in the 1970s, I had to learn the gangliocerebrosides and other minutæ associated with inborn errors of metabolism. Predictably, these appeared on examinations. It is impractical to memorize all the intricacies of chemoarchitecture, and I do not recommend that you try. You should, however, appreciate that volume transmission is part of the brain's multiplexing and that the relation between neuro-anatomy and chemo-anatomy is an area of inquiry that is developing vigorously. Already, a text exists that summarizes a little of what we know regarding how cellular components are assembled into functional entities (Strange, 1993).

In the late 1950s, only acetylcholine and norepinephrine were known, and it was taken on faith that the brain could get by with one excitatory and one inhibitory transmitter. Times have changed, and classic synaptic transmission has been displaced. We now know that more than one transmitter can reside in a single neuron and that excitatory and inhibitory receptors exist for the same transmitter (so much for the binary analogy that a neuron's only possible state was either "on" or "off"). An impressively large number of transmitters and peptides reside in the limbic system. Because this topic is rather specialized and because its study benefits from accompanying anatomic diagrams, I refer you to Rudolf Nieuwenhuys's *Chemoarchitecture of the Brain* (1985) for the anatomy and to Philip Strange's *Brain Biochemistry and Brain Disorders* (1993) for some biochemical correlates of gross behavior.

Our knowledge, however, remains meager. Clinical psychopharmacology (like psychoanalysis) is not yet based on a deep mechanistic understanding, and advances have come about more by chance than by elegant deductions based on knowing how an agent whose primary action is to block serotonin reuptake, for example, produces sustained and coherent effects on behavior. There are at least fourteen serotonin receptors in the brain, many with distinct distributions. Explaining the molecular chain of events leading to behavioral change is a daunting challenge (Jacobs, 1994).

ADVANCED CONCEPTS

Hopefully, as newcomers to the neurological foundations of neuropsychology you have grasped some of the fundamental concepts of what nervous tissue is. Now let us consider some deep issues that are currently exercising the minds of biologically-oriented neuro-scientists (bottom-uppers). Among these are the problems of inherent limits to what we can know, the nature of consciousness, the relationship between entropy and mental work, and the apparently declining role that logic plays in reasoning. These topics are being presented as an overview, so I have not cluttered this section with references for every statement, although I have tried to indicate where my comments are speculative.

Free Lunch and Imagination

The human limbic system enhances cortical processes and, by extension, reasoning, because it is surprisingly energy-efficient. Its ability to reduce entropy[1], act on incomplete information, and create order from a continuous and incoherent sensory stream is what gives us an æsthetic capacity. Without emotion, our behavior would be altogether predictable and unimaginative. One can, for instance, demonstrate that the characteristic theta rhythm of human limbic activity drops out when newly learned actions become mere unthinking habits.

It is one thing to argue that we are the most rational of animals but quite another to conclude that we are therefore "rational animals," as if reason were the only thing that made us tick. Up to the level of reptiles, brains evolved into increasingly complex neural systems that were still hard-wired, thus yielding predictable behavior despite increased complexity. The limbic system first appeared in its *developed form* in early mammals and is most richly redundant in humans. By *sharing* components and pathways for such different functions as attention, memory, emotion, and consciousness, it is able to act on incomplete information. Its ability to determine valence and salience yields a more flexible and intelligent creature, one whose behavior is unpredictable and even creative.

It is unusual for neurologists to consider engineering principles in their domains, but thinking about the energy costs of mental work leads to some surprising results. We are indebted to the American neurosurgeon Ayub Ommaya for opening up this line of inquiry. The limbic brain's use of common structures for different functions *in the same system* is not an accident at all but the optimal development of evaluating incomplete information and initiating actions at the least energy cost. Earlier assumptions of "bigger is better" failed to distinguish human brains from those of other species in any important way. What appears unique about the human brain is its high energy consumption coupled with remarkable efficiency in producing mental work. The brains of rats and dogs, for example, consume five percent of total body energy, monkey brains use ten percent, and human brains expend a whopping twenty-five percent, far greater than what is expected for their relative size.

Authorities on brain metabolism tell us that, remarkably, hardly any energy is used for mental work. Instead, nearly all the energy is consumed for housekeeping, mainly the pumping of sodium whereby electrical charges are maintained within nerve cells. The energy cost of mental work itself is minuscule compared to that consumed in just keeping up the physical structure. Getting something for practically nothing makes mental work almost the only free lunch in the universe. Mentation that needed much more additional energy would produce a brain that consumed so great a proportion of bodily fuel that life might not be possible.

It is the organization of the limbic brain that permits human cognition to occur with only slightly more energy use than is required to sustain the brain's physical structure. As incredible as this free lunch sounds, it does comply with Planck's principle of least action. In 1922, Max Planck, the Nobel laureate physicist, formulated a rule to predict which of several alternate paths a given event would take. Planck's principle states that among all possible paths, the one actually taken is always the one that uses the least energy. Such a general principle finds itself exquisitely expressed in the efficiency of the human brain.

All creatures maintain their lives by consuming organic matter in the food chain, a process that ultimately goes all the way back to the conversion of solar energy by photosynthesis in plants. The energy cost of each conversion in the food chain is enormous, and the exceptional efficiency of the human brain is again noteworthy in this context. With injuries such as trauma, burns, surgery, or infection, the body becomes hypermetabolic, consuming more nitrogen and other essential nutrients. Strikingly, when the brain alone is injured, the body's hypermetabolism increases proportionately to a greater extent and the rest of the body will be starved if necessary to protect the brain.

Not surprisingly, there is a mental cost for this inefficient hypermetabolism. The greater the body's hypermetabolism, the less efficient cerebral energy consumption becomes, resulting in greater cognitive impairment. As cognition returns to normal, so does the efficiency of cerebral energy utilization. The point is that energy efficiency is a product of how the limbic brain is organized, and this in turn influences the analytic processes of the cortex. In determining salience and valence, what we might call *qualitatively significant information*, the emotional brain acts like a valve, regulating the flow of nervous information throughout the body, integrating both the direct wiring and volume transmission systems.

In addition to these impressive facts, there are some advanced proposals, and the supporting calculations of irreversible thermodynamics, that suggest that all life forms, but particularly brains, play a large role in slowing down the rate of entropy increase and the degradation of energy in the universe (Dyson, 1971; Hess & Mikhailov, 1994). Such profound possibilities suggest that we should direct our efforts not toward controlling our emotions but toward gaining better insight into them and into the fundamental role they play in our lives. For such reasons as these, I have been increasingly drawn to the premise that emotion, not reason, frees us from the tyranny of predictable, reptilianlike thought and behavior.

I indicated that were it not for emotion, our mentation would largely be predictable and unimaginative. The ability to pluck qualitatively salient information from the passing stream and to act efficiently on fragmentary information is what leads to imagination and an æsthetic capacity. Intuition, for example, is the expression of a decision based on the efficient use of partial information. Humans excel at this, which is a blessing given that human thinking is neither inherently logical nor inherently clear.

Because the anatomy of emotion is also partially the anatomy of memory, increased clarity comes from the capacity to look at and to remember previous actions. The reasons that we develop when talking to ourselves become clearer as we gather and retain more knowledge about our motivations, the way we make decisions, and how we rationalize our actions. Seemingly irrational things such as contradictions are a natural part of this process. We develop dichotomies, such as good versus evil, to clarify our thoughts. It probably is impossible to understand anything without such polarities. Some polarities are true and have a physical basis—for example, positive and negative. Others are elusive and resolved only by perseverance. When we eventually fathom a linkage, we call it *insight*.

Some people are blessed with an intuitive grasp of relationships among huge numbers of variables without having to "reason" their way through them. Such a person was Ramanujan, the Indian boy who invented mathematical theorems. Because the proofs were so obvious to him, he wrote down only the theorems. The British mathematician Hardy declared that Ramanujan's ideas had to be true because no cheat could have fabricated such sophisticated work. Though few of us possess intuition this grand, we do possess this uniquely human type of creative thinking that brings order to a jumble of variables and somehow gives us meaningful pleasure.

When faced with a totally new problem in a new context, we somehow come up with a creative solution. This happens all the time in ordinary human situations. We solve myriad daily problems that involve our relationships with the world and with other people. It would be difficult for a logical machine operating by specific rules to deal with such problems, no matter how detailed the rules were. If we could define emotions in terms of rules, then perhaps we could stick them into such a machine and make it intelligent in the sense hoped for by AI enthusiasts. However, emotions cannot be set down in formal terms; they can be understood only by living life and feeling our way through it.

(Proponents of what is called *affective computing* suggest that wearable computers such as body nets, watches wired to a global network, and cameras with holographic displays in our eyeglasses might help us discern our various emotions by amassing data as we feel our way through life. By analyzing the information and correlating consistent patterns with our physiological responses, these ultimate mood rings will purportedly increase our communication bandwidth and alert us to whatever emotions we appear to be expressing, consciously or not [Picard, 1995]. While affective wearables might clarify feelings and provide welcome feedback to individuals eager to don them, affective computing does not change the fundamental truth that emotional understanding is a first-person issue ill-suited to formal rules.)

Creative people who do original work do it with an emotional charge, and the greater the charge, the better they seem to work. This kind of emotional tone seems to be the guiding force in any new creation. Emotion not only makes our brain strikingly efficient but also bestows our intuitive sense of what is correct and what goes together. This is, of course, an æsthetic capacity, a sense of what is beautiful and what is not. Without such a capacity, we probably would not have higher realms of creative thought, such as literature, architecture, or mathematics.

While pointing out the overlap between emotion and memory, I must emphasize that memory is not simply a fixed look-up table, like pulling a book off a shelf to locate some unchanging, indelible record. Memory is a *creative and dynamic process* too, during which the state of the brain's electrical fields changes. According to nonlinear models, the sensory cortices generate a distinct pattern for each act of recognition and recall, no two being ever exactly the same (Freeman, 1990; Barton, 1994; Freeman & Skarda, 1990). Yet they are close enough to create the illusion that we understand and have encountered the event previously. This is never quite true, however, because each time we recall something, it is tainted by the circumstances of the recall. When it is recalled again, it carries with it a new kind of baggage, and so on. So, each act of recognition and recall is a fresh creative process and not merely a retrieval of some fixed item from storage. These facts are relevant to the spate of current lawsuits claiming injury from sexual abuse, satanic cults, and the like that rely exclusively on putative "recalled memories." Such memories are almost certainly newly created fantasies, because memory is a fluid, creative act; it is not like a video camera that records every moment "as it really happened" (Barrie & Freeman, 1994; Freeman & Barrie, 1994). (Though there is some evidence that, during moments of great fear, the amygdala might impede the integration of memory that is carried out by the hippocampus and entorhinal cortex, any putative sensory fragments left are still grist for an unreliable interpretation because they lack context.)

Furthermore, persons, objects, and events are not perceived in their entirety but only by those aspects that are, have been, or can be experienced and acted on by an observer. An example of this fragmentary nature of perception is found in any mundane object such as a disposable plastic cup. Everyone knows that you drink from it, but we can comment on little else—for example, its tensile strength, translucency, thermal coëfficient, chemical composition, or what is stamped on its bottom. By such an analysis, a physical universe is contained in that cup, yet all we really know about it is *what you do with it*. This limited aspect of knowing is peculiar to humans, the observers and manipulators. All that we can know about anything outside ourselves is what the brain creates from raw sensory fragments, which were actively sought by the limbic brain in the first place as salient chunks of information.

This view of perception and memory does not appeal to the idealism of philosophers because it speaks to the *limits of our knowledge and what we really know:* That is, conscious knowing is restricted by the possible interactions we have with events and things. Conscious knowing is based in direct, hands-on experience.

Put in a more familiar context, people such as artists and writers look at the world in a certain way. It is the same world that everyone else sees but seen differently. Contemporary people often call such individuals *weird* because they do not seem to be seeing the same things that the majority sees. It is critical to realize that the sensory gateways that feed into the brain establish their own conditions for the creation of representations and knowledge. Artistic giants knew full well that their visions were not shared by most people. Even when persecuted or abandoned because of their vision, artists persist. That is all they *can* do because their visions are their reality and, for many of us, their reality subsequently becomes our reality when we experience their art.

Consciousness as a Type of Emotion

What is *consciousness?* Anyone who has surveyed the philosophy of mind or biological explorations of consciousness knows that consciousness is most often identified with reason. I would like to present a radical alternative—that consciousness is a type of emotion.

Consciousness is firmly tied to emotional drive and goal-directed behavior. We are interested not just in whether a wakeful state or self-awareness is present (typical definitions of consciousness) but in whether a creature is capable of purposeful action. Studies of natural and deliberate brain lesions clearly indicate that the cortex is not necessary for propulsive, teleological behavior. In fact, monkeys in whom the cortex has been surgically removed can barely be distinguished from their normal cagemates, a profoundly counterintuitive observation. Animals who have had their cortex and even important subcortical motor structures removed still exhibit purposeful behavior as long as their limbic system remains intact.

This may be counterintuitive but is not really surprising because the limbic system contains tissue central to the formation of memory, and goal-directed behavior requires continuity over time. Something that reacts instantaneously to a given stimulus will not do. You need some sort of register, or memory, to direct behavior from within. The hippocampus is ideally situated to couple memory with motor readouts from various parts of the brain, thus enabling purposeful, goal-directed behavior.

I am not saying that the hippocampus is the seat of consciousness; it is no more so than is the cortex. Perhaps we should stop trying to put a finger on consciousness. As Sir Karl Popper suggested, *maybe it is not a thing but a relationship between oneself and the external world.* Just as gravity describes a relationship between masses, perhaps *mind, consciousness,* and similar terms refer to relationships between an organism and its environment. There is good reason to conceive of this relation as an emotional state, the calm but indescribable one that we are in most of the time: In other words, consciousness is a type of emotion. Let's explore the reasoning.

Anybody familiar with engineering knows that you cannot have an up state and a down state with nothing in between, and yet we typically describe emotions in terms of high and low, never neutral. When it comes to emotion, this in-between state always seems to be overlooked. We are *constantly* in an emotional state that can go up or down depending on circumstances. It can also remain chronically down, so that we experience clinical depression, or chronically up, as in mania and delirium. It is impossible not to be in some emotional state at every moment. Most often, we are not in one of the up or down states considered typical of emotion but are in this in-between state that happens to be fairly calm. I previously used the example of epilepsy wards to illustrate how emotion exerts a constant nervous tone.

Ommaya's recent (1994) idea that consciousness is a type of emotion and that the brain's emotional core controls the rest of the nervous system arose from powerful contradictions in existing theories that equated consciousness with reason. I discussed earlier the explicit anatomic and physiologic reasons why it has taken until now to understand that the limbic system, which is intermediate in the brain's evolution, might regulate the cortex more than the cortex regulates the limbic system.

Dr. Ommaya suggests that emotion monitors the state of conditions at any given moment, providing a continuous index of what is going on. He calls the brain's emotional organization "a fundamental strategy in evolution which enables increased efficiency in energy utilization for success in any ecological niche. This evolutionary strategy is first noted in the late reptiles, and developed dramatically in birds, mammals, and most of all humans. The mechanism for this strategy is found in the anatomy and physiology of the limbic system with its high degree of reciprocal connections within itself and with all other levels of the brain."

This formulation restates several ideas discussed earlier and also draws heavily on the brain's ability to produce mental work at the least energy cost. In evolving into the structure that it is today, the brain still had to conform to Planck's least energy principle, and many of our higher mental functions are a consequence of that conformity. In other words, consciousness, language, and higher mental functions are the *consequences of an ability to express emotion.* Emotion is fundamental to mind and what we call consciousness.

The Limits of Artificial Intelligence and Cognitive Science

In the past, defenders of humanity pointed out that AI machines were incapable of pleasure, desires, or hope—what philosophy calls *qualia*, the feelings to which we refer in describing humans as different from machines. Early AI proponents maintained that thinking was nothing more than a set of formal rules and qualia were therefore nice but unnecessary. AI's standard rebuttal asked humanists to prove why emotions were essential for thinking. Hoist by their own petard, engineers who build neural networks have recently discovered that a machine's performance can be drastically improved by giving it something like emotion. Here is what led to this reversal.

You have already read about the beliefs among proponents of strong AI that mind and brain are separate and that "understanding" the mind is really a *technical* problem of reducing it to a series of formal logic statements. You also have read my argument that, given the failure at replicating far simpler biological parts, we should be suspicious of claims that the brain can be modeled faithfully by any computational approach.

Despite considerable efforts in the last half-century, the results of which are sometimes inherently interesting but also irrelevant to mind, AI has not produced any general principles about thinking. What are called *expert systems* have indeed been impressively successful in highly specific tasks such as medical diagnosis or financial analysis. Still, a machine must succeed in general situations before we can call it *intelligent*. We still await the barebones model, the vanilla AI without qualia. We would hardly call a calculator that added only some numbers correctly but not others a formalization of arithmetic. Likewise, we cannot call the successful replication of some specific reasoning domains a formalization of general thinking.

This has not dissuaded engineers who build neural networks modeled on some of the hard-wired circuits of the human brain (AI has yet to address volume transmission). Such workers cite the brain as living proof that hardware consisting of analog distributed circuits can act as a controller. In fact, they have successfully installed neural networks to run dangerous chemical plants, manage inventory, and oversee other industrial tasks. This success in highly limited settings has made the most enthusiastic supporters of AI more certain that replicating the spectrum of human thought is not far behind. Back in 1958, the American computer scientists Herbert Simon and Alan Newell boasted that duplicating the problem-solving and information handling capabilities of the brain was not far off: It would be surprising, they claimed, if it were not accomplished "in the visible future" (Simon & Newell, 1958, p. 8).

The real surprise turned out to be the discovery that while existing neural networks do work to varying extents, giving them something like emotion makes them perform even better. There are three parts to a neural control network: (1) a model (of an assembly line, say, or whatever domain the network is to manage), (2) an action system (for welding, putting bottles in cartons, etc.), and (3) an adaptive critic. The adaptive critic concerns our argument the most.

The adaptive critic checks the result of every action taken against the model and feeds back to the action system, telling it whether it did the right thing. A yea-or-nay critic based on a single outcome measure works fine for simple, monotonous tasks such as assembly-line work. It fails at tasks with numerous variables, however, which is what humans deal with routinely. If you are twiddling dozens of dials and the critic can say only that you are performing well or poorly, how can you know which dial led to the action being criticized? The problem becomes exponentially worse as the number of variables increases.

There turns out to be only one fundamental principle on which to build a critic that addresses the problem of too many variables. The American neural network researcher Paul Werbos, of the National Science Foundation, credits the basic idea to Freud, of all people, and his model of how neurons interact biologically (Werbos, 1992, 1994). Freud envisioned an emotional charge (called *cathexis*, or *psychic energy*) that drives every action we take. The network critic assumes this role, generating an evaluation of the ongoing action. Freud argued that every object carries an emotional charge and, if A causes B, then a corresponding and proportional flow of emotional charge must propagate backward from B to A. This led to Werbos's idea of backpropagation, which is a feature of modern networks.

Werbos claims that each component of his network has a counterpart in the human brain. He sees the brainstem and cerebellum as the action component for motor output, our objective model of the world in the cerebral cortex, and the critic in the limbic system. The limbic brain and cortex perform different functions. The limbic system provides an *evaluation* of what one is doing, generating the emotional charge that Freud talked about, whereas the cortex contains a representation of reality. Memory serves as a check on both the model and the critic.

Aside from the fact that incorporating a model of emotion makes networks work better, it is surprising how closely the engineer's ideal design for a sophisticated controller matches that of human biology. Engineers say that an effective critic must have high-speed recurrence. The limbic system performs calculations at an internal cycles-per-second rate of 400 Hz but is governed by an outer clock of 5 Hz, the rate of the theta rhythm. In other words, a high-speed calculator is embedded in a low-speed clock.

The cortex also performs high-speed modular transformations governed by a low-speed clock of 10 Hz, the frequency of the alpha rhythm. This 2:1 ratio is what engineers require to adapt a critic. They need to hold, store, and reëvaluate in a way that makes the cycle time of the critic twice as long as the model's cycle. The 2:1 ratio exists between the limbic brain's evaluation and the update of the model in the cortex in the following way: The state of the world is pumped into the cortex and an evaluation comes out one-fifth of a second later, yet elements *inside* the limbic system are cycling furiously 400 times a second to carry out the intermediate steps needed to derive that evaluation. Perhaps such similarities between real human biology and efficiently engineered networks perpetuate AI's hope that truly intelligent machines are just around the corner.

Even the best device needs minor adjustments, what engineers call *tweaks*. Tweaking the parameters one way will make the system better at some things and poorer at others. It will still be a functioning network but a different one, depending on how you tweak the parameters. Humans also have parameters that are not identical, a quasi-technical way of saying that we possess inborn differences for tolerating cognitive dissonance, such as paying more attention to either emotional or cognitive events. For example, one spouse hates dirt but doesn't mind disorder; the other is oblivious to crumbs on the floor but cannot stand papers or clothes strewn about.

Far more interesting human tweaks are seen in correlations between immune disorders and learning disabilities, or among immune disorders, high mathematical ability, and left handedness in men. The top five percent of U.S. merit scholars are predominantly left-handed men with immune disorders. AI would maintain that such diversity is a technical issue, saying that we do not yet know how to account for such differences in formal language and therefore do not really understand them.

The burden of humanists to show why qualia are necessary for intelligence has been satisfied. Now it appears to be the burden of AI believers to replicate emotion before aiming for an intelligent machine that will model thinking in general.

NOTE

1. *Entropy* is the measure of that part of a system's energy that is not available to do work. More commonly, we use it as a measure of disorder. A broken glass and a scrambled egg have more entropy, for example, than do their intact counterparts.

Disorder tends to increase if things are left to themselves. (You have only to not clean house for a week to prove this.) However, you can create order from disorder (e.g., you can clean the house) by expending effort and energy. In doing so, however, you decrease the overall amount of ordered energy available. This idea is the second law of thermodynamics: The entropy of irreversible processes (breaking glasses or scrambling eggs) of enclosed systems always increases.

SUGGESTED READINGS

Anatomy

Nieuwenhuys R. 1985 *Chemoarchitecture of the Brain*. New York: Springer Verlag

Nieuwenhuys R, Voogd J. van Huijzen Chr. 1988 *The Human Central Nervous System: A Synopsis and Atlas*, 3d ed. New York: Springer Verlag

Ramón Y Cajal S. Swanson N (transl.), Swanson L, ed. 1994 *Cajal's Histology of the Nervous System* (2 vol.) (Reprint of Cajal's historic text.) New York: Oxford University Press

Shepherd GM, ed. 1990 *The Synaptic Organization of the Brain*, 3d ed. New York: Oxford University Press

Strange PG. 1993 *Brain Biochemistry and Brain Disorders*. New York: Oxford University Press

Physiology

Barinaga M. 1995 Remapping the motor cortex. *Science* 268:1696–1698.

Becker JB, Breedlove SM, Crews D, eds. 1992 *Behavioral Endocrinology.* Cambridge: MIT Press

Brown RE. 1993 *An Introduction to Neuroendocrinology.* New York: Cambridge University Press

Kandel ER, Schwartz JH, Jessell TM, eds. 1991 *Principles of Neural Science,* 3d ed. Norwalk, CT: Appleton & Lange

Patridge LD. 1992 *The Nervous System: Its Function and its Interaction with the World.* Cambridge: MIT Press

Shepherd GM. 1994 *Neurobiology* 3d ed. New York: Oxford University Press

Other

Ader R, Felten DL, Cohen N, eds. 1991 *Psychoneuroimmunology,* 2d ed. San Diego: Academic Press

Finger S. 1994 *Origins of Neuroscience: A History of Explorations into Brain Function.* New York: Oxford University Press

Geschwind N, Galaburda AM. 1987 *Cerebral Lateralization: Biological Mechanisms, Associations, and Pathology.* Cambridge: MIT Press

Halpern DF. 1991 *Sex Differences in Cognitive Abilities,* 2d ed. Hillsdale, NJ: Lawrence Earlbaum & Associates

MacLean PD. 1990 *Brain Evolution and Behavior.* New York: Plenum Press

Sarnat HB, Netsky MG. 1981 *Evolution of the Nervous System,* 2d ed. New York: Oxford University Press

Whitaker HA, Cummings JL. 1994 *Brain and Cognition* 26(2):103–326. (The entire volume critiques the Geschwind-Galaburda model of cerebral lateralization.)

II   Clinical Assessment

4   How to Examine a Patient

Neurologists reputed to be superb clinicians are much like Sherlock Holmes: They appreciate that the most mundane occurrence may be far more than what it seems. It may be a clue to something much larger. What appears to be pure intellectual prowess actually demands acute observation, speed, and accuracy in drawing inference and deduction from seemingly no more than a cursory glance at the patient. Like Holmes's companion, Dr. Watson, others marvel at the "subtlety" of the diagnostic clues once the master points them out. As another fictional sleuth, Hercule Poirot, would say of this process, "it is a game for the little gray cells." And yet powers of reasoning and deduction will avail you nothing unless you can observe accurately and separate observation from judgement.

A simple example is the common contest of one-upsmanship that involves diagnosing neurological illness from the sound of an approaching patient's gait. Actually this is fairly easy because the footfalls, once learned, are characteristic. The scrape-and-shuffle of the circumducted gait that is typical of hemiplegia sounds entirely different from the scrape of a spastic paraparesis, which in turn is nothing like the slap of a footdrop or the slap-stomp-and-stick of a tabetic gait (the *stick* here is British English for the cane such patients use to steady themselves). The manifestations of cognitive dysfunctions lend themselves to a similar kind of analysis. For example, the utterance of three words may be sufficient for an aphasia aficionado to diagnose the type.

I have used the metaphor of sleuthing not to encourage besting your peers but to point out that quirks of behavior that seem subtle to an uninformed observer, or those that are dismissed altogether, are the stuff of intellectual satisfaction once you have learned to make accurate inferences from minimal data (Wilbush, 1992). Such talent is also practical. Good clinicians are known for their skill and efficiency. Inferences made from the examiner's observations quickly shape the approach to the examination. An odd or tangential response to, "Good morning, how are you?" may immediately suggest a dementia, aphasia, or a thought disorder. The *unexpected remark* is exactly the kind of clue that should be followed up instead of being dismissed as merely odd. Your approach to patients must be flexible yet thorough. A systematic, cookbook approach applied without deviation will get results but never as efficiently or as accurately as will a flexible one.

A flexible approach is not easily taught. Rather, it is developed individually through experience and practice. The best I can offer are some guidelines.

A broad point of view: It is easy to become constrained by the perspective of whatever discipline you are presently studying. Strive to develop a broad scope of knowledge rather than inculcating narrowness. Read widely in other disciplines. Psychology students should not be afraid to read medical texts, nor should medical students shun psychology books. Both will gain from reading philosophy. Learn which systemic medical illnesses cause mental symptoms. If you are not aware of Huntington's disease, porphyria, substrate deficiencies, or inborn errors of metabolism, for example, then your diagnoses will be faulty. Throughout medical history, lack of knowledge and too narrow a vision have caused unnecessary suffering.

Practice: Examine a patient whenever the opportunity presents itself. Try to examine a broad range of patients, even those who do not appear to have any cognitive problems. By this, you will come to understand what to expect as a "normal" response. Practice both the mental and physical parts of the examination until they become automatic. Once you have mastered clinical examination, you can then practice formal neuropsychological assessment, with all its bells and whistles.

Process of elimination: Make a diagnosis in your mind as soon as possible. Allow no more than three alternatives. Let your examination and any subsequent testing prove you right or wrong. If you were right, analyze which features were the strongest clues that led you to suggest the correct diagnosis as a possibility. If you were wrong, analyze why. Expect to make mistakes.

Understand that everything is interrelated: This is a holistic metaphor. If your only tool is a hammer, then everything looks like a nail. Having a wide assortment of tools means being able to look at things in more than one way. Medical subspecialists, for example, often view the body through their particular organ (heart, brain, kidney, etc.). Psychoanalysts do not want to hear about biology. Sociologists shout about understanding culture and the environment. Any point of view that is narrow and egocentric won't do.

You might ask whether proposing a diagnosis as soon as possible is backwards. Doesn't one need to take a detailed history, examine the patient, do neuropsychological testing, and perhaps obtain a scan or some other machine test before making a diagnosis? Bear in mind that any fool can pick a winner after the race is over. Waiting until all the facts are in is no way to sharpen your diagnostic skills. Such a question also confuses clinical judgment with actuarial judgment (Dawes et al., 1989).

You will never learn to localize a lesion if you first always look at a scan. What people are going to pay you for is your opinion, and if you cannot develop the skill of rendering one, perhaps even with charm, then you will have nothing to offer. The approach I suggest requires commitment and risk taking; then you must determine whether subsequent facts prove you right or wrong. By playing a pedagogical game with yourself you sharpen your analytical and observational acumen as well as your ability to offer decisive opinions.

Always remember that the word *diagnosis* means "through knowledge." It refers to *your* knowledge—knowledge gained through cumulative reading, examining patients at every opportunity, analyzing your mistakes, and engaging in experiment. It does not mean "through machines," "through testing," "through guessing," or "through passivity" (the time-will-tell approach). There is a medical saying that if you do not know what is wrong after taking a history, you will be no wiser after you have examined the patient. This adage understands that diagnosis means "through knowledge," which is to say your own ability to reason. The point of any examination—whether a physical exam, a mental status exam, or a formal neuropsychological assessment—is to support or refute a hypothesis. Without a hypothesis, you are just groping in the dark, and it shows.

THE CLINICAL METHOD

First contact with practicing neurologists, physiologists, or pathologists is enough to intimidate anyone. The mysterious maneuvers of the neurologic examination actually conceal the very intellectual process by which diagnosis is obtained. Turn to a textbook and you find a laundry list of rare, barely pronounceable diseases described in mind-numbing detail. It takes courage for beginners not to run away.

You must become facile in the clinical method. Diagnosis involves inference, deduction, and integration of all possible interpretations, followed by selecting the *one interpretation* most compatible with all facts. Some conditions are so striking as to be instantly recognizable—Parkinson's disease or myxedema, for example. Once these conditions jump out at you, you can spend your time looking for the cognitive problems that sometimes are associated with them. In most cases, however, the following steps are taken:

Symptoms are ascertained through the history, both that which is spontaneously given and that which is specifically elicited by the examiner. Taking a history is not passive listening: You actively guide the patient without asking leading questions. Remember this.

Signs are found by observation and examination. The neuropsychological exam has a physical component and a mental one. Pen-and-paper neuropsychological assessment is properly a test that I will refer to as *formal assessment*.

Syndromes emphasize patterns of derangement. The word is Greek for "concurrence" and refers to a set of symptoms that occur together, the sum of signs of any morbid state. Certain combinations of symptoms and signs occur regularly and constitute a syndrome that helps determine the anatomic location and etiology of the illness. For example, a nonfluent aphasia with a dense right hemiplegia is a common combination of symptoms.

Anatomic diagnosis is made from the preceding deductions. In the example just given, aphasia and hemiplegia indicate a left frontotemporal disorder. This is the anatomic diagnosis, also known as *localizing the lesion*.

Pathological diagnosis is made by noting the mode of onset and speed of the illness's development and integrating this with involvement of any other organ systems and any test results. Tumors and strokes in the same location, for example, can produce radically different results because their pathology differs (see, e.g., Anderson et al., 1990). The pathological diagnosis can be *confirmed* by tests or autopsy.

The *etiology* of the illness is the knowledge of its mechanism and cause. This information can not always be determined. Age matters, and knowing the relative frequency of various diseases helps, of course (table 4.1). The peskiness of not always being able to pin down an etiology reflects a truth that diseases are not discrete biological conditions but manifestations gathered together in our minds. Ziporyn (1992) has written a compendium of "nameless diseases" that do not fit neatly into conventional categories.

You are not expected to elicit this fundamental data accurately at first. Just do the best you can. You will have plenty of time to refine your skills. When in doubt, even experienced clinicians know to examine the patient again, particularly in those conditions in which symptoms and signs fluctuate in relation to activity, time of day, emotional stress, or other factors (e.g., Parkinson's disease, encephalopathy).

The boundary between normality and pathology is not always distinct. For example, there exist people whose culturally normal behavior would be classified as pathological in Western society. Another complicating factor is that a single disease can cause multiple symptoms. Likewise, different diseases can cause identical symptoms. However vexing this situation may be, it is the frequent combination of certain symptoms that makes syndromic diagnosis useful. The anatomic localization is almost always known once a syndrome is recognized. At the same time, the possible etiologies are narrowed considerably. The first step is to localize, as all else follows from this.

Interpreting the Data

No matter how well you may be able to gather reliable clinical data, your interpretation is handicapped if you lack knowledge

Table 4.1
Average Annual Incidence of Disease per 100,000

Disorder	Rate
Herpes zoster	400
Migraine	250
Brain trauma	200
Stroke	150
Concussion	150
Epilepsy	50
Dementia	50
Ménière's disease	50
Transient ischemic attack	30
Bell's palsy	25
Single seizures	20
Parkinsonism	20
Alcoholism	20
Cervical pain	20
Meningitis or encephalitis	15
Sleep disorders	15
Subarachnoid hemorrhage	15
Metastatic brain tumor	15
Peripheral nerve trauma	15
Blindness	15
Benign brain tumor	10
Deafness	10
Cerebral palsy	9
Congenital malformations	7
Mental retardation	6
Malignant brain tumor	5
Metastatic cord tumor	5
Tic douloureux	4
Multiple sclerosis	3
Functional psychosis	3
Spinal cord injury	3
Motor neuron disease	2
Down syndrome	2

Table 4.1 (continued)

Disorder	Rate
Guillain-Barré syndrome	2
Hereditary dystrophies	1.2
Intracranial abscess	1
Benign primany spinal tumor	1
Hereditary striatopallidal disease	0.5
Progressive myelopathy	0.5
Polymyositis	0.5
Syrinx	0.4
Hereditary ataxias	0.4
Myasthenia gravis	0.4
Transverse myelopathy	0.2
Malignant cord tumor	0.1
Spinal vascular disease	0.1

Terms to Know

Pretend to explain neuropsychology to a friend. Aloud, explain these terms.

Symptom	Anatomic diagnosis
Sign	Pathologic diagnosis
Syndrome	Etiologic diagnosis

Why are the terms *symptoms* and *signs* especially confused?

of neuroanatomy and physiology. A minimum working knowledge of neuroanatomy includes the corticospinal tract; the motor unit of the spinal cord, nerve, and muscle; motor connections of the basal ganglia, cerebellum, and cranial nerves; spinothalamic, lemniscal, and cranial nerve sensory pathways; hypothalamic and pituitary connections; reticular system of brainstem and thalamus; the limbic system; cerebral cortex topology and connections; the visual system; the auditory system; the autonomic system; and cerebrospinal fluid pathways. Though the burden may seem great, *these things must be learned.*

Working knowledge of neurophysiology should include the nerve impulse and neuromuscular transmission; spinal reflexes; central transmission; the processes of excitation, inhibition, and release; peptide, hormonal, and chemical messengers; and cortical activation of seizures.

One can reach an anatomic diagnosis in most patients. The anatomic diagnosis limits possibilities and may itself suggest the cause of an illness; the differential diagnosis requires knowledge of an entirely different order. Because it includes the etiology, the differential diagnosis is more difficult to propose than the anatomic one. Here, one requires intimate knowledge of disease process and physiology, an aptitude for thoughtful use of laboratory tests, and a working knowledge of formal neuropsychological assessment. Even the most experienced clinician is often unable to render an etiologic diagnosis (see table 4.1).

Differing Modes of Analysis

Mental symptoms pose a special problem in that variations in personality, behavior, and culture make it difficult to say where normality ends and pathology begins. Methods of studying and diagnosing the life of the mind are quite subjective, and most disorders do not have the kind of third-person objective associations that routinely occur in other fields of science: That is, no conclusive test or postmortem evidence exists to confirm the clinical picture.

Two diametrically opposed approaches to cognitive disorders are the medical-scientific and the psychological. These terms refer to two distinct modes of thought that a clinician may employ. The medical-scientific mode interprets clinical manifestations in terms of neurophysiology and anatomy. Classically, symptoms are conceived of as positive or negative.

Positive symptoms are due to excitation of a structure and negative ones to that structure's destruction or loss of function. A visual hallucination, for example, is interpreted as excess activity in some part of the visual system. The involved part can be deduced by the nature of the hallucination. A negative symptom such as aphasia arises either from destruction of left perisylvian tissue or from this tissue's inhibition by, say, a seizure causing speech arrest (an example of epileptic aphasia). To complicate matters, lesions causing negative symptoms (loss of function) often remove inhibition also. This *disinhibition* results in overactivity of other parts that formerly were inhibited. Negative symptoms can stem from release of facilitation too. Function is thereby lost because the removal of facilitation no longer counterbalances concurrent tonic inhibitory influences. Hence there are at least three causes of symptoms: (1) loss of competence, (2) disinhibition with occlusion of function, and (3) defacilitation with suppression of function. There still remain cases, however, that cannot be reduced to this simple concept of positive and negative forces.

One's education, intelligence, level of vocabulary, and facility of expression coupled with a unique stamp of personality and emotional temperament are all revealed in symptom, action, and word. These multiple facets can be grasped by an astute observer. While the examiner seeks to elicit symptoms and observe signs, the patient can also provide subjective data via introspection. Lack of insight and impaired introspective ability caused by illness, however, is always a confounding possibility.

In short, the medical-scientific approach to mental disorders assumes no difference between what are commonly called *functional disorders* and organic ones. Every disorder must have a physical basis, whether it be molecular, chemical, or at the gross tissue level. It may be congenital (genetic and hereditary) or acquired, or a combination of factors may permit specific environmental or social conditions to interact with a genetic disposition.

By contrast, the psychological approach assumes an additional category of physically expressed maladies that are wholly determined by psychodynamic forces. The growing thrust of biological psychiatry, which searches for molecular mechanisms of classic "functional" diseases, suggests that progressively fewer people adhere to this position. Moreover, after producing voluminous literature for fifty-five years, psychosomatic medicine has offered pathetically few facts to support conclusively its contention that certain diseases are engendered by emotions. Typical diseases labeled *psychosomatic* include peptic ulcer, ulcerative colitis, asthma, angioneurotic edema, rheumatoid arthritis, and migraine. Emotional stress is claimed to develop, exacerbate, or prolong these illnesses, yet each one has an easily demonstrated physiologic cause, and treatment is routinely symptomatic rather than psychological.

While advocates of psychosomatic medicine emphasized the psychological aspects of these illnesses out of all proportion to their somatic components, good clinicians—who, by definition are also compassionate and sensitive people—understand that a holistic perspective of illness is always desirable. Mind and body are united, and it is important to consider the diseased person rather than an illness in isolation. Patients are people, not interesting cases. My adjuration of the medical-scientific mode of analysis should be clear.

HIERARCHIES IN EXAMINATION

Some steps in examining the patient are more important than others. The use of medical technology often is the least important step, despite impressive advances in this area, particularly brain imaging. Save it for last. Clear reasoning should guide your use of technology to confirm a diagnosis that was made "through knowledge."

The mental status or neuropsychological exam is not a long and arduous ordeal. Although a comprehensive survey of the heart, lungs, abdomen, and other structures may take hours, most practitioners learn to get vital information in a few minutes. The same holds for the examination intended to reveal cognitive disturbances. Few patients will get the whole treatment. The order of examination is as follows.

- Observation and first impression
- History
- Examination including a mental component and a physical component
- Tests

    Formal neuropsychological assessment

    Machines (e.g., cerebral blood flow, scans, EEG)

    Blood chemistry analysis

    Consultation

- Experimental analysis
- Pathological examination
  Biopsy
  Autopsy

Taking the History

Take succinct notes during the history. Develop abbreviations that are privately meaningful. Extensive writing in their presence is awkward and makes patients uncomfortable. Do not ask leading questions: Patients are eager to please and tend to give the answers they think the examiner wants to hear. Keep the patient and yourself focused on the issue at hand; politely interrupt tangents and redirect them. (Later, you will recognize when tangents and irrelevancies are diagnostically important.) You are in charge of the interpersonal interaction, but remember that your attitude strongly influences it. Many texts have been written on nuances of this interpersonal dynamic alone. What you say, how you say it, your attitude, tone of voice, body language, and how you balance personal warmth and professional distance all matter.

Aim to extract the most useful information efficiently. You will learn with experience what is useful, especially if you analyze your data gathering after the case is closed. You cannot take all day extracting the history because patients fatigue, particularly if they are confused or very sick. Learn to go immediately to the heart of the matter; otherwise you will have to come back and examine the patient over several sessions. Sometimes this is unavoidable; generally it is poor form.

Quite often, a diagnosis suggests itself from the mode of onset and course of illness. Find out Who, What, When, Where, and How. Determine the PQRST factors:

- When are symptoms *p*resent or absent?
- What is their *q*uality?
- Are there any *r*elated symptoms?
- What is the *s*everity and *s*peed of their development?
- Do symptoms occur at any particular *t*ime of day, and what is their *t*emporal course?

Elicit answers in terms of functional ability—what patients can or cannot do compared to their capabilities prior to being ill.

The reliability of all histories is automatically suspect since everyone you are asked to consult must be assumed to harbor some potential cognitive dysfunction. It is astounding how often family and physician *overestimate* a patient's mental capacity. People have no difficulty recognizing that something is wrong with a person who urinates on the carpet or babbles incoherently, but most impaired patients appear normal in daily circumstances. You must probe to uncover their deficits. One reason for this is that vocabulary is particularly resistant to many forms of brain damage and so, superficially, patients often sound normal. Retention of a pleasant affect and an intact social demeanor means that most disturbed patients do not act like degenerates. Therefore, gross dysfunctions can be overlooked for a long time until individuals completely break down (e.g., by urinating on the carpet). Though it would seem pointless to attempt taking a history from persons so confused or feebleminded that they have no idea of what is going on, it happens all the time.

Observing how the patient relates the history is important. You must ask about intimate or deeply personal activities without embarrassing either yourself or the patient. Be nonjudgemental in acquiring the facts and ruthlessly judgmental once you have them. As Charles Darwin supposedly stated, "It is a fatal flaw to reason while observing. But so desirable beforehand and necessary afterwards." Never be so polite as to let inconsistencies slip by: Such errors may be the major symptoms of the disorder.

Special Considerations in Psychiatric Illness

In psychiatric conditions, a past history is common, with one or more visits to mental hospitals, an insidious onset, and often a family history. There are usually few physical signs and a thought disorder often is present. In fact, a thought disorder may be the solitary symptom of mental illness. Other features strongly suggestive of mental disorders include auditory hallucinations, mania, hypervigilance, paranoia (except in the elderly), humming, rocking, grunting and other stereotyped behavior (called *stereotypies,* a pleural usage of the term *stereotyped behavior*). The type of hallucination, if present, may help: Auditory ones usually are psychiatric, olfactory ones organic, and visual hallucinations may be either organic or psychiatric.

Whether delirium is a manifestation of neurological or psychiatric disease may be particularly difficult to differentiate, because accompanying neurological signs are relatively uncommon, with the exception of tremor, asterixis, and autonomic signs. Psychiatric patients rarely are "confused" in the strict sense whereas confusion can be profound in medical conditions.

Speech structure is more often aberrant in neurological disease (aphasia, failure to repeat, anomia, paraphasias [slip of the tongue]); speech content is more often faulty in psychiatric cases. Repeating the same question over and over (termed *viscous behavior*) is more often a psychiatric manifestation; among medical problems it is only seen with any frequency in dementia and temporal lobe epilepsy.

The Physical Examination

General Principles
The physical examination should be orderly but flexible, depending on the problem. It is pointless to test complex sensory discrimination in a patient who is confused, for example. Fundamentally, a clinical test is a maneuver to uncover disordered nervous function. There are a hundred clinical tests that can be employed in the neurologic examination, and just as many for testing higher functions. Most of them are variations on a few basic themes. The guidebooks of the Mayo Clinic or of William DeMeyer are recommended as monographs on the technique of the neurologic examination.

I said in chapter 1 that physician neuropsychologists are more likely than their doctoral counterparts to rely on a clinical impression rather than spend time proving closure via formal testing. The basis for this distinction lies in the physical exam. Clinicoanatomical relationships have been proven long ago, give strong localizing signs, and save time. If one is capable of performing both a physical exam and a formal assessment, why spend hours testing to discover what can be determined in a few moments by a physical sign?

A large part of the so-called physical exam actually involves observing. Astute clinicians are careful observers. How the patient walks into the room tests pyramidal, extrapyramidal, and cerebellar pathways; the patient's ability to stand stationary with feet together and eyes shut (the Rhomberg test) judges proprioceptive and labyrinthine functions; looking for asymmetry of facial movement and listening to articulation is really an examination of cranial nerves 7, 9, 10, and 12. Noting dexterity of movement, strength, muscle bulk, tone, and coördination yields far more information than a reflex hammer ever can. Although many texts separate the exam into motor and sensory components, most maneuvers involve some of each. We split things into components to make them easier to understand but, again, you should think holistically.

For the purposes of neuropsychological assessment, perhaps the most revealing sensory function is a complex sensory discrimination task such as fingertip graphesthesia, wherein patients correctly recognize letters and digits written on the index finger. The ability to discern this by sensation alone means that the following structures are intact: Peripheral nerve, spinal lemniscus, ventral thalamus, primary somatosensory cortex, posterior parietal cortices, and corpus callosum (because a number written on a left fingertip requires spatial and temporal summation in the right posterior parietal lobe and then transfer to the left angular gyrus to interpret its symbolic identity as a numeral). Hence, this simple act tests the integrity of a big chunk of nervous tissue. Any errors in this task permit immediate inferences about the side of impairment and level of lesion.

The physical maneuvers that yield the most information from a neuropsychological point of interest, in order of greatest yield, are as follows:

- Fingertip graphesthesia
- Strength and dexterity testing in the upper extremities
- Visual field testing
- Coördination and alternating movements (ability to change sets)
- Other pyramidal and extrapyramidal motor signs
- Any reflex asymmetry or Babinski sign

Details of the Physical Examination

The rationale behind fingertip graphesthesia has already been given. Other complex sensory tasks, such as stereognosis or two-point discrimination, could also be used.

Testing strength and dexterity can inform you of three things: (1) the side of the lesion, (2) the level of the lesion (e.g., a hemiplegia from a hypertensive pontine infarct where corticospinal fibers have been interrupted as opposed to the hemiplegia of a capsular infarct resulting from embolism of an atherosclerotic plaque in the neck), and (3) whether it is superficial in the cortex or deep in either the white matter or central gray tissue.

It would seem logical to use a dynamometer or some other kind of force meter to measure strength, yet the arcane and highly subjective 1-to-5 grading system still is used routinely by neurologists. Normal strength is notated as 5/5, the ability to overcome gravity as 3/5, and the barest flicker of movement is recorded as 1/5. The scale is obviously sensitive to only the grossest weakness. Overlapping innervation of myotomes and dermatomes make motor signs more reliable in the arms, whereas sensory signs are more reliable in the legs. Therefore, the neuropsychologist could concentrate only on the arms. (This is beginner's advice, because you are trying to get maximum information in minumum time. With experience, you will know when carefully examining the legs also is important.)

Gross paralysis is easy to detect but, for less obvious weakness, a finger tapper or small hand dynamometer (my preference) is useful. Either gives an objective measurement that can be repeated and compared over time. These two inexpensive tools are available from commercial vendors and are far more useful than are reflex hammers. In general, more than a ten percent difference between dominant and nondominant hands is significant.

Table 4.2 summarizes the different motor effects between upper and lower motor neuron lesions. The lower motor neuron is the anterior horn cell of the spinal cord or its axons in the anterior root and peripheral nerve. *The upper motor neuron is not synonymous with the corticospinal tract.* It also includes thalamocortical and extrapyramidal fibers, and the cortico-thalamic, cortico-striate, cortico-rubral, cortico-pontine, cortico-olivary, and cortico-reticular fibers, among others. Upper motor neuron paralysis refers

Table 4.2
Differences Between Upper and Lower Motor Neuron Weakness

Upper Motor Neuron	Lower Motor Neuron
Muscles always affected in groups of flexors and extensors	Individual muscles affected
Deep lesions—trunk and proximal muscles affected	Not applicable
Superficial lesions—distal muscles and fine coördination affected	
Atrophy slight, from disuse	Marked atrophy to 80% of bulk
Spasticity, brisk reflexes, extensor plantar reflex	Flaccidity, lost reflexes; if present, the plantar reflex is flexor
No fasciculations	Fasciculations present after time
Normal NCV and EMG	Abnormal NCV; denervation potentials in EMG

NCV = nerve conduction velocity; EMG = electromyogram.

collectively to all the descending fiber systems that influence and modify the lower motor neuron.

An example of the fine distal coördination referred to in table 4.2 would be rapid, repeated opposition of the thumb to each of the digits in sequence. Patients with large, superficial cortical lesions may show this clumsiness and no other motor weakness. Deep lesions, on the other hand, often cause dense paralysis.

Confrontation visual field testing should include detection of moving fingers in all four quadrants plus testing for desaturation of red color across the vertical meridian in each eye. The technique of field testing is given in standard texts. Given the immense spread of the visual system, neuroöphthalmological testing alone can yield a wealth of information.

Coördination is tested by the finger-to-nose and heel-to-shin tests. These are largely test of the cerebellar hemispheres, whereas tandem walking is more a test of the cerebellar vermis (hence, alcoholics *often* do well on finger-to-nose testing but fail the tandem gait test because alcohol is selectively neurotoxic to the vermis). The term *rapid alternating movement* (diadochokinesis) usually applies to cerebellar function. What one looks for is clumsiness and slowness. Another type of alternating movement, however, is the ability to *change sets*. In the fist-palm-side test, for example, you demonstrate the repetitive sequence of hitting a surface first with your fist, then with your open palm face down, and then with the ulnar edge of your hand. After one or two demonstrations, normal persons have no difficulty in mimicking this cycle of sequential movements. An obvious disruption of smooth performance of these alternating movements suggests prefrontal impairment.

Other motor signs such as spasticity, synkinesis, rigidity, festination, ballism, dystonia, chorea, akinesia, tremor, athetosis, gegenhalten, myoclonus, and ataxia all have localizing value, with respect both to the affected side as well as to the level of lesion. Readers unfamiliar with these entities can consult standard neurologic texts for further explication.

The extensor plantar response, called the *Babinski sign*, classically indicates a lesion of the corticospinal tract and usually indicates the side of the lesion. Reflex asymmetries also serve the same purpose, although spinal reflexes all involve connections below the foramen magnum and therefore rarely are helpful when one is interested in cerebral problems.

The Mental Status Examination

Most people are comfortable recognizing the physical signs of brain disease, but those that alter the life of the mind and are expressed as changes in intellect, behavior, or character can disquiet even the most experienced practitioner. Yet the acute alteration of mental status is an increasingly common event in medical illness, in complications of its treatment, in an aging population that lives longer, or as a product of trauma and a violent civil society.

Imaging technology often is not helpful in explaining changes in the mental status. Except in a few structural diseases—cerebral hemorrhage, subdural hematoma, and those that have damage at the tissue level—scanners and other devices are uniformly disappointing in their ability to disclose gross abnormality. This is because mental changes take place at the systems or cellular level and the diagnosis of such derangements, therefore, remains largely a clinical one.

Table 4.3
Higher Cerebral Functions

Manipulation of well-learned material

Arithmetic and allied analytical abilities

Abstraction

Memory (visual and verbal)

Language

Perceptual-motor ability

Problem solving

The *neuropsychological assessment* is the identification, quantification, and description of changes in behavior associated with brain failure. It is a third-person, comprehensive assessment of a wide range of intellectual, adaptive, and emotional behaviors that reflects adequacy or inadequacy of cerebrocortical functioning. It does this by testing higher cerebral functions. Complex mental functions depend on the integrity of more basic processes and are highly susceptible to neurologic and systemic illness. Numerous medical, surgical, environmental, and sociological events can precipitate a change in mental status and table 4.3 gives examples of higher cerebral functions. Table 4.4 lists some common acute changes.

It is important that we clarify what is meant by mental status. At its most fundamental, the mental status exam is the synthesis of the examiner's observations during the initial interview. It is something we actually do all the time in an informal, almost automatic way, and the best assessments are the result of basic training, a lot of experience dealing with people, and a touch of wisdom. It is part of one's bedside manner.

The mental status exam takes only three to five minutes and is a useful screening tool. Any abnormalities are an indication for further investigation (table 4.5).

Some Details of Terminology

Overall Gestalt   The gestalt itself is sometimes sufficient to suggest that something is wrong.

Table 4.4
Common Acute Changes in Mental Status

Confusion
Delirium
Encephalopathy
Psychiatric states
Hysteria (unconscious)
Fictitious mental changes (deliberate)

Psychomotor "retardation" does not mean that the patient is stupid: It means a general slowing of reaction, movement, speech, and cognitive processing. Lengthy, sometimes disquieting, pauses before answering a query is a typical manifestation of psychomotor retardation. The opposite picture is excited or agitated behavior that is driven from within; that is, the agitation has no causal relation to external stimuli.

Stereotypical movements (stereotypy) include any purposeless, repetitive action such as rocking, grimacing, finger rubbing, shouting, humming, or grunting. Rocking is particularly common in psychiatric diseases but is seen also as a toxic effect of neuroleptic medication (Cooper & Dourish, 1990).

Negativism is a resistance to following commands or toward being moved. For example, the request, "Open your mouth" results instead in clenched teeth.

Catatonia is unresponsiveness to surroundings coupled with either rigidity (maintained against all efforts to be moved) or waxy flexibility (voluntary holding for a long time of bizarre postures that are molded by the examiner). Although they appear superficially catatonic, hypervigilant patients are fully aware. Signs of excess autonomic activity are evident.

Level of Consciousness   Wakefulness is generated by the brainstem reticular activating system, but attention is focused, directed, and maintained by other brainstem and cortical circuits. Unless the patient is alert, can sustain consciousness, and has a clear sensorium, there is little point pursuing further aspects of the mental status exam. Fundamental abilities must be intact before more complex ones can function well.

Table 4.5
The Mental Status Exam

Overall Gestalt

Appearance: Neat, disheveled, perplexed, healthy, sick, frightened, bizarre.

Psychomotor behavior: Retarded or excited; presence of tics; gestures; stereotypies; "catatonic" posturing, hypervigilance.

Attitude: Coöperative, avoiding, interested, negativistic, seductive, defensive, wary, passive.

Level of Consciousness

Note fluctuations and describe meaningfully. Does the patient alert to and orient to the examiner's presence? Respond to voice only, or only to touch and shaking? Is alertness sustained only on continued stimulation?

Orientation

Time, person, place, circumstance.

Mental Control and Concentration

Count from 20 to 1; ABCs; shifting tasks (1A, 2B, 3C, etc.); recite days of week backward. Can the patient "hold" something in his head?

Speech

Structure and content (see section on thought disorder): Normal, pressured, slow, dysarthric.

Repetition and naming (quickly identifies some aphasias).

Comprehension of simple and multistep commands: Be sure patient is not responding to gesture. Answers may be given by pointing.

Memory

A combination of attention, mental control, recall, and learning: Immediate repetition (digits forward/backward) is really a concentration test.

Current information (related to IQ, culture).

Intermediate recall of three object (e.g., Dr. Victor, Saturday, eight o'clock) versus learning (use paired associates from the Wechsler memory scale).

Emotional State

Affect : Mood :: Weather : Climate.

Mood is a pervasive, sustained emotion; in extreme states, it can color perception of the world. Note depth, intensity, and fluctuations: Depressed, irritable, angry, fearful, elated, ecstatic.

Affect is the emotional expression as judged by the examiner:

Normal: A broad range, with variable expressions and gestures.

Constricted: Reduced range of expression.

Flat: Lack of any emotional expression.

Inappropriate: To the content of speech and person's culture.

Labile: Repeated, abrupt shifts without apparent reason.

Table 4.5 (continued)

Anxiety Level

Patient's description: Generalized or specific.

Examiner's description: Sweaty hands, restlessness, pressured speech, tense voice, etc.

Thought Disorders

Abnormalities are almost always psychiatric.

Structure of thoughts:

> *Productivity:* Pressured speech (can't be interrupted), slow thinking, responds only when asked, poverty of ideas.
>
> *Relevance:* Do answers really answer questions? Tangential and circumstantial thinking, confabulation.
>
> *Associations:* Flight of ideas (usually an understandable association based on word play or environmental distractions), loose associations (illogical, frequently bizarre, abrupt changes in topic), word salad (incomprehensible), neologisms, blocking (interruption of train of thought before idea is completed).

Content of thoughts:

> *Preoccupations:* Obsessions, compulsions, phobias.
>
> *Thought disturbances:* Delusions, ideas of reference, depersonalization.
>
> *Perceptual disturbances:* Illusions (misperception of stimulus) and hallucinations (no external stimulus).

Abstraction, Judgement, and Insight

Tested with proverbs, similarities, and appropriateness of responses. Is patient aware of his illness and is the emotional response to it appropriate?

Orientation Only in the movies do patients with "amnesia" forget who they are. Patients who lose their identity probably have a conversion reaction or fictitious amnesia. A more useful test for orientation to person is whether the patient knows who other persons are, even if only generically (e.g., "the doctor," or "the nurse").

Mental Control Mental control is the ability to keep one's thoughts together, to attend to more than one thing at a time, to keep track of the purpose or intention of what one is doing at the moment. It is easily interfered with by anxiety and often is one of the earliest deficits in both structural and systemic neurologic disease. Reciting the days of the week backward is a sufficiently novel and difficult task to test mental control at the bedside (try it).

Speech Speech and language are customarily divided into components: Spontaneous speech, the ability to repeat something heard, and comprehension of spoken and written language. The following encapsulated comments will be amplified in chapter 13.

In testing speech, be sure that the patient is not responding to gesture. (Comprehension should be tested without requiring any speech output whatsoever on the patient's part. For example, patients may answer spoken or written questions by pointing). *Avoid confounding by restricting both input and output to language only.* This refers to the fact that we communicate through additional means other than language. For example, in naming objects presented visually, a patient may not recognize a comb or be able to name it until the moment you unthinkingly run your thumb over the teeth. Being able to recognize it after this auditory clue is not the same as visual recognition. Your mistake would be an example of a confounding error.

Confounding factors include asking open-ended or vague questions instead of ones that require specific and relevant answers. Accepting yes or no answers at face value is a particularly common error, as you may assume that nodding affirmatively equals true comprehension. Of course, this is not true. Accepting any *overlearned information,* such as saying or writing one's name or address as evidence of retained speech or lexical skill, are equally common mistakes. Overlearned responses are generally not useful for drawing conclusions, and should be discarded. Overlearned behavior is not the same as *automatic behavior*, which can be extremely revealing of brain function (e.g., preservation of some speech gestures in some kinds of aphasia and impairment of them in others). *Automatisms* are also different, referring to well-coördinated motor actions that seem purposeful to an uninformed observer but for which the patient has no awareness or recollection. The point is to be precise in your terminology.

The issue of confounds is important enough to warrant an anecdote. A medical resident I shall call Dr. Lacy handled the emergency admission of a Chinese man whom I shall call Mr. Lee. This patient spoke poor English to start and was now globally aphasic from a cerebral hemorrhage. The next morning on rounds, Dr. Lacy reported that Mr. Lee had dramatically improved and could now understand. Being suspicious that this patient's speech could return in one day with so severe a lesion, I asked Dr. Lacy why he concluded that Mr. Lee could now comprehend spoken language. "He answered my questions," was the reply.

We marched into Mr. Lee's room for a demonstration of his remarkable recovery. He was a polite man, flattered to see so many people interested in him. In keeping with his culture, he bowed to each of us. Dr. Lacy fired off a series of questions. "Mr. Lee, are you feeling better?" "Did you eat your breakfast?" "Was your wife here yet this morning?" Mr. Lee smiled and nodded vigorously several times to each question. This nodding was Dr. Lacy's proof.

"He's responding to the enthusiasm in your voice and to your body language," I explained. I stood behind Mr. Lee so he was unable to see me and repeated the same questions, articulating clearly but without inflection. Mr Lee made no response. I then stood in front of him as Dr. Lacy had and asked "Mr. Lee, is it snowing in this room?" He smiled and nodded vigorously. The point of this anecdote is to be sure of what it is you are testing. If you doubt that a patient understands you, test your theory with a nonsense question.

Memory Memory is a complex and incompletely understood brain function. Memory impairment usually is insidious and chronic. The few conditions in which it is acutely deranged include cerebrovascular episodes such as a transient ischemic attack involving the hippocampus and medial temporal lobes; head trauma, with contusion to the temporal lobes; complex partial seizures, where the acute amnesia is brief; and intoxications and poisonings. Only in psychogenic amnesia is personal identity lost.

Emotional State   Various terms describing affect are listed in table 4.4. You need to correlate the patient's introspection with your own opinion based on observation. Some people have little appreciation that emotions and the circumstances of everyday life do cause physical, bodily sensations. Some individuals are even incapable of understanding this association. The term for this is *alexithymia*, meaning "having no words for feelings." Depression is discussed in chapter 8.

Anxiety Level   We all experience anxiety. Only when it is unusually prolonged, persistent, or severe do we call it pathological. *State anxiety* refers to anxiety caused by a particular event whereas *trait anxiety* refers to nervousness that is part of a patient's lifelong character.

Thought Disorders   Disorders of the content and structure of thought almost always signal a psychiatric condition (see table 4.5).

Abstraction, Judgement and Insight   Neurologically, concreteness is seen only with stupidity and persons with chronic temporal lobe epilepsy (where one often finds a *viscous personality* as well). Otherwise, concreteness is a classic sign of schizophrenia. Neuropsychologically, one wants to know whether patients have appropriate insight into their disability. If not, a right parietal impairment must be assumed until proven otherwise.

Frequently Confused Terms for Specific Mental States
Table 4.6 lists nine features commonly seen in what is called *organic brain syndrome*. A given patient will not have all nine features, of course. I have singled out the following specific terms used to describe various derangements of mental function because they often are so confused or used inappropriately. Practice describing a given clinical picture precisely and accurately.

Table 4.6
Nine Features of Organic Brain Syndrome

Delirium	Dementia	Intoxication
Hallucinations	Withdrawal	Amnesia
Delusions	Affective syndrome	Personality syndrome

Global Confusional State   A quiet confusion with profound disorientation, apathy, and deranged memory characterizes a global confusional state. Patients are indifferent and inattentive, unable to concentrate on the simplest task, and easily distracted. Spontaneous speech is minimal, and questions frequently go unanswered or else there are long pauses before a response is uttered. Comments are irrational and inconsistent, and betray a profound lack of insight. Meaningful evaluation of memory rarely is possible.

Delirium   Delirium constitutes reduced clarity in awareness of one's environment. The onset is rapid, the course fluctuating, and the duration brief.

Attention is difficult to focus, sustain, and shift. Wandering attention makes conversation difficult or impossible. The patient is easily distractible.

Perception is disturbed. Delirious patients may perceive a banging door as a gunshot (misrepresentation), rumpled sheets as animals (illusion), or voices commenting on their behavior (hallucination). There is often a delusional conviction of the reality of hallucinations and an emotional and behavioral response that is consistent with their content.

Thinking is incoherent, fragmented, and disjointed. Reasoning is defective, and goal-directed behavior is poor. Perseveration may be present.

Sleep-wake cycles are disturbed, ranging from drowsiness and coma to hypervigilance and mania. Vivid dreams and nightmares may merge with hallucinations. Patients may not be able to distinguish wakeful reality from dreaming.

Psychomotor activity is altered. One sees restlessness, hyperactivity, formication, and bizarre postures. Psychomotor retardation and stupor may occur, usually with abrupt shifts from hyperactivity to catatonia.

Dementia Dementia is multifaceted loss of intellectual abilities that interferes with social or occupational functioning. Diagnosis cannot be made in the presence of delirium, though the two may coëxist. Only one symptom—most often a decline in memory or language—usually predominantes early in the course. With time, many skills become impaired. Except for Jacob-Creutzfeld disease, dementias do not present acutely; whereas encephalopathy frequently does.

Memory is often the worst disturbance, particularly as time wears on. Test for recollection of immediate events, ability to learn new material, and remote events.

Impaired abstraction takes many forms. Novel tasks are failed, especially if the patient is pressed for time. Proverbs and similarities are poorly understood.

Other higher cortical functions—praxis, language, object recognition, spatial discrimination, other integrative tasks, right-left confusion, and so forth—are disturbed.

Personality changes include indifference, suspiciousness, irritability, short temper, apathy, and withdrawal.

Encephalopathy Encephalopathy is a reversible, fluctuating state marked by poor orientation, mental control, and alertness. Psychomotor activity tends to be normal in encephalopathic patients unlike in delirium. At most, one finds formication (the illusion that ants or bugs are crawling around), repetitive picking at the sheets, or aimless wandering if patients are not restrained. Unlike dementia, higher functions are intact. Encephalopathic patients can do serial seven's or arithmetic given a lucid moment.

The basic deficit is an altered sensorium with preserved higher functions—essentially the opposite of demented patients, who have a clear sensorium but are feebleminded. Encephalopathy is seen routinely with organ failure, so we speak of hepatic or uremic encephalopathy, for example, each of which has characteristic physical signs such as peripheral neuropathy, headache, asterixis, myoclonus, or telangiectasias.

Delirium and encephalopathy can each be called an *acute confusional state*. Acute changes are most often medical rather than psychiatric and are caused by metabolic imbalances (e.g., acid-base, electrolyte), a toxic or withdrawal reaction to a drug or substance (e.g., X-ray contrast), sepsis, and organ failure (e.g., heart, liver, lung) with its specificically deranged physiology.

These states can be acute but more often they begin subtly, finally becomming apparent to everyone only when the patient fully decompensates. Neuroleptics and sedatives such as *haloperidol* (Haldol), *chlorpromazine* (Thorazine), and *diazepam* (Valium) are commonly given symptomatically. However, drugs are the frequent culprits of acute mental changes.

Metabolic encephalopathy is a useful term, although many tend to think it a catchall. It implies only that the derangement is on a substructural level and that there is no grossly visable anatomic lesion within resolution of our current imaging technology; physiological measures, however, such as the EEG, often are abnormal. Some examples of the dynamic, subcellular neuropathology involved include the existence and toxicity of free radicals; the differential responses of neurons and glial cells to metabolic derangements; failures of cycle metabolism such as glycolysis, citric acid oxidation, or urea; perturbations in neuronal and systemic osmolality and the ionic exchanges and fate of organic osmols that dampen such perturbations within the central nervous system; differential pathology in the brain's gray and white matter; and the unique biochemical properties that are highly conserved across evolution and that defend the central nervous system as an isolated organ.

Mistakenly, subdural hematoma is high on everyone's list of conditions that cause an acute change in mental status. Accordingly, scans are ordered like a knee-jerk reflex. The time wasted could be better spent pondering the vastly more common causes of acute mental change.

SUGGESTED READINGS

Adams RD, Victor M. 1993 *Principles of Neurology*, 5th ed. New York: McGraw Hill (see also the companion handbook to this edition)

Arieff AI, Griggs RC (eds). 1992 *Metabolic Brain Dysfunction in Systemic Disorders*. Boston: Little, Brown

DeMyer W. 1993 *Technique of the Neurologic Examination*, 4th ed. New York: McGraw Hill

Jefferson JW, Marshall JR. 1981 *Neuropsychiatric Features of Medical Diseases*. New York: Plenum Press

Mayo Clinic and Mayo Foundation. 1991 *Clinical Examinations in Neurology*, 6th ed. St Louis: Mosby Yearbook

Rosenberg RN, et al., eds. 1993 *The Molecular and Genetic Basis of Neurological Disease*. Stoneham, MA: Butterworth-Heinemann

Stoudemire A, Fogel BS. 1993 *Psychiatric Care of the Medical Patient*. New York: Oxford University Press

Tartner RE, Van Thiel DH, Edwards KL, eds. 1988 *Medical Neuropsychology: The Impact of Disease on Behavior*. New York: Plenum Press

Ziporyn T. 1992 *Nameless Diseases*. New Brunswick, NJ: Rutgers University Press

5 Formal Neuropsychological Assessment

By formal assessment I mean a detailed and systematic inquiry of the patient's mental state. Strictly taken, formal neuropsychological assessment means sitting down and putting the patient through a series of standardized paper-and-pencil tests or physical maneuvers. More broadly, it means anything that can be done at the bedside or in the exam room with objects at hand, as long as the intention is to reveal specific aspects of the patient's cognition.

Much energy has been spent arguing about whether a fixed battery of tests or a flexible approach is best; a reasonable approach is to combine the virtues of each (Benton, 1992a; Levin, 1994). Standardized batteries exist mostly for the practitioner's convenience. Neuropsychological assessment best contributes to clinical diagnosis and treatment when it clearly defines the patient's cognitive state. The point of tests, given singly or together, should be their validity and sensitivity to a wide range of skills within specific cognitive domains. Remember that a test can only be as good as the person who administers it and that not everyone who has mastered its administration is well trained in brain-behavior relationships, nor may they even be a competent clinician.

I make this point because weekend workshops on test administration are popular, despite their potential danger to patients. Implying that a ready-made battery, rigidly applied, can detect— let alone characterize—brain damage invites unsophisticated attendees to mischief. Competent neuropsychologists must call on wide knowledge of brain-behavior relationships when undertaking formal assessment and rarely rely on a *single* test to draw conclusions. Such knowledge cannot be gained in a semester, let alone a weekend. As is true in acquiring any skill, you will learn the nuances of testing and interpretation with time and practice.

THE ASSESSMENT OF HIGHER CEREBRAL FUNCTIONS

If, with each patient, you were to systematically go through the comprehensive mental status exam outlined in table 4.5 and write down the results, you would start to capture the spirit of formal testing. Such a habit, though conscientious, would soon become tiresome and prove not very useful, given both the gamut of neurological conditions and the diversity of patients. The scope of referral questions is also broad and might vary all the way from a child not doing well in school to issues of legal competency to malingering. A rigid approach is out of the question.

What you want is a flexible instrument whose elements can be added or deleted as required. You should also be able to test either at the bedside or in the office. The following skeleton is a reasonable place to start, and I trust that you will enrich your knowledge with specific course work and practical experience in administering and interpreting formal tests.

Though the modified Halstead-Reitan battery I'm about to explicate is my own jumping-off place, the point I want to emphasize is that you must query a *variety* of cognitive functions. There is no perfect or best collection of tests. Pigeonholing cognition into categories such as language, memory, and visuospatial domains is done for our convenience. Mental functions are far from unitary, and patients seek help or are dragged in by others because of difficulties in everyday life—not because they fail to assemble block designs or draw clock faces correctly.

For practical reasons, you start with a broad assessment of cognition and zero in on domains where deficits are encountered by branching to more focused tests. Confounds must always be considered. As your experience increases, you will face novel problems that oblige you to improvise. Only with firm knowledge of brain organization and brain-behavior relationships can the clinician invent, execute, and interpret a useful test of cognitive facets.

Scope of Tests and Report Format

Here follows a suggested format for both proposed tests and the structure of your final report. First I'll indicate the overall gestalt by briefly reviewing the report categories, and then I'll consider

HCF, CPT, and ICD

Almost all neuropsychologists with a PhD speak of *neuro-psychological testing*, whereas medical doctors are likely to engage patients in a *higher cerebral function assessment* (HCF). This cumbersome name is the official term for neuropsychological testing that is found in the fifth edition of *Current Procedural Terminology* (CPT-5), a handbook containing five-digit codes for every procedure a physician can perform. Clerks of third-party payers, who are indifferent to your report and the details of your evaluation, merely determine whether the code is a "covered procedure."

For example, the CPT code for an HCF is 95880. A bureaucracy fond of numerical reduction also codes diagnoses according to the *International Classification of Diseases* (ICD-9), a compendium issued by the World Health Organization. In deciding to accept or reject your HCF done on a patient with a concussion, for example, insurers consider only procedure 95880 and diagnosis 951. All else is irrelevant.

The Halstead-Reitan Battery

Whence this name? One of the goals in the 1950s was to find a test that accurately identified frontal lobe injury. In pursuing this goal, Ralph Reitan modified a set of intelligence tests developed earlier by Ward Halstead. Through the years, Reitan and others endlessly modified these tests, and the name *Halstead-Reitan battery* was attached to various collections of them. These offspring are accurately called *modified Halstead-Reitan batteries.* Although the original collection of Reitan's tests is no longer used, Reitan's name is remembered because he demonstrated the need for neuropsychologists to sample a broad variety of behavior.

Halstead's tests included the (1) category test, (2) critical flicker fusion, (3) tactual performance test, (4) Seashore rhythm test, (5) speech sounds perception, (6) finger tapping, and (7) the time sense test. Reitan added (8) trail making, (9) the aphasia screening test, (10) a sensory-perceptual exam in multiple modalities, (11) the Wechsler intelligence scale, and (12) the Minnesota Multiphasic Personality Inventory. Total administration time was six to eight hours.

each test in detail. We start with the report title, some identifying information, and a list of what we have done.

Higher Cerebral Function Assessment

Name:

Referred by: (physician, attorney, agency, etc.)

Test date(s):

Place: (hospital name [if inpatient] or neuropsychological lab [if done in the office])

Hospital no.:   (or other identifying information such as birthdate, Social Security number)

Tests Administered

Interview

History and physical

Wechsler Adult Intelligence Scale, revised (WAIS)

Wechsler Memory Scale, revised (WMS)

Aphasia Screening Test (AST)

Drawings on Command

Tapping Test

Grip dynamometry

Form Board

Sensory-Perceptual Examination (Reitan-Kløve)

Trail Making parts A and B

Minnesota Multiphasic Personality Inventory (MMPI)

Report Headings

Tests administered

Background information

Behavioral observations

Intellectual and cognitive functioning

Memory functioning

Language functioning

Perceptual-motor functioning

Personality assessment

Summary and diagnosis

Recommendations

Closing

Your signature

Details of the Report

Now let's flesh out what to say under each of these headings. You will need a greatly expanded Greek and Latin vocabulary to write a report. See the box, "Neuropsychological Terms to Know." These should now be part of your lexicon.

Background Information   First, state the patient's age, race, handedness, education, occupation, and any notable chronic illness or social achievements, if relevant. (A parenthetical comment on handedness: Examiners rarely ask about more than the writing hand when trying to determine handedness. We assume that individuals who perform all *skilled* functions—such as combing, slicing, scissoring, throwing, dealing, and painting—with their right hand are right-handed. Individuals who perform some skilled actions with the left hand are probably not strong right-handers. They should be called *mixed* or *left-handed* because they have a non standard pattern of *cerebral dominance* that could influence your interpretation of their test performance. Quantitative questionnaires are available when needed (Oldfield, 1971), but inquiring about social activities is usually sufficient and often all that is feasible.

Nonstandard cerebral organization is typical also in persons with chronic disease of early onset, such as epilepsy or cerebral palsy. The Wada test shows that such persons who appear outwardly right-handed do not posess strictly lateralized left-hemispheric speech as often as do unaffected individuals. Therefore, the presence of chronic neurologic illness can be relevant. Be mindful that patterns of cognitive deficits that help to localize lesions in typical

Neuropsychological Terms to Know

You should be able to explain each of these term effortlessly.

Aphasia
  Expressive
  Receptive
  Conduction
  Anomia
  Agrammatism

Agraphia
  Pure agraphia
  Apraxic agraphia
  Spatial agraphia

Apraxia
  Ideomotor
  Ideational
  Constructional
  Dressing

Acalculia
  Asymbolia for mathematical signs
  Spatial acalculia
  Transcoding errors (lexical-to-digit and digit-to-lexical)

Agnosia
  Visual object agnosia
  Prosopagnosia
  Color agnosia
  Somatognosia
  Anosognosia
  Astereoagnosia
  Auditory agnosia

right-handers may lead you astray in persons with anomalous cerebral dominance.)

Next, give the chief complaint and its history as succinctly as possible. Patients frequently have no idea why they are seeing you, and their idea of what is wrong (provided they have some insight into their difficulty in the first place) often is radically different from why the referring source seeks your opinion. Try to speak to the referent beforehand. Families are only somewhat less notorious for their unreliability in explaining what the problem is. They cannot be expected to distinguish constructional apraxia any more than patients with denial should tell you that they suffer from anosognosia.

You must appreciate that laypersons usually have only two words for *all* cognitive impairments: They complain either of their "memory" or that they "can't think." Very often, they will be able to say only that "something is wrong," leaving you to dissect out the nature and degree of impairment through the systematic observation that the HCF affords. It is often helpful to ask what the patient cannot do now that he or she was able to do previously.

Here is the place to say whether the patient was coöperative and understood the instructions and whether you consider the results valid.

Behavioral Observations   If you think the patient is too demented or confused to understand your questions, here is where you say so. If the patient eats the tests or urinates on the Form Board, you might say that the results may not be fully reflective of this individual's true ability because of inappropriate behavior. Any other *noteworthy* behavior—seductiveness, disjointed or irrelevant thoughts, a flat affect, psychomotor retardation, or a catastrophic reaction when confronting failure—should be mentioned here very briefly.

Intellectual and Cognitive Functioning   If you made it through the Wechsler Adult Intelligence Scale (WAIS), interpret it here, stating the verbal IQ, performance IQ, and full-scale IQ. What if you did not or could not give the WAIS? (Perhaps this was a bedside exam and the patient had both arms in a cast, or maybe it was a place where nobody could possibly concentrate, such as the ICU. Occasionally, we have to do the best we can under trying circumstances.) Some neuropsychologists would stop, while others are comfortable giving an opinion as long as it is based on something concrete.

In ad libbing, you might write, for example, "The patient's verbal functioning seemed adequate for her educational and occupational achievements. Her vocabulary was rich, language appeared normal, and she had no apparent difficulties with math or other abstractions. Nonverbal cognition was judged to be adequate based on her ability to draw and perceive shape and dimension. No cognitive deficit is suspected, and I judge this screening to be sufficient."

Alternatively, if you encountered problems, you might write "The patient's vocabulary seemed limited for his education and occupational history. His difficulty with simple math and poor insight require that a more formal appraisal of his intellectual skills be performed when circumstances permit." Then arrange for a WAIS and other sit-down tests.

Obviously, your judgements about vocabulary, perception, and so forth are formed during the interview and overall engagement of the patient. With experience, you will learn what to ask, show, and read to patients to form such judgements.

Memory Functioning   Your interpretation of the Wechsler Memory Scale (WMS) goes under this heading. David Wechsler designed the IQ and MQ tests so that someone whose IQ equals 100 should have an MQ of 100. If there is a discrepancy between the two greater than one standard deviation (15 points), say so and explain why. Comment on both verbal and visual memory, as well as delayed recall. If you gave additional visual memory tests, such as the Rey figure, interpret that here as well.

Language Functioning   You give the Aphasia Screening Test, Drawings on Command, and part of the Sensory-Perceptual Examination for this section. State your conclusion based on their results here.

By this time, you know whether the patient has dysarthria, dysprosody, alexia, agraphia, or any of the aphasias, agnosias, or apraxias (ideomotor, ideational, or constructional). You have also judged psychomotor speed, content of thought, affect, and many other aspects of the mental status exam that I outlined in table 4.5. Any right-left confusion (allochiria) or finger agnosia should be mentioned here.

Perceptual-Motor Functioning   The finger-tapping test gives you an idea about manual dexterity while grip dynamometry tells you about strength: The dominant hand should be about ten percent faster and stronger. As a general rule, superficial cortical lesions may be revealed by a loss of fine dexterity with preservation of strength. Conversely, deep or transcortical lesions often cause gross paresis (British neurologists emphasize this superficial-deep distinction).

The Form Board informs you about post-central parietal integrity. If cross-transfer has taken place via the corpus callosum, the hand that performs the task second should complete the task approximately ten percent faster than the hand that does it first.

Trail making reveals visual psychomotor speed (assuming the patient has reasonable dexterity to hold the pencil and connect the dots). You already know by this stage (from all that you've evaluated so far) whether the patient knows the alphabet, so slow performance on part A indicates poor search skills (perhaps a lesion in the frontal eye fields, inattention, or global confusion) or poor motor performance (look at tapping speeds or for corroborating motor problems such as apraxia). Slowness on part B or the inability to *change sets* is a qualitatively different shortcoming and suggests a frontal lobe disorder.

Personality Assessment   This is the place to talk about the MMPI. Or, you can describe any noteworthy behavior here and forego the MMPI if the reason for evaluation is a straight neurological question: For example, is this person's stroke causing any higher cortical deficits? As another example, your opinion and basis that the patient suffers a catastrophic reaction can be given here.

When one is asked such questions as whether a patient's pain is as bad as the individual reports it to be, or whether the anxiety attacks and insomnia the patient is experiencing are secondary to a concussion received six months ago, or whether this person is antisocial and perhaps acting out, then an MMPI can be a useful first step. Patients who act bizarre or whose psychiatric scales are elevated should be considered for psychiatric referral.

Projective testing—such as Rorschach ink blots and the Thematic Apperception Test—are fascinating and even interesting to administer, but they are best left to those trained in projective techniques.

Summary and Diagnosis   Succinctly summarize the *relevant* results of your interaction. This part of your report will be read first, so keep it brief and relevant. List your one diagnosis with contributing factors, or your multiple diagnoses, as appropriate.

Recommendations   Providing a recommendation is what will earn (or lose) you your reputation as a worthwhile consultant. The patient was sent to you, the expert, for an opinion. Practice the art of giving one. Get to the point and be concrete. Don't hedge, try to cover every possibility, digress, or show off your erudition. Above all, do not make conclusions beyond what the facts warrant. Be helpful—to the patient, the family, and your referring source.

A few general words need to be said about the consultation note. Most hospitals have one-page consultation forms. The students and residents who rotate through the consult service use to convey their opinions always stand in stark contrast to the few lines penned by the attending physician. Eventually, you want to be able to say everything vital on a single page. Your important message will be buried—and surely will remain unread—if you leave nine pages behind. If you cannot state the problem succinctly, then you really don't understand the problem yourself.

The following is a sample of what you might write on the chart after seeing a young adult with a head injury who is eager to go home:

This thirty-two-year-old right-handed white man with a doctorate in music seems odd to the nursing staff. His brief confusion following a fall from a ladder 2 weeks ago occurs in context with a ten-year history of daily drinking without recreational drug use.

Physically, he complains of headache and blurry vision, performs tandem walking with difficulty, and has a mild peripheral neuropathy in the legs. He now shows naming and repetition errors along with loss of right-hand dexterity and complex tactile discrimination. Judgement and impulse control also seem poor. This points to acquired left temporal and frontal injury, with possible preëxisting alcoholic degeneration of the cerebellar vermis, at least. Given that he lives alone, discharge planning should begin immediately to address the degree of supervision that may be necessary while he convalesces.

Full report to follow.

This report gives the vital information in a few sentences, alerts everyone that something is amiss, and raises the danger of leaving this fellow alone. Your complete report will be attached to the chart after it is typewritten. It should lay out the grounds for your conclusions and give a numbered list of recommendations. The different purposes that the formal record and the consultation note serve should be evident.

When in doubt about what to say, think of the murder mystery. Experienced novelists or filmwriters open the murder scene with the killer's hands around the victim's throat; novices introduce the murderer eating breakfast and fill up pages with other extraneous antecedents to the crime. Get straight to the point. State the problem and your recommendation each in one sentence, and be mindful always of the audience for whom you are writing. This report is not for a specialist like yourself or your teacher but for the primary physician, family, attorney, or social service agency. The report of your consultation will be used by those who have little understanding of what neuropsychology is. Save the clever stuff for your dissertation; attempts to impress usually have the opposite effect.

The end user will seldom be interested in your raw data. File it. (If your referents knew what to make of your raw data, you would be superfluous.) The end user wants your *interpretation* and your *opinion*. You will have noticed that in each of the preceeding sections, and in the sample HCF at this chapter's end, you are not to write, "On the aphasia screening test, the patient did . . ." nor "The patient couldn't recognize a key in the left hand." Such comments are usually meaningless to your referent. An interpretation would be saying something like "This patient's linguistic and spatial deficits suggest a diffuse cerebral degeneration. . . ." If your report is likely to be used by colleagues in neuropsychology, then it may be appropriate to attach an appendix with the raw data so that those who want to can see how you reached your conclusions.

Order of Test Administration

The following test sequence is not sacrosanct, but it is the order I use. To help you remember to do a complete examination, lay out your scoring sheets and equipment in the following order and put each aside as you finish it. When nothing remains, you will have completed the entire HCF assessment. For the purposes of our exercise, I assume that our first patient is "with it" enough to sit through the entire battery (at least two hours, even for the most adept tester).

Equipment	Use
1. WMS form, stopwatch, and visual figure cards in an envelope to keep them from view	Wechsler Memory Scale (revised)
2. WAIS form and kit	Wechsler Adult Intelligence Scale (revised) and its eleven subtests
3. AST flip booklet, two sheets of blank paper on which the patient can copy and write, and your scoring sheet	Aphasia Screening Test for linguistic and paralinguistic disturbances
4. One more blank sheet for drawing	Drawings on Command to look for constructional dyspraxia and neglect
5. Sensory-Perceptual Examination scoring sheet and three or four small objects (key, large paper clip or screw, small ball, comb, pipe, hairpin, screwdriver, coins)	Assessment of stereognosis and other parietal functions, as well as confounding sensory loss of lemniscal or spinothalamic pathways
6. Trail Making, forms A and B	Visual psychomotor speed, attention, and frontal lobe function
7. Finger tapper	Manual dexterity
8. Squeeze dynamometer	Difference in gross strength between the sides
9. Form Board, cloaked in a pillow case	Posterior parietal complex sensory discrimination
10. MMPI booklet	Personality assessment

Test Features

Wechsler Memory Scale
15 minutes. I administer the WMS first because nearly everyone can get the first question (How old are you?) correctly and there-

fore it helps the patient relax. If a patient cannot get the first question right or is addled by the orientation section, you will have to improvise. Confused patients tire easily and you will have to be extremely flexible in extracting as much information as possible in the shortest time. Again, you learn how to do this sort of thing with experience. In such a situation, it will be impossible to complete the WAIS or the WMS. Administration and scoring instructions come with the test. The WMS is the *most frequently given* neuropsychological test (Piotrowski & Lubin, 1989).

A parallel form of the WMS (called Form II) exists for the purpose of comparative retesting at a later date. (Some experts question the validity and the rigor of the norms for these parallel versions. Discussion of whether one scores tests based on actuarial principles or individual pattern analysis is appropriate for a dedicated course in testing.) Using different stories and visual stimuli in the parallel form prevents a confound known as the *practice effect*, wherein the patient shows an "improvement" the second time around only because that individual has already seen the test material.

Form II can also be pressed into service for a quick screening: One story is read for understanding, the other for immediate recall. At the end of the session, ask the patient to repeat both stories to get a sense of delayed recall. Of course, you do not warn the patient that you are going to pull this stunt. The visual figures can be used similarly. Any indication of a deficit is grounds for a formal WMS Form I and a WAIS, thus checking whether there is a true discrepancy between IQ and memory, or whether the decreased memory is due to a low IQ.

WAIS, Revised

1 to 1½ hours. The WAIS test takes up a sufficiently long time to allow you to check delayed verbal and visual recall from the WMS at its end. The six WAIS verbal subtests are (1) information, (2) digit span, (3) vocabulary, (4) arithmetic, (5) comprehension, and (6) similarities. Age-adjusted scores are assigned. From these, one derives the verbal intelligence quotient (VIQ). The five performance tests are (1) picture completion, (2) picture arrangement, (3) block design, (4) object assembly, and (5) digit symbol substitution. From these, the performance intelligence quotient (PIQ) is derived. The VIQ and PIQ combine to yield the full-scale IQ (FSIQ). The test is designed so that a standard or normal IQ is 100. *Moron* and *imbecile*, once acceptable medical terms heard at every State hospital, are no longer uttered. Official IQ ranges are as follows:

120+	Superior
110–120	Bright normal
90–110	Average
80–90	Dull normal
70–80	Borderline defective
<70	Defective

The notion of general intelligence and its testing has generated a rich literature, and standard texts delve into the theoretical issues. Despite criticism and unquestioned limitations of general IQ tests, the WAIS is a classic and remains widely used. In an ideal world, you would give the WAIS yourself. In common practice, practitioners farm it out to a psychology assistant or graduate student.

A scoring form, such as that depicted in figure 5.1, is handy for summarizing not only the raw and scaled scores of the WAIS subtests but also the rather large data set from all the tests. A compact summary facilitates interpretation and report writing.

Aphasia Screening Test
10 minutes. The AST is the most widely used aphasia test. People are usually glad to finish the WAIS and, because the AST is easy, they enjoy getting things right for a change. You will already have noted any gross errors of language production or comprehension by this time; the AST discloses less obvious defects by forcing the patient to read, write, name, repeat words and sentences, and silently follow written and spoken commands. The AST is simply a structured way to quickly probe a number of language functions. It is a *qualitative* test, helping one diagnose linguistic problems by the nature of the errors.

Additionally, the AST screens for dyscalculia, right-left confusion, and constructional apraxia. Figure 5.2 and table 5.1 illustrate the stimuli and give instructions for test administration. Photocopy figure 5.2, paste it on an index card, and carry it with you. You can paste the abbreviated instructions from the bottom of figure 5.1 on the reverse side as a reminder to yourself.

Name: _____	Education: _____	Age: ____	Sex: ____	Race: ____
Occupation: _____	Date & place tested: _____			
Referral question:				

		Raw	Scaled		Raw	Scaled
VIQ: ____	Information	____	____	Pict completion	____	____
PIQ: ____	Digit span	____	____	Pict arrangement	____	____
FSIQ: ____	Vocabulary	____	____	Block design	____	____
	Arithmetic	____	____	Object assembly	____	____
	Comprehension	____	____	Digit symbol	____	____
	Similarities	____	____			

MQ: ____	Information	____		Digits forward	____		
	Orientation	____		Digits backward	____		
	Ment control	____		Visual repro	____	____	____
	Story A ____	Story B ____		Paired associates	____	____	____
	A + B/2	____		(easy, hard, total)			

Language: (AST and DOC) 1 = mild, 2 = moderate, 3 = severe

	# errors	Nosology & Description
Naming	____	Aphasia
Spelling	____	Agraphia
Reading	____	Agnosia
Repetition	____	Acalculia
Arithmetic	____	Apraxia (ideational, ideomotor, constructional, dressing)
Commands	____	Alexia

Allochiria (personal space, extrapersonal, cross-commands)

Drawing performance (neglect, apraxia):

AST: Mark errors

1. Copy square, name it, spell	2. Copy cross, name it, spell	3. Copy triangle, name it, spell
4. Name baby	5. Silently write *clock*	6. Name fork
7. Read "7 Six 2" (letter and number agnosia and alexia)	8. Read "MGW" (letter agnosia)	9. Read "see the black dog"
10. Explain "friendly animal, etc."	11. Repeat/write words/ sentence.*	12. Silently write *square*
13. Read and repeat "seven"	14. 85 − 27; 17 × 3 in head	15. Name key, draw from memory, then demonstrate use
16. L hand–R ear: read and do	17. More R-L instructions	18. Ad lib

* Repeat "triangle"; "Winter freeze hits Florida"; "I would go if he could come"; "No ifs, ands, or buts." Write select sentences.

Figure 5.1
High cerebral function assessment scoring sheet

Bilateral Simultaneous Stimulation: H = hand, C = cheek, E = ear, B = both
Tactile combinations (eyes closed; cheek items missed)   **Handedness:** R L Mixed

		Continue if errors	
Rh ____	Rc ____		
Lc ____	Rc-Lh ____ ____	Rh ____	Rc ____
Rh-Lh ____ ____	Rh ____	Lc ____	Rc-Lh ____ ____
Lh ____	Rc-Lc ____ ____	Rh-Lh ____ ____	Rh ____
Rh-Lc ____ ____	Lh ____	Rc-Lc ____ ____	Rh-Lc ____ ____

Auditory combination   Visual (x = target quadrant; circle omissions)

Re ____	Be ____ ____
Be ____ ____	Le ____
Re ____	Le ____

Finger Agnosia:
(Name, or touch pairs & ask how many in between.)

Right	Left
1–3 ____	9–10 ____
2–4 ____	7–9 ____
1–2 ____	6–9 ____
2–5 ____	6–7 ____
2–4 ____	8–9 ____

Finger-Tip Graphesthesia

Right Index	Left Index
8 ____	0 ____
1 ____	6 ____
3 ____	7 ____

Stereognosis: (Indicate which hand fails recognition.)

Key ____	Ball ____
Comb ____	Nickel ____
Pipe ____	Hairpin ____
Paper clip ____	
Other ____	

Summary of Sensory Perception:

	Sensory loss	Right	# of errors Left	Bilateral
Vision	_____	____	____	_____
Hearing	_____	____	____	_____
Touch	_____	____	____	_____
Finger agnosia		____	____	
Agraphesthesia		____	____	
Astereognosis		____	____	

Form Board:

	Right	Left
Time	____	____
# in	____	____
Recall	____	____
Totals		
Average		

10-Sec Tapping:

Right	Left
____	____
____	____
____	____
____	____
____	____
____	____
____	____

Grip Strength:

Right	Left
____	____
____	____
____	____
____	____
____	____
____	____
____	____

Trail Making:

	Time	Errors
A:	____	____
B:	____	____

MMPI scales: L ____ F ____ K ____ Hs ____ D ____ Hy ____ Pd ____ Mf ____ Pa ____ Pt ____ Sc ____ Ma ____
Welch code: ____   Critical questions:

Figure 5.1 (continued)

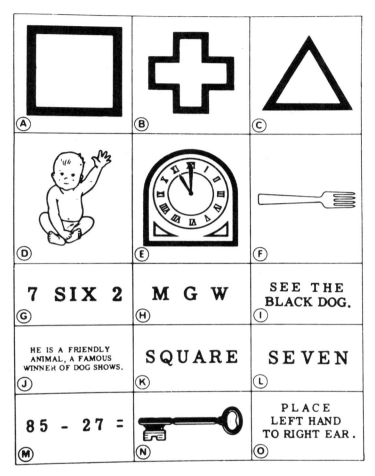

Figure 5.2
The majority of the aphasia screening test's stimuli. Paste this on a card and carry it with you. The test is available as a small flip booklet, with stimuli on one side and instructions facing the examiner. See table 5.1 for admininstration guidelines.

Table 5.1
Instructions for Administering the Aphasia Screening Test

What patient does	What you say
1. Copy square	Draw this on the paper without lifting the pencil. Make it the same size.
2. Name square	What do you call this shape?
3. Spell square	Please spell that word.
4. Copy cross	Now draw this one without lifting the pencil. Make it the same size.
5. Name cross	What do you call this shape?
6. Spell cross	Please spell that for me.
7. Copy triangle	Draw this shape for me.
8. Name triangle	What is this called?
9. Spell triangle	Spell that word for me please.
10. Name baby	What is this?
11. Write *clock*	Don't say anything aloud but simply write down the name of this next picture.
12. Name fork	What do you call this?
13. Read "7 six 2"	Please read this aloud.
14. Read "M G W"	Read this aloud also.
15. Read "black dog"	Now read this sentence aloud, please.
16. Read "famous"	Read this please. What does it mean?
Repeat words and sentences	Repeat after me: "Triangle"; "Winter freeze hits Florida"; "I would go if he could come"; "No ifs, ands, or buts." Write down the sentence about Florida, please [you may repeat it].
21. Write *square*	Please don't say anything but silently write the name of this.
22. Read "seven"	Now read this aloud.
25. Compute $85 - 27$	Here's a little math problem for you to figure.
26. Compute 17×3	Now figure this one in you head: What is 17×3?
27. Name key	What is this called?
28. Show use	Pretend you had a key like this in your hand. Show me how you would use it.

Table 5.1 (continued)

What patient does	What you say
29. Draw	[Take the picture away.] Can you draw the key from memory?
30. Read hand to ear	Please read this and do what is asked.
Additional right-left commands	Ad lib requests to identify right and left body parts, then segue into testing for finger agnosia.

Note: The numbers refer to the items in the Reitan-Indiana flip booklet. Unnumbered items are my elaboration. You don't have to be a slave to the test, but you do need to be thorough in testing for all language functions: Anomia, dysarthria, the apraxias, agraphia, alexia, agnosia, acalculia, and allochiria.

Drawings on Command

10 minutes. The AST seques seamlessly into drawings on command. Patients are asked to draw simple to complex shapes, whereby the test can assess constructional skill and visual-manual manipulation. Because they have already drawn a square, a triangle, and a cross in the AST, request a clock face, a house, a person, a bicycle, and a three-dimensional Necker cube (copied from your model). Visual neglect to one side of the midline varies in degree from squeezing in to complete absence.

Constructional apraxia is the inability to join elements manually into a meaningful whole. The patient can be asked either to draw or manually to assemble sticks, puzzle pieces, and the like. If present, constructional apraxia will usually show up in the drawing of the bicycle. Avoid prompting or commenting about the quality of the sketch. If the patient hesitates or stops, ask "Are you finished?" in a neutral voice, and gently coax toward completion if not. Patients with constructional apraxia often show a dissociation between knowledge and performance: That is, they may know that their mangled drawing is wrong and can even name all the parts of the supposed bicycle, but they are unable to correct their performance.

This is a good place to give the Rey-Osterreith Complex Visual Figure test if visual errors were encountered in the WMS and you wish a more *qualitative* analysis of the types of errors made.

Sensory-Perceptual Exam

10 to 15 minutes. Reitan gathered several neurological maneuvers together in one package that he called the *sensory-perceptual examination.* These are tests for finger agnosia, fingertip agraphesthesia, stereognosis in each hand, and sensory extinction in visual, tactile, and auditory modes. *You must ascertain that basic sensation is intact before testing for extinction on simultaneous bilateral stimulation.* The skills assessed are summarized on the second page of the HCF summary form (see figure 5.1).

Sensory extinction is a standard neurological sign for hemispatial neglect, especially if bilateral simultaneous stimulation causes extinction in more than one modality. For this reason, visual, tactile, and auditory modes are tested. The other type of test for hemispatial neglect involves systematic scanning of the extrapersonal space, such as a cancellation test in which patients must cross out a target letter or shape that is equally distributed in all four visual quadrants but surrounded with nontarget stimuli (Mesulam, 1985b, p. 101). Neglect is clinically more common on the left side.

Neglect may also be evident during reading, writing, and drawing. Patients may read material on only one side of the vertical meridian; generous margins while writing or copying are another sign, as is failure to copy one side of a figure or omission of the left-hand side of a clock face or flower petals.

Stereognosia, agraphesthesia, and *finger agnosia* are different types of agnosia. The root *gnosis* means "knowledge," which is why *diagnosis* means "through knowing" and *prognosis* means "foreknowledge of an outcome." *Agnosia* means "not knowing," and by attaching various prefixes we may specify what it is that the patient does not know. In general, agnosia is the failure to understand the significance of something previously known, even though the sensory pathways and sensorium are intact. The patient must perceive and acknowledge the stimulus, yet fail to understand it as a result of a cerebral lesion.

Stereognosia is tested by placing objects such as a safety pin, pipe, clothespin, or paper clip in each hand and asking the patient to name them. (Pointing to a picture of the object in a selection array would be a nonverbal way of answering.) This is done out of sight and without giving any inadvertent auditory cues (which would be another confound).

Agraphognosia or *agraphesthesia* (either is correct) is the failure to identify letters or numbers traced on the skin. For the sake of consistency and because of their dense innervation, I prefer to use the index fingers, drawing 8-1-3 on the right, and 0-6-7 on the left. Choose what you like, but use letters or digits of varying complexity and don't use the same one over and over (that would be yet another confound).

Finger agnosia is the inability to identify one's own fingers. This odd deficit is famous because it is a characteristic of Gerstmann's syndrome—a constellation of agraphia, acalculia, finger agnosia, and right-left confusion that specifically localizes to the left inferior parietal lobule when the cluster is seen in isolation. Loss of finger identity would be utterly irrelevant were it not for this handy fact.

Testing for finger agnosia, however, is a matter of some confusion. First, finger agnosia can be said to exist only in the absence of aphasia or, if aphasia is present, only if it is way out of proportion to the language deficit itself. Second, not all normal persons can readily name their fingers. If this is the case, then your demonstration of a numbering system from one to ten will help. Thus giving the fingers a verbal label. Patients can then be instructed "show me your second finger," and so forth. The idea is to associate *some* verbal label to fingers.

An alternative method is indicated on page two of the HCF scoring sheet (see figure 5.1). This method does not require any verbal label but relies on touch, proprioception, and an intact body schema. The patient closes his or her eyes and places the hands palms-down on the table. You touch various combinations of two fingers and ask the patient to tell you how many fingers are between the ones you are touching. For the examiner's sake, the right fingers are numbered 1 through 5 and the left fingers 6 through 10.

The sensory-perceptual exam is a good place for additional probing depending on what your maneuvers have revealed so far. Further testing of right-left orientation with crossed-hand positions, or the naming of body parts, may be useful. Though interesting, right-left confusion—also called *allochiria*—rarely occurs

The Knowing and Feeling Sensations

Neurology distinguishes between sensory discrimination in terms of either feeling (*esthesia*) or knowing (*gnosia*).

A sensory pathway lesion placed anywhere from the receptor to idiotypic cortex prevents a patient from knowing what sensory data mean because those data cannot be felt. Because the prefix used to negate is *a* before a consonant and *an* before a vowel, we say that the lesion causes *an*esthesia. Reduced sensation is *hypo*esthesia (contracted to *hyp*esthesia); the opposite case of heightened sensation is *hyper*esthesia. If the sense in question is pain, then the analogous terms would be *an*algesia, *hyp*algesia and *hyper*algesia.

In contrast, a lesion of association cortex produces *agnosia* in rendering the patient unable to appreciate the significance of the sensory impulses that reach it.

Therefore, a host of sensory talents—or lack of them—can be described by combining a positive or negetive suffix for either feeling or knowing with a variety of medical roots. For example,

grapho- means "writing,"

noso- means "disease,"

stato- means "position" or "station,"

stereo- means "form,"

topo- means "place," and

autotopo- means "self place."

Topognosia is the ability to localize skin stimuli, and autotopognosia the recognition of one's body parts. Graphognosia is the ability to recognize letters or numbers written on the skin, whereas agraphognosia is the loss of this capacity. One's sense of position or Euclidean orientation is termed statognosia, its loss, astatognosia. Absent position sense due to a spinal cord lesion, however, is properly termed statanesthesia, just as the loss of form sense due to a peripheral, spinal, or thalamic lesion is called stereoanesthesia. Stereognosia requires that all pathways from receptor to cortex be intact.

The prefixes *hypo* and *hyper* are not used in describing gnosias. *Hyper* is inappropriate because an elevated sense of knowing does not exist, and terms such as hypostereognosia are too much even for neurologists. In place of *hypo*, the prefixes *a* or *an* denote either absent or reduced gnosis.

by itself and, if present, one must first ascertain whether the patient ever was able to apply the verbal labels "right" and "left" appropriately. A surprising number of people never could. Allochiria typically signifies a dominant hemisphere lesion at the parieto-temporo-occipital junction.

Trail Making

5 to 10 minutes. Trail making tests visual psychomotor speed, attention, and the ability to shift sets. In part A, one times how long it takes the patient to connect a series of scattered dots numbered from 1 to 25. In part B, the patient must connect a similar set of dots alternating sequentially between numbers and letters (1 to A, 2 to B, 3 to C, and so on). Maximum norms are 60 seconds for part A and 120 seconds for part B.

Finger-Tapping Test

10 minutes. Finger tapping is a further test for laterality as well as frontal lobe integrity. A numerical counter with a ratchet key is mounted on a board. With the palm held flat against the board, the subject taps as quickly as possible for ten seconds. This is repeated with each hand until five consecutive trials are within five taps of each other or for a total of fourteen trials per hand. (If the first three trials are within five taps of each other, stop and take the average.) The score for each hand is either the average of five trials or the average of ten trials after discarding the two highest and lowest scores. Thirty-five to forty-five taps in ten seconds is typical. Twenty-second breaks are given between trials.

Grip Dynamometry

5 minutes. The average grip strength for each hand is measured with a squeeze-type dynamometer over three trials for each hand. You can establish your own normal values for grip strength if you like, although it is the *difference* between sides, not the absolute force, that matters for neuropsychological purposes. The dynamometers typically used in the Halstead-Reitan battery are large and expensive. Small aneroid squeeze-bulb dynamometers with an indicator dial, calibrated in either kilograms or pounds per square inch of pressure, are available from physical therapy suppliers.

Form Board

15 to 25 minutes. Also called the Tactual Performance Test, the Form Board is a boring test both to give and to perform no matter what one calls it. Nobody enjoys it, but at least you and the patient can leave when it is finished. The Form Board further evaluates the post-central and posterior parietal areas. In a patient with slow tapping, for instance, it will tell you whether the lesion extends rostrally or caudally. Hence, the finger-tapping test and Form Board should be evaluated together. The Form Board is a complex test of sensory-motor integration, psychomotor speed, nonverbal problem solving, and cross-transfer between the hemispheres.

Blindfolded, the patient feels the perimeter of a board and the geometric indentations carved in its surface and then is timed while placing the differently shaped blocks into their respective indentations. Three trials are given for (1) the dominant hand, (2) the other hand, and (3) both hands together. Ten minutes is the maximum time allowed per trial, no matter how few blocks have been placed. After the equipment is removed from view, the patient's blindfold is removed and the patient is asked to draw the block shapes and their relative position to one another on the board. (Nobody I know performs this last part of the test, and I do not believe that drawing the shapes from memory says anything useful that I don't already know by this time.)

The MMPI

The MMPI is a self-administered actuarial questionnaire containing several hundred true-false questions, most of them seemingly innocuous. However, now you know that nothing is what it seems. Four validity scales and ten clinical scales are derived from the responses to such vapid statements as "I would like to be a librarian," and "My father was a good man." The *validity scales* indicate whether the individual is answering randomly, is striving to look good or bad, is hoping to receive help and understanding, or is defensive and closed. They reveal the overall mood and test-taking attitude. The *clinical scales* compare the patient's responses against a normative population as well as different categories of psychiatric patients. The overall interpretation is based on the *pattern* of the scales and has an actuarial basis.

The MMPI was not originally developed for neuropsychological assessment when it appeared in the 1930s. Since then, it has been revised and extended to various settings, from school counseling to industrial employment. The names of the ten clinical scales reflect its older origin and are (1) hysteria, (2) depression, (3) hypochondriasis, (4) psychopathic deviate [sic], (5) stereotypical male and female interests, (6) paranoia, (7) psychasthenia (a clever parallelism, I suspect, to neurasthenia), (8) schizophrenia, (9) mania, and (10) social introversion. Critical questions may bring some unsuspected problem to the fore: Examples are answering true to such statements as "I hear and see things that nobody else around me does," "I am sure I am losing my mind," and "I am dizzy most of the time." In addition to the official scales, dozens more research scales have been developed for various purposes with varying success.

A low-average reading level or better is required and subjects work at their own pace. Speedy persons may complete the test in thirty minutes whereas others take more than ninety. The MMPI has been translated into many languages, and several computer interpretation programs are available in addition to standard code books that spell out the meaning of a particular pattern of elevated scales (Duckworth & Anderson, 1986; Graham, 1993).

The MMPI is a useful test in many general medical situations if you wish to know more about a patient's mood, energy level, and overall affect. I tell patients, "These questions will help me understand you better, particularly how you feel about yourself and about being sick."

Here are a few kinds of comments that one might make in interpreting the MMPI.

Example 1. This patient's profile is consistent with an agitated depression, and patients with similar profiles are emotionally bottled up and overcontrolled. They often are fatigued, nervous, filled with self-doubt, and fully aware of reduced mental coping. They may increase their activities in an exhausting attempt to disguise their reduced abilities. This patient was worried about losing her mind. Typical coping strategies include overcontrolling the environment with structured daily plans. Changes in these everyday rituals often are upsetting and cause more anxiety.

Example 2. This patient is very depressed and concerned about his physical ailments. Along with a somatic preöccupation, he is tense, anxious, and confused. Given the extent of his brain injury, this response is judged to be appropriate.

Example 3. This profile is typical of people who have a lot of mental energy but are unable to direct it appropriately—essentially spinning one's mental wheels. This individual seems in acute distress and is reaching out for help. Yet other elevated clinical scales indicate that she is likely to be distrustful and wary of forming interpersonal relationships. Ambivalence and distractibility are likely to be part of the clinical picture, such as frequently changing the topic to avoid dealing with anything substantially relevant to her current distress.

Example 4. After working on the MMPI for two days in his hospital room, this patient managed to answer only a fraction of the questions, although he did ruin the booklet and ate part of the answer sheet. His behavior is consistent with frontal lobe damage.

Additional Tests and Improvisation

One or two tests should be waiting in the wings for special circumstances. A typical special circumstance is an aphasic patient with impaired expression, a situation that makes administering the WAIS untenable. To get a *fair* estimate of such an individual's premorbid IQ, you might employ the Peabody picture vocabulary test.

In normal persons, the Peabody and WAIS IQs will correlate; in brain-injured persons, the Peabody often overestimates the WAIS IQ. For example, an aphasic college professor whose Peabody IQ is 75 probably has a large lesion involving posterior speech regions. On the other hand, an expressive aphasic who does well on the Peabody probably has a good prognosis.

Other common tests that you might wish to explore and which can be substituted for or added to the ones I have explicated here are the Wide Range Achievement Test, Wisconsin Card Sorting, Benton Visual Retention, Benton Facial Recognition, Porteus Mazes, Paced Serial Addition, Raven's Progressive Matrices, and the Rey-Osterreith Complex Visual Figure.

Some of your teachers will be horrified at the suggestion of using parts of tests or their parallel forms in a nonstandard fashion. For example, I might use the parallel version of the Anna Thompson of South Boston story and the visual reproduction figures from Form II of the WMS to flesh out my clinical suspicion that a memory

The Cowboy

> Sentences and paragraphs are more naturalistic for testing memory than are word lists or digit strings. The cowboy story that follows dates from 1919 and contains twenty-seven verbatim memory units and twenty-four content units (italicized words), which may be paraphrased and still be considered correct. The average person recalls eight verbatim units and ten content units. You may use this story to get a sense of a patient's attention and recall.
>
> A *cowboy*/ from *Arizona*/ went to *San Francisco*/ with his *dog*/ which he *left*/ at a *friend's*/ while he *purchased*/ a *new* suit of *clothes*./ Dressed finely,/ he *went back*/ to the *dog*,/ *whistled* to him,/ *called him* by *name*/ and *patted* him./ But the dog would *have nothing to do* with him,/ in his new *hat*/ and *coat*, / but gave a *mournful howl*./ *Coaxing* was of no effect,/ so the cowboy *went away*/ and donned his old *garments*,/ whereupon the *dog/immediately*/ showed his wild *joy*/ on seeing his *master*/ as he thought he ought to be.

deficit really exists. Alternatively, I might use the cowboy story (see box) for the same purpose. Rather than being a half-hearted approach to formal testing, such improvisation reflects the different approaches between medical and philosophical doctors of neuropsychology. You may profitably discuss the virtues of these different approaches in class.

The idiosyncratic use of the Form Board is another example of these differences. The three official scores of the Form Board are (1) total time, (2) the number of shapes correctly remembered, and (3) the number of shapes recalled in their correct position. The time taken by *each* hand and the *difference* between hands reveals more useful information than that given by the official total time, however. Because the task is done blindfolded (see the box, "Those Notorious Blindfolds"), the patient relies on tactile discrimination and shape recognition, reafference, proprioception, and visual imagery (we assume). These factors must all be considered in interpreting any abnormal performance. Suppose the dominant right hand performs first, getting all blocks inserted in five minutes (written as 5:00), whereas the left hand repeats the task in four minutes and ten seconds (4:10). What can we conclude?

Those Notorious Blindfolds

Most readers probably are too young to remember the TV quiz show "What's My Line." At the end of each program, the blindfolded panelists had to guess the identity of a celebrity mystery challenger. Because Dorothy Kilgallan and Arlene Francis guessed correctly so often, many people suspected them of peeking through their blindfolds.

Though we may never know whether these two ladies were really in the dark, it's nobody's secret that blindfolds are notoriously unreliable. Having patients see what they are not supposed to see is one to the worst confounds of all.

Blindfolds are uncomfortable when worn for long periods, are not always opaque, and tend to slip. If you don't believe this, try wearing whatever you propose using on patients yourself. Standard alternatives to using a blindfold are putting an opaque pillowcase over patients' heads (a bit much, I think), taping their eyes shut, or having an assistant hold their eyes closed. The best, and least uncomfortable, choice is using an opaque screen under which patients can reach to manipulate test items out of sight.

With experience, you will learn that most normal people can do this task within 3:30 to 6:00 minutes. Therefore, our subject not only performed in the normal range, but the right hemisphere, guiding the active hand the second time around, has learned from the left hemisphere's execution of the first trial and turns in a speedier performance. This is called *cross-transfer* or *callosal transfer*. A rule of thumb is that the nondominant hand, performing second, should complete the task faster by ten percent. We would expect this to be thirty seconds in our hypothetical subject [5 minutes = 300 seconds × 10% = 30 seconds]. The actual performance of 4:10, therefore, is better than the minimum expected amount of cross-transfer.

Conversely, what do you conclude from the three examples given in table 5.2? The table lists the number of blocks correctly inserted for each hand as well as the time required for each hand to accomplish this. In each case, the right hand performs the task first. In patient 1, the fact that the right hand ran out of time at ten minutes while the left hand inserted all the blocks in less than half this time allows you to conclude the existence of a left-hemispheric

Table 5.2
Callosal Transfer

Pt.	No. Placed	Right-Hand Time	Left-Hand Time	No. Placed
1	6	10:00	4:00	10
2	10	10:00	4:20	10
3	10	4:00	6:20	10

lesion. You should therefore look for corroboration elsewhere to narrow down the lesion's locus. If this patient further demonstrated decreased tapping speed with relatively normal strength, then he or she could not have a lesion compromising the frontal motor strip nor a deep one in the white matter affecting the corticospinal tract. Therefore, the lesion is most likely posterior and superficial, which would explain both the decreased dexterity in tapping and the poor tactile discrimination of the right hand on the Form Board.

Patient 2 shows nearly the same situation except that the right hand inserts all the blocks in the maximum allotted time. You might reach the same conclusion as for patient 1. If, however, I revealed that the patient had a peripheral neuropathy or a cast on the right hand, then this poor performance could be attributed solely to decreased speed and, in the absence of any confirming signs, no further conclusion about the possible presence of a cerebral lesion is warranted.

Patient 3 displays a typical failure of cross-transfer, with both hands completing all blocks well within the time allowance, though the left hand fails to turn in a speedier performance. In this instance you would look for corroborating evidence of a right-hemispheric lesion or callosal impairment. Corroborating evidence might be poor fingertip graphesthesia on the left index finger or astereognosis and extinction on that side.

These brief examples illustrate the necessity of having *internested tests* in any neuropsychological battery. This term means that cognitive functions are evaluated by more than one instrument in order to prevent simplistic analyses or erroneous conclusions. In our three examples from the Form Board (see table 5.2), a slow performance with the right hand could be due to a motor

deficit, a failure of sensory feedback and reafference, proprioceptive loss, or mechanical interference. In each case, the examiner
must ascertain whether there is an external impediment, a peripheral nerve lesion, or a central lesion responsible for the abnormal performance. Additional confirming or disconfirming signs are
sought to bolster or reject the conclusion.

*Simplistic localization of a lesion based on a single test is
fraught with error. The better habit is to correlate patterns of behavior with neural organization and to rely on internested tests.*
Some commercially available neuropsychological packages (dis-
paragingly called Doc in the box) are not very useful for exactly
this reason. For example, kits that spit out global assessments (e.g.,
"There is a visual processing impairment") or force binary choices
regarding the presence or absence of an organic impairment don't
tell us very much. Clinical acumen is always more important than
the choice of test.

For example, an acquaintance who attended a weekend workshop was impressed with himself at having administered his newly
purchased battery. He concluded that his patient had an occipital
lobe lesion because the occipital lobe subserves vision and the
test battery had indicated a "visual processing impairment." I
pointed out that there was more to visual perception than just
connecting the eyeball in the front of the head to the occipital lobe
in the back of the head. To understand what the nature of this
putative "visual processing impairment" might be, one needs to ask
whether patients have sufficient visual acuity to see the test stimulus. If so, are there adequate search skills and are the frontal eye
fields intact so that they can move the eyes and look at the stimulus? Is language sufficiently intact for them to say what it is that
they see? Is there an agnosia that prohibits recognition, and is the
synthesis of extrapersonal space adequate to know where the thing
being viewed is located? Can they take in more than one thing at a
time or are they bound by single elements (simultagnosia)? Are
there visual field defects or achromatopsia? The list goes on. These
types of questions must be answered before one can conclude that
a visual impairment actually exists and what its cause is.

Though neurologists are accustomed to testing the visual fields
and other sensory modalities for extinction, or checking stereognosis and graphesthesia for parietal lobe function and naming, they

have been trained to consider such maneuvers as flexible parts of the overall neurologic exam, to be included or omitted as the case dictates. Graduate students, on the other hand, are likely to have first encountered such maneuvers as part of the Reitan-Kløve sensory-perceptual examination and therefore develop a sense that these tests must always be performed as a unit.

Tests are not holy relics, and there is no law against using tidbits. Such a practice does raise the related issues, however, of validated test norms and whether one uses a normal distribution (nomothetic) or idiotypical approach. Factors that make the content of tests valid, the use of appropriate normative samples in developing them, cross-validation, and sensitivity to specific cognitive functions are all topics for dedicated course work (Mapou, 1988; Cicchetti et al., 1991, 1992).

Another issue is determining when research protocols, which may take half a day or more, are appropriate or even necessary. The elucidation of early cognitive change in those infected with human immunodeficiency virus is such an example. Here, a half-hour screening or even a brief battery of tests with high sensitivity but limited specificity is inadequate. The National Institute of Mental Health (NIMH) battery is a good example of a research testing instrument that covers a broad scope of cognitive ability and in which quality control and psychometric precision are emphasized (Butters et al., 1990). The ten areas covered in the NIMH battery are (1) indicators of premorbid intelligence, (2) attention, (3) speed, (4) memory, (5) abstraction, (6) language, (7) vision, (8) construction, (9) motor skill, and (10) psychiatric assessment. The NIMH battery places heavy emphasis on divided and sustained attention as well as speed of processing and retrieval from working and long-term memory. The purpose of other test assemblies will determine their unique focus.

TYPICAL KINDS OF CONSULTS

The nature of the most frequently asked referral questions will vary depending on the complexion of one's practice. In general, however, common evaluations center on acute change in mental status; memory loss; change in personality; hyperactivity or learning disability in children; cognitive loss and persistent symptoms following closed head trauma; mental decline in the elderly; and the general aptitude of children having difficulty in school. Testing to identify deficits and plan rehabilitation is common in strokes, brain tumors, and illnesses that feature lengthy coma.

One is sometimes asked, especially within a psychiatric setting, to answer the functional-organic question: That is, is the problem "real" (neurological) or "in the head" (psychiatric). Note the value judgement in this request. Those who ask you to distinguish among, say, depression, dementia, and psychosis betray their own confusion about what neuropsychologists do.

In truth, there is great overlap between what are typically classified as functional and organic illnesses, and psychiatric patients often do show cognitive impairments (Mapou, 1988; Stoudemire & Fogel, 1993). For example, the cognitive profiles of chronic schizophrenics and persons with neurological injury may be indistinguishable. Conversely, "pure" psychotic patients are occasionally found to have structural brain pathology at autopsy. Because organic findings frequently occur in psychiatric patients, accurately describing their cognitive dysfunction in order to understand how it relates to the psychiatric disorder is more fruitful than just labeling it and may actually assist treatment.

The worst case ensues when the treating physician interprets *organic* to mean that no treatment is possible and then writes the patient off. Even in progressive disorders such as Alzheimer's dementia, an accurate and clear analysis of the patient's difficulties may help caregivers improve that patient's quality of life. For example, it might be used to determine how much structure the patient requires to maintain some level of independence.

Malingering and hysteria are other issues that confront the neuropsychologist. These are difficult areas and the available data on deliberate faking of neurologic or mental illness is not illuminating. The three points that most help to distinguish these two conditions are *attitude, persuasion,* and *unconscious intent.* The hysteric patient appears truly ill at first and invites examination, usually responds to persuasion, and has a largely unconscious motivation. The malingerer seems less ill and evades examination, is resistant to persuasion, and deliberately intends to deceive.

A particular type of repetitive malingering with an open intent to deceive is called Munchausen's syndrome, named after the fictional Baron von Munchausen who invented incredible tales of adventure and derring-do. These interesting but exceedingly rare patients have had multiple hospitalizations, visited scores of specialists, appear unexpectedly with dramatic illnesses of pending emergency, have an abdomen full of scars, and perhaps even have multiple cranial burr holes. From time to time, they are caught in the act of tampering with diagnostic tests. They are far more dramatic than the hysteric, producing convincing bouts of sudden fevers, fits, or bleeding, and they almost always vacate the hospital against medical advice.

Ganser's syndrome of approximate answers is another uncommon but impressive show of pseudodementia. Its functional nature is soon apparent by the patient's consistently inconsistent answers to all questions. Though rare, it has most often been described in prisoners. Patients feign having become insane, acting in the loony manner that they assume someone who has lost their mind would act. The term *Ganser's syndrome* is erroneously applied to the occasional patient who does have a true neurologic illness but who embellishes it with additional fantastic symptoms.

Bernard (1990) recently showed that several popular memory tests are vulnerable to faked deficits. Given the increased use of neuropsychology in worker's compensation cases, disability determinations, and personal injury lawsuits, this issue begs further study. Although malingerers are able to match the overall cognitive impairment of head trauma patients, for example, different patterns of strengths and weakness do emerge. Dissimulators have better recall and worse recognition memory than would be expected in natural amnesias. Unfortunately, recognition memory tasks are not widely employed in popular memory tests.

Lastly, you should expect to see at least one case of Hollywood amnesia during your distinguished career. This total wipeout of identity occurs only in the movies. Postictal epileptics, concussed accident victims, or those who suffer from acute confusional psychosis do not show up at hospitals desperate for help in finding out who they are or what that gun is doing in their pocket. Total amnesia for one's past life in someone who otherwise acts normal is unknown in any medical condition.

DISCUSSING RESULTS WITH PATIENTS

Because patients rarely request evaluations of themselves, one develops an instinct to avoid discussing the results of their tests directly with patients. Is this instinct misplaced? True, it is most often appropriate for the requesting physician or agency to discuss and explain the purpose and results of testing with the patient, but you will discover that they rarely do, either beforehand or after the fact. A happy condition occurs when the treating physician is also the neuropsychologist. However, it is a sad comment on the state of medical practice when the neuropsychologist is the only person who ever gives a coherent explanation of the patient's predicament.

This happens often and not just in neurologic illness. For example, neuropsychologists noticed that patients who undergo coronary artery bypass or heart valve replacement surgery may have visual hallucinations for several months after their operation. The typical surgeon's response is, "Well, my patients don't have it. If they were seeing things, they would have told me." This anecdote reiterates my earlier point that the medical history is not passive listening: It is something that you skillfully extract from patients. For such reasons, one should not deny a patient's direct request for explanation. This situation holds true most often in tertiary medical centers, where patients see the nursing and house staff much more often than the attending physician or consultant.

Patients also have a hard time immediately grasping the nature of neurological illness and its consequences. Few things frighten a person more than the possibility of losing one's mind and, though patients seldom acknowledge such concerns, fears of sudden death and brain damage are common. Neuropsychologists should appreciate that they are in a unique position to allay the fears that patients have about their illness. Patients are understandably reluctant to voice their fears—lest they be confirmed. You might probe for such ideas and reassure patients that they are not alone in harboring them.

Epilepsy inflicts unique psychological trauma. Persons whose power and influence may reach around the globe may find themselves utterly helpless during a seizure and plagued by dread of sudden death or fantasies that their brain is rotting in between fits. Unless vented, these fears can drastically impair psychosocial functioning. *Persons with epilepsy are commonly and deeply frightened by the imagined consequences of their seizures.* In fact, more than half of all epileptics say that fears of having a seizure or its possible consequences are worse than the social stigma customarily associated with epilepsy (Mittan, 1986).

A SAMPLE HCF REPORT

Let us now go through the exercise of testing a patient, recording the results, and writing a report to the referring physician.

Higher Cerebral Function Assessment

Name: *Non compos mentis*
Referred by:
Test date(s):
Place:
Hospital no.:

Tests Administered
Interview
History and Physical
Wechsler Adult Intelligence Scale revised
Wechsler Memory Scale revised
Aphasia Screening Test
Drawings on Command
Tapping Test
Grip Dynamometry
Form Board
Sensory-Perceptual Examination (Reitan-Kløve)
Trail Making, parts A and B
Minnesota Multiphasic Personality Inventory

Background Information

This thirty-nine year-old right-handed white man with eighteen years of education has an MBA degree in finance, is the managing partner of a CPA firm, and suffered a closed head trauma eight weeks ago in a car accident. He was wearing lap and shoulder belts while waiting at a stop light when a tractor-trailer plowed into the left rear of his vehicle, sending the car forward into a storefront after causing it to spin several revolutions counter-clockwise. Abrasions indicate a right frontal impact, and tenderness of the greater occipital nerves indicate a probable rebound against the headrest. He was unresponsive when found but was conscious on arrival at the emergency room 80 minutes after injury.

Physically, he has constant daily headaches, worst on awakening, blurry vision OD > OS, and brief spells of sudden vertigo several times daily. He is tired, and his sleep is fragmented with poor onset and frequent awakenings. He has noted vivid dreams that began just two weeks ago. He is uncharacteristically irritable, complains of photophobia and sonophobia, and prefers to be alone. He has lost interest in sex and has declined social invitations and going to church, both of which he formerly enjoyed. He startles easily and says that scenes of the accident pop into his mind for no apparent reason.

He has attempted to resume a full workload at his firm but is now anxious and depressed about his surprisingly inability to "get anything done." He complains of difficulty concentrating, forgetting the names of old employees and associates, and generally of being unable to do work of which he was unquestionably capable before. He becomes confused if distracted from a task and has trouble resuming it. He has trouble reading, particularly spreadsheets, and has twice gotten lost in the building where he has worked for eight years.

Medications include Xanax (alprazolam), Flexeril (cyclobenza-prine), Tylenol no. 4 (with codeine), and a transdermal scopolamine patch. He is receiving physical therapy with dynamic traction for neck pain.

The referral questions what to do about his work situation. Colleagues say he is disorganized.

Behavioral Observations

Mr. Mentis was coöperative, understood directions, and performed diligently. Because of fatigue, testing was done in two sessions.

Intellectual and Cognitive Functioning

He obtained a verbal IQ of 107 and a performance IQ of 85, for a full-scale IQ of 96. While this places him in the average range of overall intellectual ability, it is almost certainly below premorbid ability given his education and occupational achievements. There is greater than one standard deviation between the VIQ and PIQ and his performance on subtests is extremely uneven, showing inter-test and intra-test scatter. These are often features of acquired brain injury.

He had difficulty with vocabulary and arithmetic as well as more abstract aspects of both verbal and nonverbal problem solving. Mental control and the ability to sustain attention were poor. He would blurt out wrong answers to computations and then try to correct himself, not always successfully. There was particular difficulty with visuospatial analysis and manipulation.

Results are consistent with bilateral cerebral impairment that is worse on the right side.

Memory Functioning

His MQ is 90, placing him in the low average range of overall mnestic ability. There is a discrepancy between verbal and visual memory, the latter being worse. Recall of logical, sequential material was variable but adequate, as was his ability to learn new verbal information. Delayed verbal recall was inadequate, however, and delayed visual recall was nonexistent. Visual memory showed retention of some details with loss of the overall gestalt.

In brief, Mr. Mentis has a mild decrease in general memory, with severe deficits in visual memory.

Language Functioning

There was no dysarthria, but the patient's speech lacked a normal prosody and seemed flat. Spontaneous speech had a rich vocabulary, but his responses were not always relevant to the question asked and he has mild to moderate difficulty comprehending reading material and a frank error in repetition. Naming and reading errors were present, as were acalculia and finger agnosia, the latter on the left hand only. Right-left confusion was not seen. There was no motor apraxia, but there was a severe constructional apraxia.

Results are consistent with biparietal impairment.

Perceptual-Motor Functioning

There was no deficit of any sensory modality with single stimulation, but extinction was present on the left side to vision and touch. Errors in fingertip graphesthesia and stereognosis were also present on the left side.

Manual dexterity speed was slow on the right, and grip strength also failed to show the usual advantage of the dominant right hand. Performance on the Form Board, a test of posterior parietal sensory discrimination, showed generally slow performance and no transfer learning. The left hand had difficulty recognizing and manipulating shape and dimension.

Visual psychomotor speed was adequate on a nonshifting task, and one error was made on the shifting task.

Personality Assessment

MMPI Welch Code 0000. This is a valid profile, suitable for interpretation.

The patient's profile is consistent with this examiner's observations. Someone with this profile prefers to be with others rather than by himself; currently avoiding social and intimate contacts is atypical for him. There is a great deal of psychic energy being expended, but it is not effectively being channeled. Such persons are prone to exhaustion as they attempt to take on more and more. Valid concerns about his physical condition are present.

Depression, agitation, and concern about physical problems are significant. This profile is compatible with post-traumatic stress syndrome.

Summary

Two months after a closed head trauma with significant torsional forces and physical evidence of right frontal and bi-occipital impact, this patient is functioning in the low-average range of general intellectual abilities. This is almost certainly below his expected premorbid capacity and is likely acquired and due to the head injury described. There are definite islands of impairment, however, which are serious given the referral question.

Evidence of *biparietal injury* includes linguistic deficits (comprehension, repetition, anomia, and reading difficulty), along with mathematical failure (acalculia) and general signs localizable to the region of the left angular gyrus. *Right temporo-parietal injury* is evidenced by a severe constructional apraxia, the history of getting lost in familiar surroundings, and a visual memory failure in which the overall pattern is lost more than are the details (this is a pattern of memory disturbance typical of right temporal injury).

His method of coping is counterproductive, and signs of posttraumatic stress syndrome are present (startle response, sleep fragmentation, social withdrawal, and flashbacks).

Diagnoses

1. Closed head trauma, grade II, with right temporal and bilateral parietal brain injury.

2. Post-traumatic stress syndrome, acute and secondary to item 1. [Add the DSM-III code here if you like.]

[If you were a neurologist and did a physical examination, you could add the following.]

3. Chronic headaches secondary to traumatic neuritis of the greater occipital nerves, bilateral.

4. Probable sedation and possible contribution to amnesia secondary to drug interactions (codeine, cyclobenzaprine, scopolamine, benzodiazepine).

Recommendations

Discontinue drugs, especially scopolamine, except for Xanax (Cytowic et al., 1988) and consider nerve blocks (Cytowic, 1990) for his headaches instead of codeine and Flexeril, both of which are sedating. The physical therapy regimen could also be altered. Some of his confusion, lassitude, and memory loss should clear after detoxification. Drug treatment for concussive vertigo is almost always ineffective, and the scopolamine probably is contributing only adverse effects.

On the cognitive side, it is too early to return this gentleman to his demanding, multifaceted work. This will only cause further frustration. A possible target date six weeks hence could be set to help allay frustration, and then a part-time load in a setting that minimizes distractions should be arranged. This will help his self-image. Symptoms should settle out over the next several months, and we can then reassess which problems might be permanent, if any. His post-traumatic stress syndrome should be addressed because there is the risk that it may become chronic. Increasing his dose of xanax may help multiple symptoms as well; an alternative is perphenazine alone if symptoms are severe.

Psychotherapy would help provide structure for this man, who is accustomed to being in control. His comprehension deficit is an obstacle, however. I will discuss the pros and cons of speech therapy versus psychotherapy with you. The severity of the visuo-spatial difficulties is worrisome, but it is too early to say more without certainty. Reëvaluation in the near future is warranted and improvement is expected. In fact, his vivid dreams following a post-accident phase of dreamlessness (REM suppression) is a favorable indicator that the patient is improving at present.

Nullius in verba, MD, PhD
Ace Neuropsychologist

That's how it's done. I have picked a complicated example and even included two references, breaking my own rule (even though I did it for your benefit). Degreed examiners would not include medical recommendations here as I have, but the suggestions are provided here to illustrate what a neurologist neuropsychologist might do. This example raises the issues of exogenous complicating factors (this patient's polypharmacy; always determine what drugs patients are taking), time factors in symptom resolution, a psychiatric complication on top of his cognitive impairment (the post-traumatic stress syndrome), and obstacles to counseling (the aphasia), which possibly is what would be most helpful in the short run. Other clinicians will, of course, have different priorities or suggestions, but it is hoped that this exercise has illustrated the overall manner in which a person's *individual* circumstance is tested, analyzed, and reported.

SUGGESTED READINGS

Benton A. 1992 Clinical neuropsychology: 1960–1990. *Journal of Clinical and Experimental Neuropsychology* 14:407–417

Franzen MD. 1989 *Reliability and Validity in Neuropsychological Assessment.* New York: Plenum Press

Lezak MD. 1983 *Neuropsychological Assessment.* New York: Oxford University Press

Reynolds CR, Fletcher-Janzen E. 1989 *Handbook of Child Neuropsychology.* New York: Plenum Press

Rourke BP, Fisk JL, Strang JD. 1986 *Neuropsychological Assessment of Children: A Treatment-Oriented Approach.* New York: Guilford Press

Spreen O, Strauss E. 1991 *A Compendium of Neuropsychological Tests: Administration, Norms, and Commentary.* New York: Oxford University Press

6 Localization: Symptoms Caused by Focal Lesions in the Cerebrum

The division of the cerebrum into frontal, temporal, parietal, and occipital lobes was done so long ago as to retain no validity. Yet the names of the four lobes still are used as a general point of reference despite today's more sophisticated divisions of the cerebrum. In chapter 3, we learned that the entire cortical mantle can be divided into just five highly ordered types of tissue (see figure 3.8). These five topologic zones, however, are neither consistent with nor mutually exclusive of the fifty-two Broadmann areas (see figures 3.6 & 3.7).

Based on this knowledge and what we also learned about the distributed system and multiplex information transfer, we obviously do not now use the term *localization* in its strictest sense. In table 6.1, I have organized the usual laundry list of focal symptoms according to topology, but because the boundaries of the lobes are ill-defined, the decision to label a symptom of sensory heteromodal association cortex, for example, as *temporal*, *parietal*, or *occipital* nearly becomes arbitrary. I try to follow conventional usage.

A few general points before we begin may help you stay mindful of the several confounds that can easily hamper the method of lesion analysis. A loss of function associated with a lesion does not mean that the function resides there; a lesioned part is not necessarily *solely* responsible, because both physical and behavioral symptoms are possible products of either (1) lost function, (2) the under-activity or over-activity of intact cerebral regions, or (3) both. Associating a syndrome with a lesion does not imply that all its elements share some common feature.

Case series and case reports have their own confounds when one attempts to draw general inferences from single well-described cases or to characterize extensive series without possessing good

Table 6.1
Behavioral Correlations of "The Lobes"

Effects of occipital lesions

Primary Idiotypic Visual Cortex
Contralateral, congruent homonymous hemianopia
Elementary, unformed hallucinations (photisms)
Lost conscious awareness of visual perception
With bilateral lesions:
Cortical blindness with reactive pupils (Anton's syndrome)

Unimodal Visual Association Cortex
Loss of motion, shape, color, spatial orientation, steropsis, depth
perception, and other components of visual experience
Complex perceptual deficits with retention of elementary sensation
Metamorphopsia, illusions, hallucinations, release hallucinations
Visual-specific disconnections
Pure alexia (word blindness), color and other visual dysnomias, visual
agnosias, modality-specific visual amnesias
With bilateral lesions:
Prosopagnosia, simultagnosia, Balint's and Charles Bonnet syndromes

Effects of temporal lesions

Primary Idiotypic Auditory Cortex
Unilateral "cortical" deafness (detectable only by dichotic listening or
evoked potentials because A1 receives from both cochleæ)
Auditory illusions and hallucinations, paracusiæ

Unimodal Auditory Association Cortex
Homonymous quadrantanopia
Wernicke's aphasia
Impairments of auditory discrimination and retention: Some aspects
of amusia and other nonverbal auditory agnosias, amnesia for verbal
material (left hemisphere) or visual material (right hemisphere)
With bilateral lesions:
Klüver-Bucy syndrome, hypo- or hyper-sexuality
Pure word deafness (also produced by a left-sided lesion plus trans-
callosal auditory interruption)

With Limbic and Paralimbic Involvement
Stereotypical "temporal lobe" behavior: Dreamy state, autoscopy, déjà
vu/jamais vu, déjà vecu/jamais vecu, time distortion, feeling of a
presence, clairvoyance, depersonalization
Synesthesia
Psychosis and forced thinking, non-directed agitation and violence
Disturbed of drive and affect, dysautonomia, dysgeusia, dysosmia
Amnesia, modality-specific or global

Effects of parietal lesions

Primary Idiotypic Somatosensory Cortex
Loss of sensory localization and two-point discrimination, agraphesthesia, astereognosia, sensory extinction

Table 6.1 (Continued)

Mild hemiparesis and decreased fine dexterity

Unimodal Somatosensory Association Cortex
Disturbed body schema (asomatognosia)

Temporo-parieto-occipital Heteromodal Association Cortex
Lesions in angular gyrus, supramarginal gyrus, inferior and superior
   parietal lobules cause deficits in multiple modalities
On either side:
   Hemi-neglect for the contralateral body or extrapersonal space,
      homonymous hemianopia or visual inattention, absent optico-
      kinetic nystagmus with targets to the affected side
In the language hemisphere:
   Wernicke's aphasia, anomia, alexia, constructional apraxia, acalculia,
      dysgraphia, finger agnosia, allochiria, bilateral ideomotor apraxia
      and mood disturbance
In the non-language hemisphere:
   Dressing and constructional apraxias, agnosognosia, misalignment of
      body in extrapersonal space (all more common on right, but may
      occur in either hemisphere); left-sided multimodal neglect, global
      confusion, apathy and other mood disturbance, geographic amnesia

Effects of frontal lesions

Primary Motor Cortex
Loss of fine dexterity, "frontal" limb apraxia with normal axial control
Contralateral spastic hemiplegia

Unimodal Motor Association Area
Category-specific deficits of motor output without primary weakness
Conjugate gaze defects (frontal eye fields of Brodmann area 8), impaired
   visual scanning and exploration of contralateral hemispace
Broca's aphasia, other motor aphasias with agraphia and apraxia

Prefrontal Heteromodal Association Areas
Changes in personality and comportment
Disinhibition: facetiousness and shallow joking (*Witzelsucht*), puerile
   affect, garrulousness, loss of typical social restraints, distractibility
Apathy, impaired response preparation "readiness potential")
Difficulty directing attention to targets
Amnesia
Dementia
Anosmia (with orbital lesions)
With bilateral lesions:
   Pseudobulbar palsy, often with catastrophic reaction
   More intense personality and mental changes, with abulia, akinetic
      mutism, gait and sphincter disturbance, primitive reflexes

Table 6.2
Major Categories of Illness

Congenital vs. Acquired
This is the first major dichotomy. One must distinguish disorders present at birth from those that are hereditary and phenotypically expressed at some later time.

Acquired

Systemic	Circulatory (CSF)	Infectious
Endocrine	Meningeal disorders	Demyelinative
Metabolic within the CNS	Vascular	Degenerative
Toxic (exogenous)	Tumor	Developmental
Substrate deficiency	Trauma	Epileptic
		Psychiatric

pathological anatomic descriptions. As we will see in later chapters, it is a mistake to assume that all our brains are identically hard-wired. They are not. The connectivity of individual brains is malleable by experience, language, and environmental factors.

A related issue is that not all reliable signs of neurologic illness have localizing value. Those that do not are called *nonspecific signs*. Psychomotor retardation is an example of a nonspecific sign. It refers to a paucity of speech, thought, and action. The cause of impoverished speech, constricted vocabulary, and dampened prosody may be just as uncertain as that for photophobia, hyperacusis, dysosmia, dysgeusia, or disorientation to time, place, or circumstance. Dullness, uncharacteristic joking or glibness, negativity, and resistance are further examples, as are the dropping of social or moral restraints, the taking of sexual liberties, or launching into verbal tirades. Such nonspecific signs can occur alone or in the company of strong localizing deficits such as hemiplegia or a visual field cut. Whether solitary or not, they raise the suspicion of cerebral disease.

In chapter 4 we discussed establishing separate syndromic, anatomic, pathologic, and etiologic diagnoses. In practice, these factors are considered simultaneously. Table 6.2 lists major categories of illness, and table 6.3 lists some age-typical symptoms. However, as figure 6.1 shows, considering an etiologic diagnosis can help determine whether the problem can be localized within the central

Table 6.3
Age-Related Behavior and Mental Disease

GRADE SCHOOL—ADOLESCENCE
  Encephalitis
  Ictal and post-ictal behavior
  Wilson's disease
  Gilles de La Tourette's syndrome
  Sydenham's chorea

20–40 YEARS
  Alcohol or drug intoxication and withdrawal
  Schizophrenia
  Infections (meningitis, encephalitis)
  Immunosuppression (AIDS)
  Closed head trauma
  Multiple sclerosis
  Anoxia and hypoglycemia

MIDDLE AGED
  Metabolic: thyroid, uremia, hepatic, porphyria, etc.
  Complications of prescribed or multiple drugs
  Brain tumors
  Deficiencies: Wernicke's, pernicious anemia, pellegra, etc.
  Vascular: strokes, hemorrhages, coagulopathies

AGED
  Dementias and other neocortical degenerations
  Vascular: multi-infarct and lacunar states, subdural hematomas
  Parkinson's disease and other subcortical degenerations
  Increased sensitivity to polypharmacy
  Psychiatric disorders

nervous system, or whether it might be a manifestation of systemic aberration or even fictitious.

Just as the divisions of the lobes have no real validity, lesions themselves seldom respect histologic boundaries even though the conceptual neatness of table 6.1 might inadvertently suggest otherwise. At the end of this chapter I will touch on a few symptoms caused by focal subcortical lesions. Therefore, you may wish to consult your anatomy atlas regarding the rich white-matter connections among the lobes. The commissural fibers, long association tracts, and cortico-cortical fibers that join homologous areas often are clinically significant.

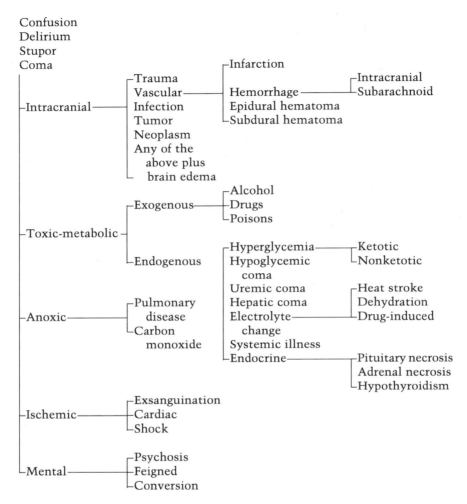

Figure 6.1
A decision tree of possible etiologies for some common expressions of alteral mental status. Modified with permission from W DeMyer, *Technique of the Neurologic Examination*, 3d ed. New York: McGraw-Hill, 1980.

SYNDROMES CAUSED BY OCCIPITAL LESIONS

It was not always obvious that a discrete part of the neocortex is devoted to vision; that discovery required more than a century (Glickstein, 1988). Only a small portion of primary visual cortex (also called *V1* or *area 17*) is visible on the brain's surface at the occipital pole: Most of it straddles the calcarine fissure. *Macular* fibers terminate here. Idiotypic visual cortex is also called *striate cortex* because of its grossly visible white band of Gennari, a thick layer of myelinated fibers coursing in layer IV.

Visual projections to striate cortex are *retinotopic*, but inverted: That is, the upper visual field maps inferiorly, downward vision maps superiorly, and right and left are reversed (consult your atlas for diagrams). The most peripheral parts of the retina project to the lingular gyrus of the temporal lobe and have rich limbic connections. Perhaps this is why we are most startled and frightened by objects that appear in our peripheral vision and why we similarly seem to catch something in the "corner of our eye" when in a heightened emotional state.

Unimodal visual association cortex has been nicknamed *VA*, *parastriate cortex*, or *areas 18 and 19*. These two Brodmann territories project to each other, the frontal *motor* areas (query: What does seeing have to do with moving?), and the angular, medial temporal, and medial parietal gyri. Vision has multiple *intermodal* associations. The fronto-occipital fasciculus is an important intrahemispheric white-matter tract, while homologous trans-hemispheric connections travel through the splenium of the corpus callosum. If you have not yet done so, go get your atlas now and review these structures.

Your review showed vision's impressive reach. Nearly two dozen functionally discrete visual areas are now known (Zeki, 1993). Once geniculate axons have synapsed in area 17, there is a multiplex branching to distinct areas of association cortex, each one presumably emphasizing a different aspect of vision such as contrast, color, size, shape, position, orientation, movement, and binocular disparity. In addition to this divergent branching, there is also an overall forward flow of visual input from striate cortex to temporal association cortex and, eventually, to limbic brain.

Limbic and paralimbic projections originate from the synaptically most downstream parts of temporal visual association cortex. The kind of impulse flow idealized in figure 3.9 might be the anatomic basis for the extraction of progressively more abstract features as visual input travels further and further downstream, and may suggest how we recognize invariant features of objects.

I will say more about the multipartite processing of vision later, leaving you for now with the fact that even though an object's shape, color, position, and motion seem mentally unified, each component is processed separately in a geographically distinct region of the brain (notice that I did not say, "cortex"). This idea seems to discomfort some people, who are never bothered by seeing someone speak; even though our perception of another's voice and mouth movements are also processed independently, and much farther apart than the components of a visual experience are. Jumping ahead a little, let me suggest that it may be the capacity for *aspects of perception to be displayed prematurely to awareness* that may explain subjective experiences such as hallucinations, synesthesia, or metamorphopsia.

In chapter 3, I noted that the highly differentiated neocortex performs repetitive transformations and is the repository of our model of reality. Neocortex is not the seat of human reason or perception, but provides only a fine grain of discrimination. Accordingly, we find that animals and people with striate ablations are not dreadfully handicapped. What they lose visually is the conscious perception of stationary objects. Because so many aspects of vision are split up as soon as input reaches area 17, abilities such as visual orientation and the accurate reaching for moving targets can be retained despite striate lesions. The ability to detect visual stimuli, discriminate shape, and localize targets in the absence of striate vision is an example of subception called blindsight (Weizkrantz, 1986; Celesia et al., 1991): Patients can accurately perform these tasks, yet they deny seeing anything. *Phantom vision*, discussed below, is a similar phenomenon, although more striking because persons who have had their eyes removed still claim to have visual experiences.

The term *subception* itself means "below awareness," and refers to an apprehension or knowledge inaccessible to conscious awareness. If you let the old hierarchical model of the brain guide your thinking, then subception seems difficult to fathom. On the other hand, the multiplex model contains many pathways for sensory inputs. As an example of their ideas figure 6.2 shows a variety of cortical and subcortical projections of retinal ganglion cells.

Anopia

The correlations among size, shape, and location of visual field defects and the locus of their responsible anatomic lesion has been known for a century. Figure 6.3 illustrates classic field defects.

The evolution and resolution of visual field defects is not studied now in the detail it once was. Instead of making firsthand observations we now let machines such as automated perimeters do our work and sometimes even our clinical thinking. Not too long ago, following the fluid course of clinical symptoms was the only tool a practitioner had. From this vast experience we know that color vision fails first, and that field defects progress from the periphery to the center and resolve in the opposite direction. Sensitivity to red is lost first, whereas that to blue goes last. Testing for subjective desaturation of a red object across the vertical meridian will, therefore, pick up early field cuts.

Cortical Blindness

Occlusion of the posterior cerebral arteries and complications of contrast myelography or angiography are the usual causes of acute cortical blindness, which implies functional devastation of both primary cortices. Because fibers of the pupillary light reflex terminate in midbrain, patients with cortical blindness have normal light reflexes (assuming intact optic and oculomotor nerves; Why? If you do not know why the third nerve must be intact, look up the anatomy of the light reflex). In contrast to preserved pupillary light reflexes, opticokinetic nystagmus cannot be induced because it depends on the ability to fixate targets. Likewise, evoked potentials and the alpha rhythm are absent. Interestingly, voluntary visual imagery and dream imagery remain. (This has to do with the sleep-wake generator in the pontine paramedian reticular formation.)

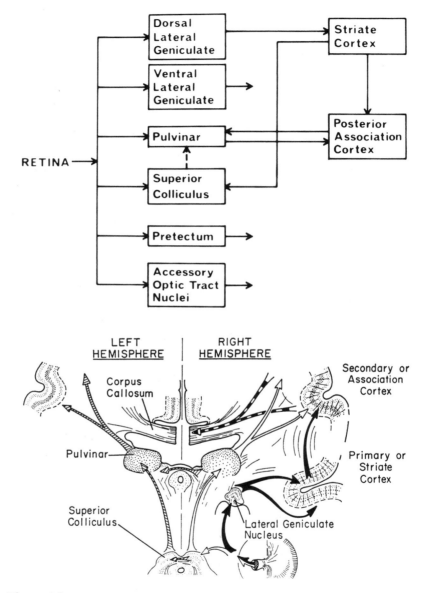

Figure 6.2
(*Top*) Retinal ganglion cells project to numerous subcortical and cortical entities. From Weiskrantz (1986), with permission. (*Bottom*) Several subcortical pathways that might explain visual subception. In this example, the corpus callosum has been sectioned. From Popper and Eccles (1977), with permission.

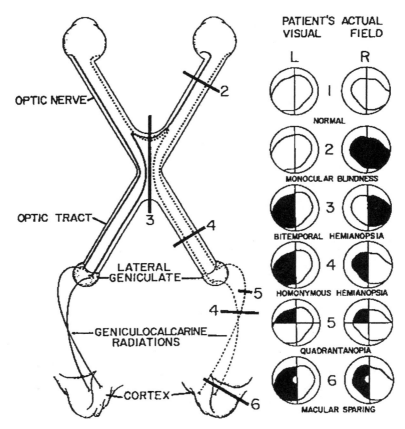

Figure 6.3
Lesions at various points along the optic pathways, together with their corresponding visual field defect. From Curtis, Jacobson & Marcus (1972), with permission. See also figure 12.8.

Visual Anosognosia

Also called *Anton's syndrome*, visual anosognosia (from the Greek, *a* ["negation"] + *nosos* ["disease"] + *gnosis* ["knowledge"]) is the denial of blindness in patients who have irrefutably lost their vision. Whether they walk into the walls under their own steam or are bluntly confronted with their disability by you or others, their response is indifference, an implausible explanation (e.g., "I lost my glasses"), or both.

Anton's syndrome is distinct from *phantom vision*, in which enucleated patients or those with severed optic nerves claim to perceive light and shape. The existence of visual subception suggests two dissociable levels of "seeing," instrumental behavioral responses to optical stimuli on the one hand, and subjective visual awareness on the other. The American neuroöphthalmologist David Cogan (1908–1993), of the National Institutes of Health, has compiled a video collection of patients with phantom vision. These patients do not readily volunteer their experiences of "seeing things." In fact, they feel ashamed at experiencing something that intellectually they know to be not "real."

For example, after fifty-year-old patient ER had her left eye enucleated because of a melanoma, she began to see geometric figures in that eye. The shapes were external, close to the face, and consisted of metallic blobs, spirals, and parallel lines. Her explanation was, "This is involuntary. My brain is doing it." (This claim is most plausible. We have long known that migraineurs who have no eyes nonetheless have visual symptoms during their aura [Peatfield & Rose, 1981].)

Patient JS, a twenty-year-old soldier, had severed optic nerves and, therefore, no light perception. Yet he experiences a feeling of brightness that varies on closing and opening his eyes. He also claims to see "objects" such as the sink when he shaves, the bed if he bumps into it, or parts of his own body. He is deeply convinced about this synthesis of an image. He claims to see the outline of his own hand when he holds it in front of his face, but not Dr. Cogan's hand when Dr. Cogan holds it up. Actions such as palpating his legs when he says that he is able to see their outline, or claiming to see his own hand in front of him, but not someone else's, suggest that sensory input such as proprioception contributes to JS's subjective visual experience.

The inverse of Anton's syndrome has also been reported (Hartmann et al., 1991)—namely, the denial of visual perception in a man with remarkably preserved visual skills in his upper right quadrant. When confronted with his success in correctly identifying colors, objects, faces, facial emotions, and words, he denied any awareness of visual perception. His explanation for his accurate performance was, "I feel it."

Visual Illusions and Hallucinations

Visual illusions and hallucinations may be either positive or negative symptoms and can be seen in drug reactions or withdrawal, delirium, epilepsy, and mass lesions. They may be elementary or formed. Epileptic discharges in Brodmann areas 18 and 19 (lateral occipital) are said to cause twinkling or pulsating lights. Striate lesions produce elementary visual sensations of dark shapes, phosphenes, and flashes that may be stationary or moving, colored or achromatic. Gowers (1893, p. 166) noted that red is perceived most often, followed by blue, green, and yellow. These visions may appear straight ahead or in the visual field opposite the lesion.

Elementary flashes of light, zigzags, or other geometric shapes are called *photisms*, and are distinct from *phosphenes*, the flashing lights one sees on firmly rubbing the eyes. Phosphenes are caused by mechanical deformation of the retina and are an example of an *entopic perception* (literally "within the eye"). These latter need to be distinguished from perceptions of cerebral origin as the eye and the occiput are poles apart.

Other entopic phenomena are the seeing of one's own retinal blood vessels, vitreous floaters, afterimages, or the muscæ volitantes. Entopic perceptions appear to move with the eyes, whereas perceptions of cerebral origin are independent of eye movement. Afterimages are produced by fatigued retinal photoreceptors and are complimentarily colored; images of cerebral origin are often chromatic. Retinal vessels and floaters look like cobwebs or blobs, are fixed in appearance, and can be viewed or ignored at will. The muscæ volitantes are the actual corpuscles coursing through vessels near the macula. You should normally be able to see your own, particularly against a bright sky or a field of snow. They travel in lines or arcs, then disappear. Awareness of your own normal retinal circulation is called *Scheerer's phenomenon* (1924). Traction of the vitreous or retina causes arch-shaped, achromatic phosphenes called *Moore's lightning streaks*. Macular edema or hemorrhage will produce distortions such as heat waves, and glaucoma causes halos and rainbows around objects. Certain maculopathies can also cause metamorphopsia.

Release hallucinations are perceptions, in any modality, that occur in a *deafferented field*. Visual and auditory ones are most common. In vision, for example, one sees elementary or categorical objects in a scotoma or hemianopic field (figure 6.4). Lance explains the term *categorical* and expresses the opinion that release hallucinations arise from association cortex. "The hallucinations are not of great complexity, suggesting that the function of the association cortex is to group images into categories of person, animal or thing, leaving the final identification to a further stage involving links with the temporal lobe and limbic system to incorporate knowledge from memory stores" (Lance & McLeod, 1981 p. 327; Lance, 1986).

Primary idiotypic cortex has no direct links with other cortical areas except through obligate relays via the unimodal association cortex that lies adjacent to it. Stimulation of association areas or their temporal-limbic projections gives rise to formed hallucinations that are "seen," "heard," or otherwise sensed in the external receptive field that is impaired by damage to the primary receptive cortex, as though the association area were released from its normal afferent input from the primary idiotypic cortex (Cytowic, 1989 p. 101).

Similar to the confound that confuses entopic visions with cerebral ones is the mistaking of formed hallucinations due to ocular disease for those of cerebral origin. In the *Charles Bonnett syndrome*, formed visual hallucinations occur in persons with visual loss but who are otherwise normal (Berrios & Brook, 1982; Rolak & Baram, 1987). The hallucinations are exclusively visual and highly detailed, such as people or scenes. They are unemotional, nonthreatening, brief, and occur in a setting of visual loss: Macular degeneration, cataracts, glaucoma, and other instances of poor acuity. Patients are not psychotic and are quite aware that they are hallucinating.

Visual release hallucinations can wander out into the normal field. They are experienced in extrapersonal space, and patients almost always appreciate their unreal nature. Elementary hallucinations tend to occur with occipital lesions, whereas formed and more complex ones emanate from the temporal lobe. *Hallucinations due to temporal lobe lesions tend to fill both visual fields, in contrast to those engendered by occipital lesions, which usually inhabit only the contralateral field.*

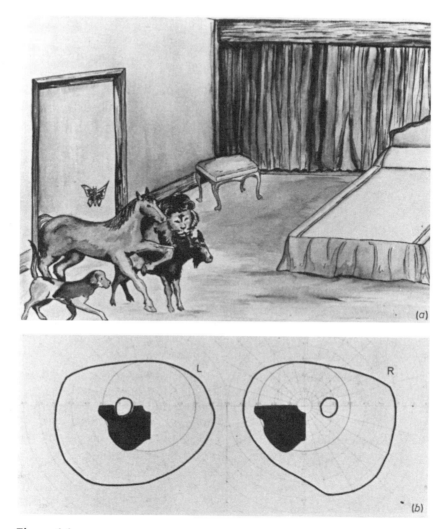

Figure 6.4
(*Top*) Categorical release hallucinations. Animals appear one at a time in the area of the quadrantic field defect (*bottom*). From Lance & McLeod (1981), with permission.

Elementary visual hallucinations have many causes, and the ground is strewn with confounds. In addition to entopic and occipital lobe causes, hallucinations can also result from lesions of the anterior optic tract. These are special, however, in that they are not spontaneous but rather are induced by another sense, most often sound (Lessell & Cohen, 1979). This is an example of an acquired *synesthesia* (see below). Figure 6.5 and table 6.4 give examples. Sounds that induced photisms in these patients included clanking of the radiator, crackling of the walls as they cooled at night, the whoosh of a furnace ignition, a dog's bark, and slamming doors.

The photisms ranged from simple flashes of white light to colored forms that looked like a flame, amoebas, oscillating flower petals, a spray of bright dots, or kaleidoscopic effects. All lasted for just an instant. The monocular visual-evoked response from the scotomatous eyes showed conduction delays and reduced amplitudes. It is curious that photisms arising in one eye are perceived to be caused by sounds reaching only the ipsilateral ear. This is, of course, contrary to our conventional understanding as acoustic localization depends on differences in the sound reaching both ears. Yet

... the click of an electric blanket thermostat induced a flashbulb photism in the right eye of patient 6 only when the thermostat located to her right clicked; the same clicking from her husband's thermostat to the left never

induced the phenomenon. A petal photism was perceived coming from the right eye of patient 7 when a nurse spoke into his right ear. The photism never occurred when the nurse spoke into his left ear (Jacobs et al., 1981).

Spontaneous visual phenomena are quite common, occurring in nearly sixty percent of individuals whose visual loss is pre-geniculate (Lepore, 1990). Yet positive symptoms must be specifically sought, because patients are reluctant to reveal "crazy" symptoms. Spontaneous visual phenomena can occur when visual loss is trivial (as in Lepore's three pseudotumor cerebri patients whose acuity remained 20/20), though its frequency rapidly increases as acuity worsens past 20/50. Elementary visual experiences are more common than complex ones (table 6.5).

I will return to release hallucinations and expand on other unusual experiences after we have discussed stereotypical symp-

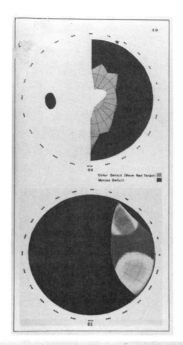

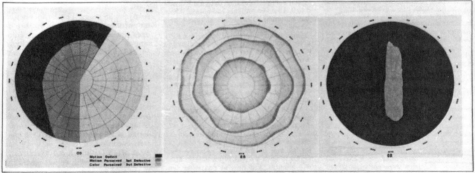

Figure 6.5
Visual fields and scotomas are indicated in black. (*Top*) Nasal defect of left
eye, and below it a flame photism induced within it by "sharp" sounds.
(*Bottom*) The entire left field is variably defective with anopsia, achromatopsia, and dyschromatopsia. The center panel shows a petal photism, the
right an ameba photism. From Jacobs et al. (1981), with permission.

Table 6.4
Characteristics of Sound-Induced Photisms

No.	Photism appearance	Color	Location	Sounds
1	Flame, flashbulb	Red-orange, white	In scotoma	Not sure (sharp)
2	Spray, pollywogs, kaleidoscope	White, pink, red, black, green	In and out of scotoma	Clap, CT gantry
3	Flash	White-yellow	In scotoma	Walls crackling, digital clock, TV crackling
4	Lightbulb	White-blue	In scotoma	Not sure (soft)
5	Flash	White	In and out of scotoma	Engines, loud sounds
6	Flashbulb	White	In scotoma	Electric blanket, digital clock
7	Petal, ameba, goldfish	Pink, white, yellow	In and out of scotoma	Furnace, dog, voices, clatter
8	Plaid	Green	In scotoma	Book or fist on desk, loud
9	Flashbulb	Pink	In and out of scotoma	Furnace, door slam, TV, radio

From Jacobs et al., 1981, with permission.

toms associated with lesions of the temporal lobe in the next section.

Metamorphopsia and Allied Experiences

Many bizarre visual experiences are subsumed under the term *metamorphosia*, the essential features of which are (1) deformation of shape, (2) change in size, (3) the illusion of movement, or (4) all three. Its locus is imprecise, being vaguely in the occipito-temporo-parietal territory, though I have listed it under "occipital lesions" in table 6.1. Indeed, as piquant as metamorphopsia is to neuroscientists, the preponderance of cases are caused by retinal maculopathy rather than cerebral disease.

In metamorphopsia, objects may appear to advance or recede relative to the viewer, their vertical or horizontal orientation may

Table 6.5
Spontaneous Visual Phenomena (SVP)

Content and frequency of SVP in individuals with visual loss				
Lesion site	No SVP	Elementary	Complex	Both	Total
Retina	4	6	1	4	15
Optic nerve	29	25	2	7	63
Chiasm or tract	1	1	1	3	6
Postgeniculate	11	5	2	2	20
SVP Content				No. of Patients
ELEMENTARY				
Mobile photopsias				
Achromatic				23
Chromatic				7
Stationary photopsias				
Achromatic				13
Chromatic				5
Diffuse color or glow				4
Geometric forms (lines, waves, ring, spots, smoke, snowflakes, egg crate, rolling bar)				13
Multiple types of elementary SVP				9
COMPLEX				
People				13
Faces or body parts				7
Animals or insects				5
TV or movies				3
Vehicles				2
Clothing				2
Palinopsia or polyopia				2
Miscellaneous objects (jars, numbers, lamp, steps)				5
Multiple types of complex SVP				12

From Lepore (1990), with permission.

suddenly skew, or objects may "break apart" as if they were painted on glass, the parts sliding over one another as in Cubism. One object may transform into another, sometimes with the two shapes alternating rhythmically back and forth. Visual field defects are frequently found in all these subjective visual experiences. Specific types of metamorphopsiæ have earned their individual terminology.

In *micropsia* and *macropsia*, objects seem too small or too big, respectively. This changing of size is well described in Lewis Carroll's *Through the Looking Glass and What Alice Saw There*. (Some authors suggest that Carroll, a migraineur, had firsthand experience with metamorphopsia, since it occasionally occurs during the aura of classic migraine.)

Umkehrtsehen is German for inverted vision, meaning that things look as if you are standing on your head. *Verkehrtsehen* denotes the reversal of right and left. These aberrations usually appear and resolve suddenly, and the experience is transitory in all recorded cases (Brown, 1984; Steiner et al., 1987). For example, one patient was walking downtown when the buildings suddenly shifted to the opposite side of the street. After a few minutes they reverted to their original positions. In another patient, everything in both visual fields became suddenly inverted: People appeared with their legs up and their heads down, and the floor became the ceiling. Color, shape, and the spatial relations among objects remained normal during this failure of egocentric visual orientation. A dysfunction of central vestibular-ocular integration is proposed. These two metamorphopsiæ always seem to be referred to by their German names and I am unaware of any standard English nomenclature.

Palinopia (also known as *paliopsia, paliopia,* and *palinopsia*) is visual perseveration. For example, a patient saw his wife leave the hospital room, and then he saw her leave again a few moments later. Aside from static cerebral lesions, antiserotonergics such as LSD and mescaline can produce it (Critchly, 1951; Abraham, 1983). LSD users speak of "trails," positive images that remain immediately behind an object as it moves across their visual field.

Polyopia signifies multiple images of the same object. For example, a patient looked at a single rose and, on turning away to look at the blank wall, saw multiple roses. "Insect vision," or *entomopia* (from the Greek *entomon* meaning "insect"), connotes rows and columns of multiple images numbering in the hundreds, as might be experienced by looking through compound eyes (Lopez et al., 1993). Polyopia is a form of cerebral diplopia.

Cerebral diplopia may be vertical or concentric. Strict terminology would limit it to only two images (the above terms of *polyopia* and *entomopia* taking care of larger iterations), yet triple impressions are especially common. Migraine is probably the most common cause of cerebral diplopia (Sinoff & Rosenberg, 1990).

Medical students often are taught that monocular diplopia is an infallible sign of hysteria based on the false assumption that all double images are caused by misaligned optical axes of the two eyes. The fact that monocular diplopia has bona fide cerebral causes is well established, yet not widely known. Patients with ophthalmic diplopia and that due to faulty extraöcular muscles describe a "real" image that is clear and an indistinct overlying "ghost" image. Refractive correction or viewing through a pinhole causes marked improvement. In bilateral monocular diplopia that is caused by cerebral disease, however, the prechiasmal visual input causes two images whether it originates from either eye separately or from both eyes together. Refractive correction in this instance is does not help.

Monochromatopsia refers to illusory coloration, such as erythropsia (red) or xanthopsia (yellow). Vitreous hemorrhage causes the former and digitalis intoxication the latter more often than do cerebral lesions. Beware of this possible confound. The painter Van Gogh is said to have suffered xanthopsia due to intoxication from digitalis, which was commonly used in his day to treat epilepsy— thus the yellowish cast to his later canvasses.

The term *achromatopsia*, indicating "no color seeing," is somewhat misleading because patients do perceive some color. The chroma that they see is pale and desaturated, however, as in a television whose color is turned down. Patients also describe a spatial "gap" between the normally saturated field and the achromatic one. The responsible lesion is in unimodal visual association cortex.

I will again note that some students are unsettled by the fact that what they had always taken for objective reality turns out to be more fluid and relative. The experience of metamorphopsia, in which objects advance or recede, change size, or freely transform supposedly stable properties in a Daliesque manner, is surprising. It may help to think of metamorphopsia as a normal mechanism operating out of context.

Suppose that you are playing tennis, accurately hitting the ball back and forth. As you play, the ball maintains a constant psycho-physical size regardless of its proximity, although the retinal image is much larger when the ball is up close than when it is in your opponent's court. As you volley the ball, you do not have an illusion that it shrinks and expands. Rather, the brain provides an illusion of constant size by contracting and expanding the psycho-physical size of the ball inversely to its actual size, which depends on the geometry of foveation on the macula. It is only when metamorphopsia occurs with objects we expect to be stationary that we think something is amiss. You can think of it as a release of a normal cognitive process in an incongruous situation.

Visual Agnosia

Instances of visual "not knowing" are rare. The patient can see, the sensorium is intact, there is no aphasia, and yet the individual cannot comprehend something seen. Clues from other modalities—such as ringing a bell, running one's thumb over the teeth of a comb, or permitting the patient to feel, smell, or taste the object—may prompt instant recognition.

Basolateral occipital lesions cause visual-verbal and visual-limbic disconnection, producing *object agnosia*.

Prosopagnosia is the inability to recognize familiar faces and is caused usually by bilateral, basal, occipito-temporal lesions. As with other visual agnosias, patients recognize their spouses, children, and other intimates by their voice, perfume, or the sound of their gait. Other visual cues aside from faces, such as a particular item of apparel, can also trigger recognition.

Simultagnosia is the ability to comprehend the parts but not the simultaneous whole of a visual scene, especially words. Looking at the word *mate*, for example, patients can read the individual letters *m-a-t-e* aloud but cannot read the word as a single object.

Hearing themselves spell aloud, they can then understand the word. The locus of the responsible lesion is not certain; possibly it is the left peristriate cortex (area 18).

Pure alexia is a visual agnosia for letters or words only.

Color agnosia is distinct from achromatopsia or color blindness. True color agnosia is the inability to designate colors by name while still being able to match them to test objects of the same chroma, hue, and saturation. A left parieto-occipital lesion is implied.

None of these agnosias typically occurs in isolation, and visual field defects are the rule. Neither of two opposing theoretical positions adequately explain agnosia. The older one assumes a distinction between sensation and perception, explaining agnosia as a failure of the latter function. The more modern theory emphasizes disconnections between association cortices and verbal areas. Nuances of visual agnosia are discussed further in chapter 12. Disconnection syndromes are discussed in chapter 7.

Balint's Optic Ataxia

Despite their capacity to make full eye movements, patients with Balint's optic ataxia cannot voluntarily fixate a visual target or accurately touch it. In addition to this *psychic gaze paralysis* or *optic ataxia*, they are inattentive to visual stimuli even though there is no inattention to other sensory modalities.

In other words, patients cannot follow the command, "Look at my finger," nor can they pursue the finger once the eyes have fixated on it. If instructed "Touch my finger," they grope as if blind, yet their visual fields are full. The failure is in peristriate projections to the frontal eye fields, causing an inability to direct oculomotor output to extrapersonal space. Bilateral parieto-occipital lesions are responsible.

SYNDROMES CAUSED BY TEMPORAL LESIONS

The sylvian fissure demarcates the anterior and superior borders of the temporal lobe, though there are no distinct boundaries between the so-called temporal, occipital, and parietal lobes. Heschl's transverse gyri comprise the primary auditory area (A1), which is tonotopically arranged. Lesions of the primary auditory cortex are not clinically apparent because A1 receives projections from both ears. Evoked potentials and dichotic listening tests will disclose an abnormality, however.

The white matter connections of the temporal lobe are rather important, given the huge fiber connections between idiotypic and unimodal visual cortex, and the inferior and medial parts of the temporal lobes. The *arcuate fasciculus* joins the posterior superior temporal lobe to Broca's area and motor cortex, and the *uncinate fasciculus* yokes the anterior temporal and orbitofrontal regions. For trans-hemispheric communication, the body of the temporal lobe uses the middle of the corpus callosum, whereas the temporal poles use the phylogenetically older *anterior commissure*, a structure belonging to the limbic system. This is an important distinction. (The anterior commissure has two major branches, one connecting the olfactory bulbs, the other joining anterior temporal lobes both directly and through the amygdala.)

Wernicke's Aphasia

Wernike's aphasia is discussed in chapter 13.

Amusia and Other Auditory Agnosias

Lesions of unimodal auditory association cortex (Brodmann areas 21 and 22) cause auditory agnosia. The left hemisphere is sensitive to speech sounds; the right is more attuned to complex nonverbal sounds such as rhythm, pitch, the prosody of speech, and environmental noises.

Musically untrained persons demonstrate a right temporal superiority for musical recognition. The situation is more complicated in professional musicians, however, where the left temporal lobe participates in the semantic and notational aspects of music. Much of our understanding of the anatomic basis of musical appreciation has come from cases of composers with various cerebral lesions.

Historically, amusia and aphasia have been discussed jointly, although we now understand that the neurologic substrates of music and language are functionally independent. The proximity of structures critical to each, however, does make a concurrent disruption of both domains likely when brain injury is either extensive or diffuse. The disruption need not be complete, as the aphasia of composer Maurice Ravel illustrates (Cytowic, 1976). Ravel was able to think musically but unable to express his ideas either in writing or performance. The lesion producing aphasia also dissociated his capacities for musical conception and realization. In other words, musical thinking was preserved, but musical expression was not. Ravel's intriguing deficit presumably depended on the interaction between a musical cognitive system (right-sided and intact), and a verbal linguistic system (left-sided and injured).

Up to now, the rarity of brain-damaged musicians willing to avail themselves to researchers has limited our knowledge of this cognitive domain. The use of positron emission tomography in healthy musicians has partly overcome this deficiency (Sergent et al., 1992; Sergent, 1993), so that we presently know that musical sight-reading and keyboard performance embrace a cortical network spanning all cerebral lobes and the cerebellum. These two skills are, of course, but a small slice of musical talent.

The spatial aspect of printed musical notation and its auditory representation call upon the superior parietal lobe—a structure *not* involved in verbal language. Keyboard playing of scales activates motor and premotor cortices (areas 4 and 6) and the cerebellum; listening to scales bilaterally activates secondary auditory cortex (area 42) and the left superior temporal gyrus (area 22); listening to a composition rather than repetitive scales additionally engages area 22 on the right.

On reading words, one activates the extrastriate cortex bilaterally and the lingual and fusiform gyri on the left; the latter areas are inactive during musical sight-reading, being replaced by activation at the left occipito-temporal junction, an area known to participate in spatial knowledge. It may be that musical notation is understood not by feature analysis of the printed notes (as occurs with printed letters), but through spatial analysis of their staff positions that correspond correctly to intervals in sound pitch (Judd et al., 1983).

Pure word deafness is an auditory agnosia for spoken language. Patients respond normally to environmental sounds as well as written language, thus demonstrating that they are neither deaf nor aphasic. A distinction is made between pure word deafness and Wernicke's aphasia. Both are discussed further in chapter 13.

Auditory Illusions and Hallucinations

The term *paracusia* refers to an alteration of volume, timbre, or some other distortion of sound. This may be both unpleasant and persistent. Unlike tinnitus and other auditory perceptions caused by end-organ disease, paracusiæ are cerebral in origin. This is analogous to the distinction between entopic and cerebrally based visual hallucinations. Auditory hallucinations may be elementary or complex, ranging from humming and buzzing to music, voices, and radio programs. Their cause is not limited to the temporal lobe, however. Ipsilateral musical hallucinations, for example, also result from lesions in the pontine tegmentum (Murata et al., 1994; Lanska et al., 1987). That such brainstem hallucinations usually occur in the context of hearing loss suggests that they may be an instance of *release hallucinations*, as previously discussed.

Olfactory and Gustatory Hallucinations

Olfactory hallucinations are customarily associated with mass lesions or epileptic discharges in the inferior and medial segments of the temporal lobe, especially the hippocampal convolution or *uncus*—hence the name *uncinate fits* when referring to the disagreeable smell that sometimes constitutes the aura of partial seizures. It is externally projected and experienced as coming from some nearby but unknown source. The smell is impossible to identify other than being described as foul, rancid, or vile. (This quality of *indescribableness* is characteristic of experience associated with temporal structures; we will return to it later.)

Gustatory hallucinations also arise from the temporal lobe. Intense and sudden hunger can be a symptom of temporal lobe epilepsy (TLE), and, paradoxically, also of lobectomy. Fisher (1994) reported a boy who experienced two episodes of right anterior temporal intracerebral hemorrhage, each preceded by exclamations of intense hunger. It is not clear why hunger is not noticed more frequently as a clinical sign. An anterior temporal localization is reasonable given that other gastrointestinal experiences commonly constitute the aura of TLE and also are experienced during electrical stimulation of this region.

Synesthesia

The term *synesthesia* derives from the Greek *syn* (meaning "union") and *aisthesis* ("sensation"), and refers to an involuntary joining of one or more senses (Cytowic, 1989, 1993, 1995). That is, perception in one sense is accompanied by a parallel perception in another sense. Synesthesia's medical and psychological history reach back 300 years.

Idiopathic synesthesia is not a disorder per se, but a perceptual curiosity found in roughly 1 in 25,000 individuals. Women outnumber men by at least two to one, and left-handedness or mixed dominance is more common than expected. Psychophysical testing reveals mild left-hemispheric deficits, and pharmacological manipulation and measurement of cerebral blood flow further implicate the temporal lobe and hippocampus on the left. Additional well-chosen cases await detailed study of exactly how synesthesia occurs, so I will focus here on describing its rich phenomenology.

Though permutations of the five senses yield twenty possible pair-wise combinations, some synesthetic combinations are much more common than others. The yoking of sight with sound is by far most frequent, touch and taste less so, and smell is least often involved. Color, movement, and geometric shape are typical properties of the parallel sensation(s). Replication and either radial or parallel symmetry of the percepts are usually present (figure 6.6). In colored hearing synesthesia (*chromesthesia*), words, voices, environmental sounds, or music will trigger the perception of an involuntary photism that is perceived in extrapersonal space. In a case that I called geometric taste (i.e., taste-touch synesthesia) the taste of mint caused subject MW to palpate a cold, smooth, curved shape in front of him.

We often emphasize the yoking of just two senses when speaking of idiopathic synesthesia, though polymodal synesthesia occurs as well. Individuals mention that a third or fourth sense sometimes participates, but "not as often" as the main two that are

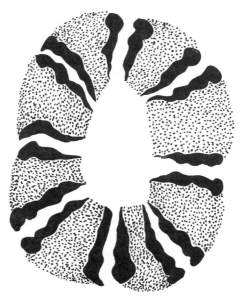

Figure 6.6
Patient's painting of a visual synesthesia: In this instance a large circular radiation with radial symmetry, and replication of amorphous blobs whose elements are both colored and black and white. The small dots represent scintillation, a sense of movement.

joined. It is important to distinguish that synesthetic percepts are neither metaphoric nor pictorial. They are concrete, generic, and unelaborated. By *generic*, I mean that synesthetes see blobs, lines, spirals, and lattice shapes; palpate smooth or rough textures; agreeable or disagreeable taste flavors, such as salty, sweet, or metallic. They do not see pastures and temples, taste chicken soup, or feel a sponge or some other *specific object*. Sensations never go beyond this elementary, unembroidered level to become specific exemplars. If they did they would no longer be synesthesia but rather well-formed hallucinations or figurative mental images.

Acquired synesthesia is classically seen in TLE, head trauma, and mass lesions involving the medial temporal lobe. Synesthesia may also be *induced* by sensory deprivation, antiserotonergic hallucinogens such as LSD and peyote, or direct electrical stimulation of subcortical limbic structures (Adams & Rutkin, 1970).

Epileptic synesthesia occurs in 4% of temporal lobe seizures and appears to be due to the actual discharge. In one case my own experience (though not part of the 1989 series) both the temporal focus and the synesthesia were inhibited by carbamazepine. Visual, auditory, tactile, gustatory (and, much less often, olfactory) sensations may combine with visceral sensations, vertigo, and involuntary movement, as in the following examples:

1. A taste of bile, dysesthesia on the left wrist, abduction of the left corner of the mouth, and clonic contractions of the left side of the body

2. Epigastric pain, shivers, a bitter taste, nausea

3. A lump in the throat, oral movements, phosphenes in the right upper fields, a bitter taste

4. An intense heat that ascends from the stomach to the mouth accompanied by a disagreeable taste

5. Bitter taste, hypersalivation, swallowing, spitting (sometimes vomiting), angry outbursts accompanied by shouting (examples 1 through 5 from Hausser-Hauw & Bancaud, 1987)

6. Hearing the word *five*, seeing the number 5 projected externally on a gray background, shooting pains in all three divisions of the right trigeminal nerve (Jacome & Gummit, 1979)

Behavioral aspects of the epilepsies are discussed further in chapter 11.

Other Subjective Experiences Dependent on the Temporal Lobe

Extremely unusual subjective perceptions have been recorded in cases of TLE and in patients with other known temporal lobe pathology. These experiences are almost never casually acknowledged because most people fear being thought hysterical or insane. I have collected below a potpourri of *organic* manifestations that are bizarre or frankly incredulous on their face but that are generally assumed to arise from the temporal lobes or its limbic projections.

Time dilation or *time contraction* occurs with lesions of either temporal lobe. Changes in the perception of time are certainly cognitive and, because they emerge following temporal-lesions one would expect to find them associated with other interesting neurological conditions. Yet the fact that one rarely hears of such occurences suggests incomplete ascertainment, presumably due to our focus on more readily-apparent behavioral signs.

Autoscopy is seeing your double or having an out-of-body experience. You observe yourself from a bird's-eye view or from behind your own body with a detached curiosity. This detached calm is typical of many of the strange perceptions attributed to the temporal lobe. Autoscopy is surprisingly common though seldom mentioned, occurring in approximately 6% of partial or generalized tonic-clonic seizures. The temporal lobe is involved in eighty-six percent of those in whom the focus could be ascertained, though the focus shows no definite preference for lateralization (Devinsky et al., 1989a).

The similarity of autoscopy to what is reported in near-death experiences is evident. That this is a subjective experience generated by the brain rather than something supernatural is a reasonable assumption, inasmuch as the brain continues to function for a while after the heart and lungs have stopped—i.e., after typical indicators of bodily death. Both autoscopic and near-death experiences induce profound changes in one's attitude toward life. They are a kind of *noëtic* experience that prompts individuals to rearrange their priorities and dispose of once-meaningful goals as no longer important. This kind of spiritual resonance in neurological conditions has intrigued and inspired the writings of a number of famous neuroscientists.

Déjà vu and *déjà vecu* mean "already seen" and "already experienced" (the latter literally means "already lived"), and refer to one's sense that something novel is extremely familiar or has been experienced exactly so at some past time. *Jamais vu* and *jamais vecu* refer to the opposite sense that a familiar setting feels nonetheless alien and strange. These are examples of *cognitive dissonance*, a discrepancy between what is felt and what is known. These conditions are most familiar from TLE but can occur by themselves without definite clinical or electrographic evidence of an ictal discharge. These kinds of experience often lead patients to believe that they are clairvoyant or possess psychic powers, a good example of how the language hemisphere *interprets* experience. Some individuals are utterly convinced that this is so, saying "I knew it would happen," or "It was like a dream, and I had seen it all happening before."

The *feeling of a presence* is not an uncommon experience, yet its occurrence rarely is volunteered for fear of negative judgement. Sensing a presence can occur in pathological states as well as be part of normal experience—in the latter case, it is most often experienced late at night or at times of great creativity. The certitude and sense of portentousness that accompanies such an experience indicate that limbic structures presumably participate in its generation; the left medial-basal portions of the temporal lobe are suspected (Persinger & Makarec, 1992).

Other odd personality characteristics that are said to be typical of those who suffer from temporal lobe seizures are a heightened interest in religion and cosmic matters, the keeping of diaries or voluminous writings, a sense of portentousness or the attribution of heightened significance to otherwise mundane events, and a viscous or "sticky" personality (Bear & Fedio, 1977).

Because these uncommon and highly unusual experiences are known only to a handful of physicians, it should not be surprising that others might interpret them in a religious or cosmic vein. Epilepsy, in fact, was known in earlier times as the *sacred disease*. It is facile to dismiss interesting human experiences with materialist explanations, particularly those experiences regarding surety and the convictions of one's inner knowledge. Reducing someone's most intimate experiences to nothing but "an electrical flurry in the brain" dehumanizes us all. (Readers interested in what Aldous Huxley called "nothing-but thinking" may wish to consult his prescient comments [Huxley, 1946, especially pp. 35–36].)

Psychosis and *forced thinking* are other fascinating manifestations of TLE, and are thought primarily due to limbic involvement. *Psychosis* may emerge if physical convulsions are controlled too well. Carefully lowering medication and permitting some seizures to occur may mollify the psychosis. As lesions extend to limbic structures in the more medial parts of the temporal lobe, one finds hyper-sexuality and hypo-sexuality, dramatic autonomic dysregulation, dreamy states, depersonalization, and violent behavior. Aggressiveness is unfocused and may increase if one tries to restrain the patient forcefully. It is considered an automatism and not voluntary.

The experience of repetitive and involuntary thoughts is called *forced thinking*. Examples such as psychosis and forced thinking suggest that the ability of the limbic brain to overwhelm rational thinking should make us question the exalted role that we have typically assigned to human reason.

Release Hallucinations (Revisited) and Form Constants

The various syndromes I have discussed do not necessarily occur in isolation, and symptoms are not always limited to one modality. Here are two cases of deafferentation with multiple symptoms.

The first patient had release hallucinations for the first two weeks after she developed a paracentral scotoma. Very restricted stimuli triggered her hallucinations (watching television or reading a book). They would abruptly disappear when she stopped these activities, only to come back when she resumed. She saw "four or five men, variably dressed (two or three in business suits, one in a cowboy's suit and hat, one in a plaid shirt), moving about, not speaking and not relating to one another."

The second patient had a large left homonymous hemianopia and a right posterior temporal lucency on CT scan. His hallucinations, which lasted for a year-and-a-half, were of three kinds: (1) *simple synesthesia* of perpendicular red and green lines, red and blue spots, and black and white pulsations, (2) *metamorphopsia*, with the right half of faces melting while turning yellow or violet, and (3) *palinopia*, such as people walking across his scotoma (Brust & Behrens, 1977).

You should now appreciate that hallucinations and illusions are quite common with sensory deprivation (deafferentation) or even simple boredom (Heron, 1957). For example, when you are surrounded by the white noise of the shower, how often have you hallucinated that the phone was ringing or that someone was calling your name? When deafferentation is mild—as it is with peripheral neuropathy, presbycusia, cataracts, or even during a long car ride (highway hypnosis) or other monotony—results are unlikely to be florid. When deafferentation is severe, psychosis may result (Gordon, 1994). Studies of sensory deprivation in normal persons have documented the progression from mild to severe hallucinations. Visual hallucinations begin with geometric patterns, mosaics, lines, or rows of dots, then become more complex and dreamlike, involving bizarre juxtapositions of people and objects. On returning to a normal environment, subjects continue to experience metamorphopsia and a heightened brightness of color.

The astute reader will have noticed by now that what people experience, in both visual and tactile modes, is often elementary. Beginning in the 1920s, psychologist Heinrich Klüver showed that a limited number of perceptual frameworks appear to be universal, possibly hard-wired and part of our genetic endowment (Klüver, 1966; Horowitz, 1975; Siegel, 1977, 1978; Siegel & Jarvik, 1975). The four types of consistent hallucinogenic images that Klüver identified are gratings and honeycombs, cobwebs, tunnels and cones, and spirals. Variations in color, brightness, symmetry, and replication provide a finer gradation of subjective experience. Given an infinite variety of stimulation, the brain seems capable of responding in finite ways.

The analysis ... has yielded a number of forms and form elements which must be considered typical for mescal visions. No matter how strong the inter- and intra-individual differences may be, the records are remarkably uniform as to the appearance of the above described forms and configurations. We may call them form-constants, implying that a certain number of them appear in almost all mescal visions and that many "atypical" visions are upon close examination nothing but variations of these form-constants (Klüver, 1966 p. 22).

Figure 6.7 shows the generic quality of Klüver's form constants. I mentioned earlier the generic quality of synesthetic perceptions (see also figure 6.6) and indeed the elemental quality of any hallucination occurring in any sense modality. You should be able to inquire about form constants or pursue suggestive comments. To convince yourself that this is so, ask the next patient with migraine to draw the aura.

Klüver's analysis was a reaction to the vagueness with which others had typically described hallucinations. Klüver suggested that the novelty and vivid coloration of the visions captured the subject's attention much more than their configuration did and that individuals were so overwhelmed by their "indescribable" nature that they simply gave in to cosmic or religious explanations. The notion of form constants caught on quickly but was forgotten when the rise of behaviorism made interest in direct experience taboo. Consequently, few of your teachers are likely to be familiar with the concept, although I think you will find it both useful and valid.

The tendency to attach supernatural meanings to hallucinations is attributable to the referential nature of the perception along

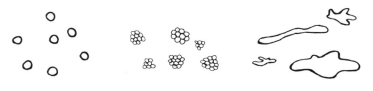

Small circles, clusters, amorphous blobs

Central radiation, radial symmetry, kaleidoscope

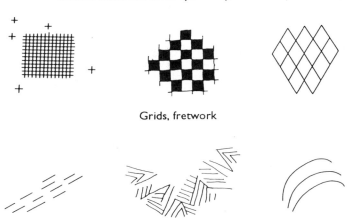

Grids, fretwork

Geometric lines: straight, angular, circular

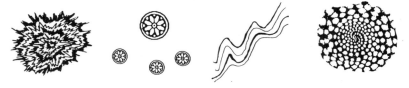

Scintillation, extrusion   Iteration   Movement   Rotation, spiraling

Figure 6.7
The generic shapes of Klüver's form constants are common to hallucinations, synesthesia, imagery, and other cross-modal associations.

with its emotional content. This likely accounts for the sense of familiarity and recognition that such experiences instill. In Adler's words (1972, p. 19), "To attach cosmic meaning to these events is a presumption. We are more likely confronting here the projection of affect onto the outside world. The response that one thinks he recognizes is his own projected and reflected image."

Both bottom-uppers and top-downers sometimes wonder why individuals with supposedly identical cerebral lesions have different subjective experiences. The primary reason is that the detailed anatomy of the cortex varies considerably among persons. Thus, lesions are never identical in the usual sense of that word. The studies of morphological asymmetry mentioned earlier showed that macroscopic differences could be measured with rulers. That microscopic anatomy is also highly variable is demonstrated by studies of the striate cortex that were undertaken as part of the visual prosthesis project: This was the surgical implantation of electrode arrays into the striate cortex of blind individuals in the hope of producing patterns of photisms that they could "see" (Brindley & Lewin, 1968; Dobelle & Mladejovsky, 1974).

Researchers found that adjacent electrical contacts may or may not produce photisms that are adjacent to one another in the perceived visual field. Nonetheless, whatever photism map is produced does remain stable in each patient even though the map differs between patients. For striate cortex, response to stimulation between patients varies greatly, but there is considerable reproducibility of responses in any given patient.

If such a degree of individual variation exists in the visual system, generally considered to be the most hard-wired, then anatomical and functional variability certainly seems likely in other cortices. As Ojemann and Whitaker (1978) suggested, "The detailed functional anatomy of our brains may be as individualized as the detailed anatomy of our faces."

Memory Disturbance

Memory is discussed in chapter 9. Right and left cortical lesions produce qualitatively different kinds of mnestic errors, whereas hippocampal lesions interfere with learning new material. Of course, frontal and thalamic lesions can also produce amnesia.

SYNDROMES CAUSED BY PARIETAL LESIONS

I listed the rich variety of clinical manifestations following parietal lesions in table 6.1. Because the boundaries of the lobes are vague and because I have also organized our explication of localization according to topologic types of tissue, we have either already touched on some classic parietal syndromes, or else we will discuss them at length in later chapters (e.g., the aphasias, visuospatial disorders). What follows, therefore, are a few of the more straightforward manifestations of parietal dysfunction.

Lesions of primary idiotypic somatosensory cortex cause loss of sensory localization and two-point discrimination, agraphesthesia, astereognosis, and sensory extinction. Because all motor and sensory processes are intimately linked (reafference), a mild hemiparesis or loss of fine dexterity can often be detected.

Critchley's *The Parietal Lobes* (1953) is a classic account of the higher disorders associated with lesions of heteromodal association cortex of the temporo-parieto-occipital region, referred to in earlier times as *tertiary association cortex* because three modalities converge here. This area does not really finish myelinating until late childhood and continues to myelinate slowly into the third decade. Large fiber systems traverse the parietal region.

Intermodal associations are the rule in heteromodal association cortex of the parietal lobe as well as in the heteromodal association cortex of the frontal lobe (discussed below). According to our topologic analysis of cortical tissue, the distinction between what is motor and what is sensory becomes lost in the parietal region. The distinction between limbic and non-limbic has become blurred, too (refer back to figure 3.9 as necessary). This point of view stands in distinction to that implied by the term *tertiary association area*, the latter implying that the parietal region is the epitome of abstract knowledge. In fact, parietal and limbic regions have strong reciprocal connections.

The major parietal functions are complex tactile discrimination and intermodal associations, the awareness of one's own body, the distinction between interpersonal and extrapersonal space, and the alignment of one's body in extrapersonal space. The grammatical and syntactical aspects of language and numerical competency, including the spatial aspects of calculation, are other parietal functions.

Cortical Sensory Disturbances

Most of these cortical sensory disturbances have already been described as part of the sensory-perceptual exam from chapter 5. Table 6.1 summarizes them.

Perversion of sensation, or *paresthesia*, occurs with lesions of the primary cortex although the term is also used to describe the same sensation that occurs with peripheral neuropathy, so you need to be clear about which meaning you intend.

Where we once were content to call the single post-central gyrus the *somatosensory cortex*, we now know that five somatosensory cortical areas exist in humans, each with its distinct somatotopic representation, cytoarchitecture, and projections. They are the primary idiotypic somatosensory cortex (S1), the ventrolateral somatosensory cortices (S2, S3, & S4), and the dorsomedial somatosensory cortex (S5). This illustrates the topologic rule that *all isocortical sensory systems have multiple cortical representations.*

Knowing what relative roles the various somesthetic cortices play in human sensation is another matter (Caselli, 1993). At present, we can say that dorsomedial lesions produce severe anesthesia and apraxia that eventually improve considerably. Ventrolateral lesions, in contrast, produce tactile agnosia that remains detectable years after brain injury. Pain, though less well understood than other sensory systems, also has multiple cortical representations. Painful heat, for example, activates contralateral anterior cingulum, S1, and S2, a pattern distinct from the predominant S1 activation caused by vibrotactile stimulation (Talbot et al., 1991). Because the forebrain usually is thought to regulate emotion, the specific cingulate representation of pain is unexpected.

Categorization of sensory loss on clinical grounds is far less confusing. Patients with loss of one or more elementary sensations (touch, pain, temperature, vibration) in a face-arm-leg-trunk pattern have inferior-anterior parietal lesions involving the parietal operculum and insula. Theirs is a *pseudothalamic sensory syndrome* in that it mimics a lesion of lemniscal or spinothalamic projections. Other individuals who lose the ability to discriminate sensation (stereognosis, graphesthesia, proprioception) have superior-posterior parietal lesions. Theirs is called a *cortical sensory syndrome* (Bassetti et al., 1993).

A somatic hallucination that bears a superficial resemblance to release hallucinations is *alloësthesia*, a condition in which a noxious sensory stimulus given on one side of the body (where a sensory deficit exists) is perceived at the corresponding locus on the opposite side (Kawamura et al., 1987). This aberration occurs with lesions in the putamen and spinal cord, represents an elementary disturbance of sensory pathways, and is not to be mistaken for a higher cortical dysfunction. Segmental sensation or pain can also be referred to a different and quite distant dermatome via spinal mechanisms (Lee et al., 1991).

Asomatognosia

Asomatognosia is a disturbance of *body schema*, the perception of one's own physical self, the relations of its parts to the whole, and its orientation and extension into extrapersonal space. (The related term *autotopognosia* is more restrictive, referring only to the capacity for recognizing and orienting one's body parts. It is the superordinate category of finger gnosia and right-left orientation for example.) The teleological importance of this capacity was suggested in the discussion of cerebral dominance, where we noted that the right hemisphere usually matures before the left (chapter 3, under the heading, "Standard Brain Development"). Though others had noted that patients with dense left hemiplegias sometimes were unaware of or else flatly denied their paralysis, it was the Parisan neurologist Joseph Babinski (1857–1932) who named this coöccurrence *anosognosia*, usually meaning "no knowledge of disease." We discussed visual anosognosia (Anton's syndrome) earlier. You can refer back to the box in chapter 5 (p. 188) if you are still uncertain about the terminology of the knowing and feeling sensations.

That limbic processes are typically integrated in parietal functions is disclosed by the absence of emotion in this disorder. The limb may hang lifeless and neglected. Requests to move the arm are met with either no response or an insistence that the requested action has been performed when, in fact, nothing has occurred. When the paralyzed arm is brought across the midline (into the intact visual field) and the individual is asked what it is or to whom it belongs, the patient may insist that the arm belongs to the examiner or someone else, or may flatly deny its existence altogether. This negation is particularly striking when the race of patient and examiner differs.

Constructional apraxia is the inability to assemble or arrange items such as puzzles, blocks, or lines in a drawing in their correct spatial configuration. We mentioned this deficit in chapter 5, and will take it up again when we discuss spatial knowledge and configurational gestalt in chapter 12.

Dressing apraxia refers to hemi-neglect in the sphere of grooming or apparel. A classic maneuver demonstrates that patients are unable to don a hospital gown or jacket whose left sleeve has been turned inside out. Their failure here likewise involves the gestalt of a spatial configuration, namely—how one's limbs fit into clothing.

Lesions responsible for asomatognosia often center on the superior parietal lobule, but frequently extend in any direction. Right-sided lesions are noticed far more frequently than their left-sided counterparts, possibly because there is often an overlying aphasia with left-sided lesions, but also because the right hemisphere (in dextrals at least) is functionally specialized for the direction of attention in extrapersonal space (Mesulam, 1981a).

SYNDROMES CAUSED BY FRONTAL AND LIMBIC LESIONS

Well into recent times the frontal lobes were called "silent" because destruction of large parts of them caused no *apparent* motor or sensory signs. We claim to know better today in speaking of their role in higher-order cognition, but we have still failed to assign any straightforward function to some segments of both the frontal and temporal lobes. We do know that parts of them are concerned with the mind in ways that are sophisticated, not readily apparent, and even less readily explained. One generalization I can make is that the frontal lobes insert attention and emotion between what has occurred in the past and what one intends in the future, or between the perception of an event and one's response to it.

The enigma of the frontal lobes is an old one. Frontal tissue accounts for nearly half the cerebral cortex, and yet extensive damage often appears to leave many neuropsychological functions intact. *Frontal Lobe Function and Dysfunction* (Levin et al., 1991) is a recent compendium of the strides we have made in the last forty years in understanding how the frontal lobes affect memory, attention, response preparation (intention), affect, personality, drive, the attainment of goals, and other higher functions of the mind. Because we still are trying to integrate experimental animal models with observations of patients, it often is not possible to state simply, let alone precisely, the mechanism that underlies these complex behaviors.

To make matters worse for the beginner, two opposing models of prefrontal function currently are being verified or refuted by fresh research (Daigneault et al., 1992). Because this competition is actively afoot I can do no more than outline it here. The standard model drawn from human neuropsychology consists of five constructs: (1) Devising and executing sequences of planned responses, (2) self-regulating behavior in response to environmental contingencies, including one's own errors, (3) sustaining a nonautomatic cognitive or behavioral set, (4) segmenting and organizing events into spatiotemporal chunks, and (5) sustaining spontaneity in mental production. The competing model is based primarily on the monkey research of Goldman-Rakic and postulates a fundamental prefrontal function of "on-line representational memory" that guides behavior in the absence of, or even despite, discriminative external stimuli. *On line* means that sensory, mnemonic, and symbolic representations elaborated elsewhere are kept activated long enough in the prefrontal area for them to influence behavior appropriately in the absence of external contingencies.

My comments regarding the variety of clinical manifestations following parietal lesions applies to frontal and limbic lesions as well (see table 6.1), the effects of which are less easy to classify than are those of sensory cortices. One reason for this is their far-reaching and reciprocal connections; another is that we simply know less about them compared to lesions of sensory cortices.

Frontal Lesions

Lesions of the primary motor cortex cause a contralateral spastic hemiplegia, a loss of fine dexterity, or a Broca's aphasia with agraphia and buccolingual apraxia. Accumulated evidence argues against the common concept of perseveration as a "frontal" sign. It is more likely that both brain-damaged and normal individuals will perseverate more on tasks to the extent that they find these tasks difficult.

As in primary idiotypic somatosensory cortex, primary motor cortex projects no callosal fibers for the hand or foot. This may underlie the hemispheric independence of hand control as well as the emergence of so-called frontal ataxia (see below) when primary motor cortex is damaged.

Regarding the unimodal and heteromodal association areas, we find that an irritative lesion in area 8 (frontal eye fields) causes contralateral deviation of the eyes and sometimes of the head as well, whereas ablations cause ipsilateral deviation. The unimodal motor association area (rostral part of Brodmann area 6) receives inputs from all sensory modalities and is involved in planning, initiating, inhibiting, and perhaps also learning complex movements. Lesions in association cortex do not cause primary weakness. Rather, they cause category-specific deficits of voluntary action.

Dominant frontal cortical lesions cause Broca's aphasia. Deeper lesions on either side can dampen prosody, make word finding difficult, and lead to a paucity of spontaneous speech. Such signs are seen frequently, for example, in hydrocephalus with its ballooning of the frontal horns and stretching of the surrounding white matter.

Lesions of frontal association cortex produce muscular rigidity and bladder incontinence, though its more dramatic changes involve personality and comportment. Generalized disinhibition is represented by facetiousness and a compulsion to make shallow jokes, often at the expense of others (*Witzelsucht*). Patients are also talkative, unbelievably distractible, and cast off typical social restraints. Overall psychomotor retardation is usually present.

Medial lesions of the frontal lobes, particularly their parasagittal segments, can severely affect gait and stance. The inability to place the feet adequately in the act of taking a step is called *frontal ataxia* or *frontal apraxia*. Both these terms are misnomers given that no weakness, sensory loss, or a true cerebellar ataxia is truly present. Some authors suggest calling the disturbance simply a *frontal gait*. The mechanism of the deficit is faulty integration between cortical and basal ganglionic control of posture and gait.

Patients with a frontal gait stand flexed, on a wide base, and walk either with petite, shuffling steps or else jerk their feet with great effort, as if their shoes were magnetized and stuck to the floor (*magnetic gait*). Turning, if possible, is done with scores of minute steps. Eventually, standing or sitting is impossible and patients will fall over unless supported while sitting. Other motor signs ensue until the result is Yakovlev's *cerebral paraplegia in flexion* (1954), in which patients are permanently curled up, akinetic, and mute.

Patients with normal pressure hydrocephalus or parasagittal meningiomas demonstrate so-called classic frontal lobe signs: The frontal gait disorder, some personality change, and incontinence. *Bladder incontinence* appears when the superior frontal and cingulate gyri are compromised. Initially, patients cannot discern that their bladder is full and thus are surprised when they wet themselves (*unwitting wetting*). As disease progresses, they no longer care about such accidents. The triad of mental change, gait disturbance, and incontinence in normal pressure hydrocephalus has lead to the three-W mnemonic: Such patients are described as "wet, wacky, and wobbly."

It is not common to see patients with a full-blown frontal syndrome. Rather, the indicators of frontal disease often are subtle, and confirmatory signs found only when deliberately sought.

The placidity noted in monkeys given frontal ablations as well as observations from human cases prompted the Portuguese neurologist Egas Moniz (1875–1955) to offer prefrontal leukotomy to the mentally ill (Moniz, 1936). At first, only violent or agitated individuals were candidates for the simple operation, which often was performed with local anesthesia. Soon psychosurgery was considered appropriate for a variety of conditions and eventually won Moniz the 1946 Nobel Prize (although that award was not without controversy). Because patients who underwent leukotomy were rarely normal to begin with, the results of ablations and, by extension, any naturally occurring, deep, bilateral frontal white matter lesions are difficult to interpret (Valenstein, 1986).

Ironically, Moniz went unsung for his far more useful and lasting invention of cerebral angiography in 1927. Nonetheless, mental disease was considered to be so unrelated to brain structure in his time that Moniz' concept of modifying it was a vital step toward indroducing the psychopharmaceuticals that eventually displaced psychosurgery.

Limbic and Paralimbic Lesions

Simple sensory disturbances such as dysosmia and dysgeusia can occur with limbic and paralimbic lesions. But because the inputs arriving there are an extensively transformed and abstracted account of the external world, we tend to think of complex alterations of drive, affect, movement, autonomic balance, and memory as more typical of limbic lesions. An amnesia, for example, may be modality-specific.

Mesulam calls limbic tissue a "synaptic buffer between external reality and internal urges. It is in these parts of the brain," he continues, "that the same stimulus can elicit very different responses, depending on the context (1985a, p. 31)." That is, behavioral relevance exerts a reciprocal influence on limbic force. The limbic system is connected to all subcortical interoceptive systems, and receives projections from all neocortical exteroceptive association areas and (via thalamocingulate projections) prefrontal heteromodal association cortex.

The limbic system's cortical members share chemical, physiologic, and immunologic features in that they (1) are rich in cholinergic neurons and opiate receptors, perhaps reflecting a limbic role in memory, pleasure, and pain, (2) easily develop seizure foci, and (3) have a special immunologic affinity for herpes simplex virus.

Dysfunction of paralimbic and limbic tissue can severely disrupt the synergy among experience, thought, behavior, and emotion. Clinically, the emotional coloration of mental life can be both unpredictable and incongruous. Experience may seem unreal, for example. Perceptual distortions, time dilation, the feeling of a presence, *déjà vu* and *jamais vu*, memory flashbacks, autoscopy, synesthesia, dissociative states, and a certitude that one is clair-voyant are some of the many subjective experiences associated with this neural entity.

The two major paralimbic efferents are heteromodal association cortex, and the most distal synaptic reaches of modality-specific association cortex. As the flow illustrated in figure 3.9 attempted to convey, the relevance of a stimulus is more important in this region than are its physical properties, given that highly abstracted qualities of the external world converge here.

In more developed mammals, the paralimbic regions interpose themselves between external stimuli and the urge to act. Para-limbic areas channel drive toward appropriate targets, emotionally shading thoughts and perception. The cingulum appears to direct motivation to spatial targets.

The context of inputs may evoke any number of possible behav-ioral scenarios. Lower mammals and vertebrates do not appear sensitive to context, as I mentioned in chapter 3. Rather, context-insensitive instinctual responses saddle them with rigidly fixed behaviors.

Dramatic and consistent autonomic responses are seen with both irritative and ablative lesions of the anterior insula, cingulate gyrus, orbitofrontal cortex, and the temporal pole. Respiratory arrest, hypertension, gastric and esophageal ulcers, lethal cardiac arrhythmias, and even multifocal cardiac necrosis in healthy sub-jects all occur in response to such brain lesions. That visceral tar-gets are prominent suggests that the paralimbic areas may provide an anatomic basis for some maladies that have historically been labeled *psychosomatic*.

Primary olfactory and gustatory relays are part of paralimbic cortex, which is why distortions and hallucinations of taste and smell are common in TLE. Aside from this, little is known about the cerebral basis of these modalities in humans. Mesulam (1985a) speculates that taste and smell are associated with the limbic and paralimbic brain because these chemical senses might have evolved from mechanisms closely related to the monitoring of the internal milieu. All other senses project to idiotypic cortices.

Medicine and psychology have often dismissed taste and smell as trivial, perhaps because their importance in daily life is so taken for granted. Yet chemosensory dysfunction appears in many diseases, and a considerable expanse of subcortex and cortex is devoted to taste and smell (Cytowic, 1983; Schiffman, 1983). Some 2 million Americans suffer chemosensory impairment and complain bitterly of it. Loss of taste (aguesia) can reflect such varied conditions as TLE, brain tumor, endocrinopathy, cancer, malnutrition, demyelination, viral infection, chemotherapy, dialysis, or radiation therapy.

Aside from its role in detecting rancidity, taste protects some species. The high concentrations of bombesin and cerulein peptides in frog skin, for example, produce vomiting and diarrhea in predators and are thus teleologically important as preservers of frog species. The Monarch butterfly possesses a similar mechanism. We have not yet pondered fully the intriguing role that taste plays in mammalian species preservation, in suckling, in the ritual importance of dining in mammals (including us), and in the evolution of the kiss.

The piriform cortex appears to have a dual function, acting as both a sensory and a limbic relay. It is the primary relay for smell and modulates feeding, sex, and defense. That it does play a non-sensory role is particularly suggested by cetaceans, mammals that are totally anosmic yet have well-developed piriform cortices.

The septal nuclei (medial septal nucleus, diagonal band of Broca, and the nucleus basalis of Meynert) contain cholinergic cell groups, numbered Ch1 through Ch4, that project to the entire neocortex. Cholinergic chemoarchitecture is essential to memory, and the basal forebrain has understandably attracted much attention, particularly its nucleus basalis of Meynert. Memory loss is prominent in patients with ruptured anterior communicating aneurysms, septal tumors, and Alzheimer's disease, in which profound dropout of Ch4 neurons is universal. Single-cell recording in primates suggest that the cholinergic neurons are pivotal in forming multiplex associations between external objects and their salience. The role of these structures in humans continues to be explored. This is an example of our continuing efforts to integrate experimental animal models with observations in humans.

Recently, damage to the dorsal septal region has been shown to produce markedly increased overt sexual behavior in two well-documented cases (Gorman & Cummings, 1992). This is an important observation, given that either increased or decreased sexual drive has been described in single case reports involving lesions in various limbic structures (inferior frontal cortex, hypothalamus, amygdala), each of which has major anatomic connections to the septum.

The amygdala associates an appropriate emotional response to an external object. In epileptics in whom depth electrodes have been implanted, one sees amygdalar discharges whenever patients feel strong emotions or have a subjective experience. Clues about what the amygdala does were first garnered from monkeys with the Klüver-Bucy syndrome (effected by amputating both temporal poles). Its three features are (1) hypersexuality aimed at any target, (2) an inappropriate loss of fear toward humans and other animals, and (3) the inability to distinguish by vision edible from inedible objects, so that the monkey examines everything by putting it into its mouth. Only after it has discriminated by taste does the monkey reject inedible objects. What these manifestations have in common is a breakdown in matching salience and context to visual targets. Drive itself is not lacking; its link with a proper object is.

The amygdala also influences autonomic, endocrine, and immune function, perhaps explaining the high frequency of visceral sensations in patients with TLE. Further, persons with TLE show hormonal changes that cause conditions ranging from dysmenorrhea and impotence to polycystic ovaries. Estrogen-concentrating and testosterone-concentrating neurons reside in several limbic structures, again suggesting a possible anatomic basis for the sensitivity of mood to hormones.

Investigation continues on the innervation of the immune system (Felton & Felton, 1991). This exciting work may illuminate the assumed relationship between mental states and immune disorders.

SYNDROMES CAUSED BY SUBCORTICAL LESIONS

Basal Ganglia

Most textbooks cite the basal ganglia as motor structures that are particularly involved in the automatic execution of movements that have been thoroughly learned. Curiously, few sources touched on the nonmotor behavior associated with the basal ganglia until just recently, though it was a lifelong interest of MacLean (1990). The basal ganglia have emerged recently as structures of particular importance in mediating emotional expression and comprehension in lesions involving either hemisphere (Cancielliere & Kertesz, 1990). They are involved most frequently in aprosodic syndromes accompanying lesions of the insula or anterior temporal lobe.

Not long ago, Parkinson's disease was similarly considered the prime example of the "movement disorders," and attention was fixed on its motor aspects relative to nigro-striatal degeneration. Now, we find that cognitive and affective disturbances are plentiful and not at all subtle in this disease. Today's neuropsychologist must consider such further variables as the alteration of cognition and affect by fluctuating levels of dopamine, the behavioral side effects of drug treatment, and the behavioral influence of adrenal medullary implantation (Huber & Cummings, 1992).

All parts of neocortex project to the striatum in the form of multiple, overlapping terminal axon fields. Thus, it is quite possible for striatal lesions to produce behavioral deficits that mimic those usually attributed to the cortex. Symptoms caused by caudate damage, for instance, can be similar to those of injured prefrontal cortex. Dementia is intrinsic to Parkinson's disease, even in those patients who fail to show cortical plaques and neurofibrillary tangles consonant with Alzheimer's pathology. Huntington's disease, in which there is marked loss of striatal neurons (caudate and putamen), also has a marked mental disturbance. The brainstem degeneration constituting the Steele-Richardson-Olchewsky syndrome (progressive supranuclear palsy) is yet another example (Gearing et al., 1994).

Obsessive compulsive disorder (OCD), both idiopathic and that associated with other neurologic disease, involves subcortical portions of prefrontal-cingulate-limbic-basal ganglionic circuits. Patients perform worse than controls on spatial, perceptual, and discriminating tasks requiring vision, as well as on tasks requiring sequencing, tracking, and shifting of sets (Aranowitz et al., 1994). Serotonin agonists seem to help.

Because the globus pallidus receives the outflow of the striatum and projects in turn to thalamus, habenula, and other extrapyramidal structures, pallidal lesions can disrupt behaviors usually

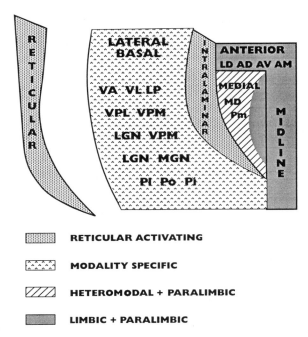

RETICULAR ACTIVATING

MODALITY SPECIFIC

HETEROMODAL + PARALIMBIC

LIMBIC + PARALIMBIC

Figure 6.8
Thalamic divisions. Thalamic lesions can mimic symptoms usually attributed to the cortex. From Mesulam (1965a), with permission.

associated with the limbic system. The most common human lesions are carbon monoxide poisoning and occlusion of the anterior choroidal artery. Human behavioral deficits associated with these lesions have not been fully explicated.

Specific neurochemical dysfunction has now been implicated in many behavioral disorders in which the central nuclei are affected. Parkinson's disease, Huntington's chorea, progressive supranuclear palsy, and OCD, for example, involve dopaminergic dysfunction. Volume 23 of *Brain and Cognition* is dedicated to the role of dopamine in cognitive dysfunction (Cohen & Cohen, 1993).

It should not be so surprising that subcortical structures are involved in thinking, comportment, and other mental aspects that heretofore have been labeled *higher cortical functions*. Many neurotransmitters are synthesized in brainstem and subcortical nuclei and are actively transported to more rostral targets.

Thalamus

Behavioral associations of the thalamus are an advanced topic. Hemihypesthesia, hemianopia, and analgesia may result from lesions of modality-specific nuclei. Nonspecific nuclei produce deficits in visual recognition and spatial capacity. Memory impairment is, of course, prominent in Korsakoff's psychosis, which destroys the medial dorsal nucleus of the thalamus. Surprisingly, there are almost no interconnections among individual thalamic nuclei (figure 6.8). It is conjectured that cortico-thalamo-cortical circuits reactivate associations under specific contextual circumstances.

The thalamus is receiving new attention in schizophrenia (Andreasen et al., 1994). Because schizophrenics manifest cognitive and emotional deficits across many functional systems, scientists speculate about a defect in a central node of information transfer and point out that the thalamus and neighboring tracts are somewhat reduced in size. The more established view explains the scope of symptoms by postulating a broad alteration between dopamine and its distributed receptors.

Electrical stimulation of either thalamus interrupts backward counting and serial subtraction (Ojemann, 1974). During left thalamic stimulation, counting rate accelerates, and is accompanied by an increase in calculation errors. Conversely, right thalamic stimulation slows counting but is still accompanied by significant errors. These findings suggest either that the thalamus is directly involved in number operations or that projections from or through it to the cortex are involved in the ability to calculate. In a similar vein, a patient with a left lenticular-caudate lesion was unable to multiply orally (Whitaker et al., 1985).

We probably know most about subcortical contributions to cognition in the domains of language and memory (Crosson, 1992). What is becoming increasingly clear is that a neocortical-limbic dichotomy is too simplistic and that neurological accounts rooted in one or the other entity must accommodate diencephalic and other subcortical systems.

Cerebellum and Higher Functions

Without hesitation, any neurologist will tell you that the signs of cerebellar disease are ataxia, dysmetria, dysarthria, and hypotonia.

Many neurologists, however, are surprised to learn that retinal neurons project to the cerebellum. (Together with collicular relays they direct the eyes toward visual targets.) Some are incredulous that the cerebellum can modulate higher behavior. That cortico-ponto-cerebellar pathways from heteromodal association cortices do modulate behavior, however, was first suggested a century ago (Schmahmann, 1991).

Clinical Observations

An empirical correlation between cerebellar disease and mental symptoms has been made frequently, although pathological analysis and neuropsychological assessment have inconsistently elucidated the meaning of that correlation. The association of intellectual deficits with cerebellar degenerations seems not to have made a deep impression, despite the prominence of cognitive dysfunction in many of the classic reports. For example, patients with cerebellar agenesis or familial cerebellar dysgenesis have been noted as mentally deficient. Individuals with ataxia-telangiectasia or Friedreich's ataxia suffer visuospatial, linguistic, mnestic, and frontal dysfunctions. Those with cerebello-olivary or olivo-ponto-cerebellar degeneration, spastic ataxia, and Marinesco-Sjögren syndrome have either dementia or some degree of psychosis (Kish et al., 1994; Berent et al., 1990).

The reverse association of feeble-mindedness and cerebellar abnormalities has also been noted. As far back as 1926, Ramón y Cajal noted amyloid plaques in all three layers of the cerebellar cortex in Alzheimer's patients. Vermian atrophy in schizophrenics has been confirmed by both autopsy and scanning. Autistic patients have both vermal and hemispheric atrophy on MRI scans, and histology shows depletion of Purkinje cells and neurons of the fastigial, globose, and emboliform nuclei. Nearly the entire neocerebellum is affected in autism. (For the biology of autism, see Gillberg & Coleman, 1993.) Because the Purkinje, granule, and fastigial neuronal loss is unaccompanied by histologic gliosis, it must occur quite early in development, perhaps in the second trimester (Hallett et al., 1993; Courchesne et al., 1994).

Explaining how a conventionally-conceived motor structure profoundly thwarts social communication in autism is explained by assigning the cerebellum a coördinating role in attention that is analogous to its role in coördinating movement. That is, individuals with normal cerebelli find the shifting of mental attention easy, accurate, and propitious. Clumsiness in this regard could be deemed an *attentional dysmetria*.

Evidence accumulates that the cerebellum does indeed participate in cognition. The dentate nucleus (one of the three major output projections) activates during solution of a pegboard puzzle, for example (Kim et al., 1994), and neurosurgeons are becoming increasingly aware that normally-speaking children can become mute following removal of a cerebellar tumor (van Dongen et al., 1994). Agrammatism and abnormal speech similar to that of Broca's aphasia are some of the linguistic disturbances seen in instances of right cerebellar lesions (Silveri et al., 1994).

Cerebellar stimulation via chronically implanted electrodes has improved some patients' mood and lessened their anger and aggression. These changes may last weeks after the last jolt of stimulation. The cerebellum, especially its vermis, has extensive projections with many entities involved in arousal and attention (Courchesne et al., 1994; Nieuwenhuys et al., 1988).

More recent neuropsychological research has disclosed impaired mental imagery and anticipatory planning in individuals with cerebellar hemispheric lesions. Their inability to correctly use temporal clues is independent of any motor deficit. Cerebro-cerebellar loops operate via neocortico-ponto-cerebellar and dentato-thalamo-neocortical circuits projecting mainly to prefrontal heteromodal cortex (Appollonio et al., 1993). It is probable that the cerebellum participates in planning (Grafman et al., 1992), language, and other cognition (Leiner et al., 1991).

Crossed cerebellar diaschisis refers to a unilateral supratentorial lesion causing hypometabolism in the contralateral cerebellar hemisphere (Fulham et al., 1992). Reversed cerebellar diaschisis is sometimes noted. The prevalent view is that diaschisis is caused by afferent interruption from the cortico-ponto-cerebellar pathway. In addition to cerebellar diaschisis in lesions of the cerebral cortex, SPECT scanning shows metabolic activation in the inferolateral neocerebellum during language processes that do not involve movement, as well as in the vermal and paravermal areas during panic and anxiety attacks. Thus, contemporary techniques are currently reappraising the earlier conjecture that the cerebellum does modulate higher behavior (Cole, 1994).

Anatomic Substrates

All heteromodal association cortices project to the pons, where they synapse and then pass through the contralateral middle cerebellar peduncle to the cerebellar cortex. These neurons of the basis pontis project exclusively to the cerebellum. Paralimbic and autonomic projections also synapse here. Therefore, it is possible that the basilar pons contains clusters of neurons that are responsive to multiple modalities. The precise termini to which cortical and limbic projections travel still needs to be determined.

Exactly how the cerebellum modulates behavior is uncertain at this point. Speculations include the possibility that it facilitates nonverbal communication and regulates the speed, capacity, consistency, and appropriateness of cognitive processes. This idea draws a parallel between dysmetria of movement and unpredictable and illogical social interaction—a dysmetria of thought, if you will.

Astute clinicians must first suspect that the cerebellum plays a role in modulation of behavior, then must specifically look for it. In this regard, you are well poised to make contributions that will shed light on this deep issue.

SUGGESTED READINGS

Critchley M. 1953 *The Parietal Lobes*. London: Arnold

Damasio H, Damasio AR. 1989 *Lesion Analysis in Neuropsychology*. New York: Oxford University Press

Kertesz A ed. 1994 *Localization and Neuroimaging in Neuropsychology*. San Diego: Academic Press

Livingston MS. 1988 Art, illusion and the visual system. *Scientific American*, 258:78–85

Nieuwenhuys R, Voogd J, van Huijzen Chr. 1988 *The Human Central Nervous System: A Synopsis and Atlas, 3d ed*. New York: Springer Verlag

III Specific Neuropsychological Topics

No book about any aspect of the brain can pretend to be complete. I have striven for practicality instead of scope since I wanted to exercise your wits, not your arms.

Part I presented conceptualizations about what we think mind and neural tissue are, while Part II guided you through the examination of mental status and briefly described the approximate cerebral loci of common symptoms. At this point, you are like a fresh medical graduate armed with a stethoscope and a copy of the Physicians' Desk Reference—competent enough to deal with common ailments, but not much more.

Part III deals with specific neuropsychological domains, problems that will often confront you in your clinical practice. This section is organized from the general to the specific. Thus, we begin with syndromes of cerebral disconnection that will encourage you, I hope, to think about how neural entities *interact* rather than encouraging your natural tendency to regard them in isolation. Similarly, the succeeding chapter on emotion emphasizes the constant tone that emotion exerts on our mental life. All mental processes have both emotional and cognitive contents at all stages of their development. Other specific neuropsychological topics are addressed in the remaining chapters.

In this third section of the text, you will gain a deeper understanding of various aspects of cognition. The danger that faces anyone studying a specialized field of knowledge is developing a myopic point of view.

At Queen Square, the British neurologists criticized American students for being too eager to whack patients with their reflex hammers. It was almost always the first thing we did. Accordingly, the faculty suggested that we save reflex testing for *last*, because the evaluation of muscular tone, power, proprioception, sensation, and cerebellar function yielded more useful information. We were less likely to forget something important, they suggested, if we saved our favorite maneuver—and the one we seemed to associate exclusively with neurology—for the end.

If you have anticipated my analogy then you may appreciate the importance of keeping the technique of the general medical and neurologic exams in mind, as well as the art of differential diagnosis that entails familiarity with the major categories of neurologic disease. In other words, before rushing in with diagnoses peculiar to our beloved sub-specialty of neuropsychology, I suggest that you mentally rehearse the major categories of neurologic disease. "What else could it be?" should always echo in your mind. You will be a better clinician and less dangerous to patients if you are both broad in your approach and unafraid to confront the limitations of your own knowledge and ability.

7 Disconnection Syndromes

You now know that dissociable factors exist in what appear to be unified mental faculties. In beginning this section of clinical topics with an explication of disconnections I hope to prompt you to think about how various parts of the brain *interact* rather than regarding them as isolated *modules*, a notion that tends to be fostered by concepts of strict localization.

Almost until 1950, the right hemisphere was regarded as a cerebral spare tire. Likewise, the corpus callosum was presumed to serve no function, even though it has more fibers coursing through it to connect the hemispheres than the hemispheres have coming in from the senses. A major reason for this mistaken stance was that patients who had their commissures surgically cut did not have obvious impairments, even on a standard neurologic exam. This is by now a familiar refrain. Only when examiners took pains to invent testing methods that restricted input and response to one hemisphere at a time were glaring deficits readily apparent.

Modality-specific syndromes arise from lesions that disrupt the unimodal projections to various heteromodal, paralimbic, or limbic targets that also serve the projecting modality. The diverse failures of interhemispheric communication that can be clinically apparent in split-brain patients are collectively called *the callosal syndrome*. Although extremely rare, the callosal syndrome is easy to comprehend, and I use it as the major example of disconnections. There are, of course, other disconnections besides those caused by callosal lesions.

Initially, it appeared that each half-brain was an independent entity. That is, we believed that each functioned the same when disconnected as when unified with the opposite side. Later work challenged this assumption and suggested that the connection between the hemispheres is not passive, like an intercom, but dynamically interactive. A specific cognitive skill, such as the ability to work block-design puzzles, is believed to be carried out through the interaction of subprocesses that can be distributed either within or between the hemispheres (Gazzaniga, 1989). This seems reasonable given that brains are inherently unstable. That is, they evolve phylogenetically and are modified ontogenetically by experience. Further research will illuminate this issue.

When we speak of the cerebral commissures we do not refer solely to the corpus callosum but include the anterior commissure, hippocampal commissure, and sometimes the massa intermedia. The following review closely follows the analysis of Joseph Bogen (1993), the American neurosurgeon who has operated on and astutely analyzed the behavior of split-brain patients for some thirty years.

HISTORICAL DEVELOPMENT

Bogen identifies five schools of inquiry into the function of the corpus callosum: (1) the humoral anatomists, (2) the traffic anatomists, (3) the classical neurologists, (4) the critics, and (5) the two-brain theorists.

The *humoral anatomists* theorized in terms of humors rather than neural tissue. This idea began with the Greeks and reached its most elaborate expression in the Renaissance. The cerebrospinal fluid was more esteemed than the brain's solid matter, and the corpus callosum was thought to be only a mechanical prop that kept the fornix from collapsing and crushing the ventricles. Because it was white and harder than the rest of the brain, it was named *tyloeides* in Greek or *callosus* in Latin, both meaning "hard."

The *traffic anatomists* hailing largely from the era of Thomas Willis, thought about traffic, or interaction, among the solid parts of the brain. For two centuries, an integrative function was inferred from the corpus callosum's central location, widespread connections, and noteworthy size. Today, we know that only part of this inference remains true. The corpus callosum fibers myelinate late, suggesting that they are involved in mature cognitive functions. That it does integrate is shown by the symptoms of those in whom their commissures are completely sectioned: A tactile anomia, hemialexia, and an apraxia (all on the left side). That is, patients are unable to name objects placed in the left hand, unable to read in their left field, and are unable to execute left-hand actions that are requested verbally.

The *classical neurologists* worked in the late nineteenth century. The German philosopher Hugo Liepmann (1863–1925) became a psychiatrist-neurologist (Kurt Goldstein called him a "theoretical neuroanatomist") who distinguished *ideation* from *action*. He developed the concept of apraxia to describe a patient who had the callosal syndrome. This patient had left-hand apraxia and agraphia. Instead of postulating direct descending pathways that we would now call ipsilateral control, Liepmann proposed that apraxia resulted from the interruption of callosal projections to the right hemisphere, so that the left hand became unable to carry out verbal commands. Note that the left hand had no weakness or sensory loss, as would be expected if there were a right-hemispheric lesion causing the apraxia and agraphia.

Today we conceive that transcallosal projections are necessary for the left hand to carry out verbal commands, whereas callosal integrity is required for the right hand to access spatial knowledge.

The critics is Bogen's phrase for all those detractors who claimed to find nothing in cases of callosal lesions. For example, in 1936 the American neurosurgeon Walter Dandy (in Bogen, 1993) spoke with the surety that only a surgeon can muster:

The corpus callosum is sectioned longitudinally ... no symptoms follow its division. This simple experiment puts an end to all the extravagant hypotheses on the function of the corpus callosum.

Failure of clinicians to find signs of disconnection most often stemmed from simple confounds arising from inappropriate testing. Indeed, one of Dandy's own patients had a hemialexia that was detected by someone else. Additionally, symptoms are not seen when commissurotomy is incomplete because unsevered remnants can still transfer information between the hemispheres. This is particularly so if the splenium remains intact. Even allowing patients to speak out loud is a confound, as the right hemisphere is able to hear what the left one says. (Some detached right hemispheres do possess an impressive lexicon and symbolic ability. Despite this, language is nearly always limited because its facility with phonology, morphology, and syntax is poor.) It is necessary to avoid cross-communication when testing patients for disconnection symptoms.

Additionally, the critics objected that special cases such as *agenesis of the corpus callosum* did not manifest the callosal syndrome. But the reason for this is that unusually well-developed ipsilateral tracts can transfer visual information via the anterior commissure, which is often hypertrophied in individuals with callosal agenesis. Additionally, transfer of somesthesis between the hemispheres is believed to be due to their unusually well-developed longitudinal bundle of Probst, which might make available to the anterior commissure information that it normally does not carry (Fischer et al., 1992).

Rather than disconnection symptoms, patients with callosal agenesis tend to show intrahemispheric deficits. For example, they have difficulty with fine finger movements, fine tactile localization, finger agnosia, or clumsiness of individual finger movements.

The *two-brain theorists* are the many investigators who have performed commissurotomies on several species and who have argued convincingly that each of the disconnected hemispheres can act independently of the other. This work grew from animal experiments begun by Nobel Laureate Roger Sperry in the 1950s, in which monkeys and cats could learn different solutions—even conflicting ones—to a problem after their commissures had been cut.

Callosum-sectioned cats and monkeys are virtually indistinguishable from their normal cagemates under most tests and training conditions. But if one studies such a "split-brain" monkey more carefully, under special training and testing conditions where the inflow of sensory information to the divided hemispheres can be separately restricted and controlled, one finds that each of the divided hemispheres now has its own independent sphere or cognitive system—that is, its own independent perceptual, learning, memory, and other mental processes . . . it is as if the animals *had two separate brains* (Sperry, 1961 p. 1749).

Perhaps one of the most dramatic illustrations of the apparent possession of two brains is the production of a unilateral Klüver-Bucy syndrome in a split-brain monkey. When the hemisphere with the intact temporal lobe sees, the monkey behaves normally. When the hemisphere with the ablated temporal lobe sees, however, it acts like a typical Klüver-Bucy monkey.

Such experiments alerted Norman Geschwind and Edith Kaplan to await a human with an appropriate lesion to test for disconnection symptoms. In 1962, they found such an individual who had *alexia without agraphia*. As long as they confined stimulation and response to the same hemisphere, the patient performed normally. However, when hemispheric transfer was required, he exhibited a unilateral tactile anomia (inability to name objects in the left hand) although he handled and retrieved objects correctly by touch. Where the right hand wrote normally, the left hand made aphasic errors that frankly surprised him. Autopsy confirmed that a callosal lesion had disconnected the left hand from language areas.

In ensuing years, the association of specific symptoms with callosal lesions, both surgical and naturally occurring ones, was demonstrated repeatedly. Geschwind summarized his ideas in his article, "Disconnexion Syndromes in Animals and Man" (1965a). For him, disconnection involved far more than callosal lesions. In fact, his entire model of language was based on the connection paradigm (Absher & Benson, 1993).

SYMPTOMS OF THE CALLOSAL SYNDROME

Commissurotomy is beneficial in well-selected cases of epilepsy. Initially, the entire length of the corpus callosum, the anterior and hippocampal commissures, and sometimes the massa intermedia were severed in a single operation. Today, surgery tends to be less extreme and the degree of sectioning varies from case to case.

Some of the obvious features of the callosal syndrome compensate within a few months so that the patient appears normal to casual inspection. Yet special testing shows that each hemisphere functions independently and has knowledge and memories that are inaccessible to the other.

Disconnection signs are seen in the four spheres of vision, hearing, movement, and touch. Dichotic listening, tachistoscopic presentation, Purkinje image eye trackers, and similar devices permit selective input to one hemisphere or the other as the examiner wishes.

Visual effects: When objects are presented to the right brain (left visual field), the patient claims to see nothing or at most a flash of light. Most patients cannot verbally identify stimuli, but can do so by touch with the left hand. (The portion of callosotomy patients who have right-hemisphere language is ten to fifteen percent, aprroximately what you would expect from a random sampling of the population.) Objects that are identified in the left visual field cannot be recognized as the same object if they appear in the right field.

Auditory suppression: Words and other sounds are correctly identified if presented to one ear at a time. During dichotic listening, however, only words spoken to the right ear are correctly distinguished.

Motor apraxia: The degree of ipsilateral hand control varies from person to person and so, therefore, will the severity of left-hand apraxia. Undoubtedly, this variation accounts for some of the negative results reported by Bogen's "critics." Motor apraxia compensates with time so that it may not interfere with daily life. However, it can be clinically demonstrated to persist to some degree for years.

Patients have difficulty with such commands as, "Wiggle your left toes" or "Make a fist with your left hand." Apraxia exists for two reasons: Poor comprehension of the right hemisphere and poor ipsilateral motor control by a left hemisphere that understands verbal commands quite well.

Somesthetic transfer: Failure of both lemniscal and spinothalamic sensory transfer is shown by (1) cross-localization failure of fingertip sensation, (2) the failure to cross-replicate hand postures, and (3) the failure to cross-retrieve objects felt by the opposite hand.

The failure to cross-localize a touch stimulus to the fingertips is demonstrated as follows. With the patient's palms up, you touch a fingertip with a pencil point and ask the individual to indicate which finger was touched by opposing the thumb to it. This is done out of sight for obvious reasons, and answering with the thumb removes language from the task. Split-brain patients can do this sensory task with either hand with nearly 100% accuracy. When the response condition is changed so that they must now indicate which finger was touched by opposing the contralateral thumb and finger, performance falls below chance level. Intact adults achieve better than 90% accuracy at this cross-localizing task; children usually are incompetent, possibly because the callosum myelinates later in life. (An unanswered question is, "When is it sufficiently myelinated to permit cross-localization?" We do not yet know if there is a discrepancy between the age at which humans can cross-localize and the age at which the callosum is reasonably well myelinated.)

The failure to cross-replicate hand postures refers to an inability to imitate hand postures that the examiner imprints on the opposite, unseen hand. This demonstrates failure of proprioceptive transfer. With the patient's hand out of sight, the examiner molds it into a certain posture—forming a circle with the thumb and fourth finger, for example. The patient is then asked to make a fist (to "erase" the posture), and then to assume the former pose. When asked to put the opposite hand into the same posture, patients are unable to do so. This failure of proprioceptive transfer can be shown in either direction.

Lastly, one can demonstrate the failure to cross-retrieve small objects hidden from sight. The right hand can name and manipulate objects appropriately, but we have already seen that the left hand has a tactile anomia. Either hand, however, can retrieve the same object from a collection of unseen objects, thereby demonstrating that each hemisphere has recognition. Split-brain patients distinguish themselves from intact persons by the inability of one hand to retrieve an object that was felt initially with the other.

Testing for Callosal Signs

The following maneuvers used to confirm signs of suspected callosal disconnection apply only to right-handed persons. The situation in non-right-handers is complex, and you should refer to secondary sources.

History
A history of conflicting bodily actions, intermanual conflict in which actions of the left hand are contrary to whatever else is going on, and patients' astonishment at the capacity of their left hands to act independently of volition are all historical points that suggest callosal disconnection.

An example of intermanual conflict would be buttoning with one hand while simultaneously unbuttoning with the other. The patient is bewildered by such behavior, and the left hand seems to act on its own. This clinical observation is old, but the relatively new term *"le main étrangère"* caught on (Brion & Jedynak, 1972) and referred specifically to individuals with callosal lesions. The inelegant translation of "alien hand" attempts to describe the patient's feeling that their left hand behaves strangely or is in fact alien. Although it is the hand that usually executes contrary acts, the entire left side of the body is capable of being uncoöperative. One of Bogen's patients complained for years of difficulty in getting his left foot to go in the same direction as the rest of him. Whether the alien hand is truly part of the callosal syndrome or a result of surgical retraction of the right hemisphere—and thus actually a manifestation of medial frontal dysfunction (namely, the supplementary motor area)—is not fully resolved (Banks et al., 1989). On rare occasions, one finds the term *alien hand* applied to the disturbance of body schema and somatosensory anosognosia of parietal lesions (Gasquoine, 1993; Feinberg et al., 1992). The two clinical phenomena should not be confused.

Examination

(1) A *right verbal anosmia* is demonstrated when the patient is unable to name smells presented to only the right nostril. The anterior commissure must be severed to produce this defect (recall that the anterior commissure connects the phylogenetically old anterior parts of the temporal lobes whereas the rest of the temporal lobe uses the corpus callosum). This is not a defect of smell but of naming. Patients can match odors presented to the right nostril by selecting objects that represent the smell.

(2) *Double hemianopia* is a way to test for splenial disconnection when you do not have a tachistoscope handy. The patient is instructed to keep both eyes open, remain silent, and sit on one hand to keep it out of the way. When you then test the visual fields by confrontation in the standard manner, the patient will point only to the field on the side of the indicating hand. That is, the homonymous hemianopia will appear to switch sides depending on which hand does the pointing. Double hemianopia is a symmetrical sign, thus distinguishing it from the simultaneous sen-

sory extinction that is seen often in parietal lobe lesions on either side.

(3) *Hemialexia* (the inability to read in one half of the visual field) is present in the left visual field if the splenium is disconnected. You must first verify that a left hemianopia is not present.

(4) *Left ideomotor apraxia* means that the individual is unable to carry out with the left hand an action that is readily done with the right. The key observation here is that the patient makes deft but incorrect movements with the left hand.

Test this by asking the patient to imitate an action, such as saluting, inserting a key in a lock, or combing the hair. The right hand will easily imitate these actions; the left will not. However, when given a real key or comb in the left hand, the patient performs correctly. Bogen feels that the inability to carry out skilled movements with the left hand is strong evidence for a callosal lesion. Unfortunately, there is often weakness or sensory loss due to extension of the causative lesion to adjacent tissue, and the apraxia may be difficult to demonstrate.

(5) *Left-hand agraphia.* Most intact right-handed persons can write adequately with the left hand, an ability lacking in the callosal syndrome. In contrast to this inability to write with the left hand, those with the callosal syndrome can readily copy even complex geometric figures with their left hand.

(6) *Left-hand tactile anomia* has already been discussed. To exclude the possible confound of astereognosis one can ask the patient to retrieve the felt objects from a box of similar objects. It is necessary, of course, to test this outside of vision. My previous comments about the unreliability of blindfolds are especially important here.

(7) *Right-hand constructional apraxia* can be demonstrated with drawing, blocks, or large puzzles. Constructional apraxia per se can occur with lesions of either hemisphere, although each hemisphere produces different qualitative errors. In disconnection, constructional apraxia is seen only in the right hand.

(8) *Spatial acalculia.* Most people perform arithmetic better with paper and pencil than they do in their heads; the opposite is true in the callosal syndrome. Because of their right-handed disability for spatial forms, patients have trouble with math on paper. Similar

spatial abilities may be seen in those who sketch regularly, such as architects and graphic artists.

OTHER DISCONNECTION SYNDROMES

Alexia Without Agraphia

Alexia can occur with or without agraphia. When it occurs without agraphia it is commonly explained as a disconnection syndrome and has been so explained since the first case of Dejerine in 1892. His patient, who had infarcts of the left occipital lobe and splenium, could write whole pages to dictation without error, but was unable to read anything he had written in his own hand! A musician, he could also no longer read notes.

The left occipital lesion produces a right homonymous hemianopia. The splenial lesion keeps information presented to the right occipital lobe from crossing to the left side. Therefore, no visual information that is necessary for reading reaches the left angular gyrus. This conceptualization involving double lesions, particularly the splenial one, explains the ability to write correctly to dictation while being unable to read the information that does reach the right occipital lobe.

This tidy explanation is not totally convincing. Alas, cases of alexia without agraphia occur in which the splenium appears intact. There are also cases in which no right homonymous hemianopia can be found. Finally, patients can often name objects but not words; one wonders how this can be if there is a splenial disconnection.

The typical analysis of why patients can sometimes recognize objects but not words is not wholly satisfactory: Incomplete splenial lesions may permit partial or degraded information to reach the left hemisphere, which may be sufficient for gross recognition of objects but not for fine discrimination of letters and words. Hence, patients cannot read because reading is argued to be a more demanding task than object recognition.

The occasional absence of right homonymous hemianopia as well as those cases in which the splenium appears intact are rebutted more satisfactorily. Anatomy shows that the angular gyrus receives dorsal and ventral inputs from the splenium as well as medial and lateral inputs from striate cortex. Splenial-occipital alexia with hemianopia is the usual type of disconnection seen, in which there is the combination of splenial and occipital lesions (left lingual and fusiform gyri).

The infrequent cases of splenial-occipital alexia without hemianopia are caused by dual lesions in the splenium and in afferent pathways from the left calcarine cortex. In this situation, the calcarine cortex is intact so there is no hemianopia, although it is disconnected from the left angular gyrus and thereby produces alexia. Lesions undercutting the subangular gyrus can either spare or involve the optic radiations, again accounting for cases either with or without hemialexia. So, some type of disconnection seems to account for all forms of pure alexia after all. Now would be a good time for you to consult your atlas and review the white matter fascicles that project to and from the occipital lobe.

Alexia without agraphia is revisited in chapter 12, where we look at its relationship to visual agnosia.

Pure Word Deafness

I mentioned this auditory agnosia briefly in chapter 6. It is a bilateral disconnection of Wernicke's area from auditory input. It is rare, because there must be a unilateral lesion in the subcortical temporal lobe that interrupts the left auditory radiations as well as those callosal fibers from the opposite side that project to Wernicke's area.

These patients recognize nonverbal environmental sounds and can read, write, and speak relatively well. In stark contrast is their inability to understand speech. The term *pure word deafness* indicates that individuals are relatively free of aphasic symptoms. Stroke is most often the cause.

Patients foremost have a Wernicke's aphasia. Even as the alexia and agraphia gradually resolve, patients still cannot comprehend spoken language. Brainstem auditory evoked responses are normal, indicating intact pathways up to the auditory radiations. The problem therefore seems to be one of discriminating sounds, and is distinct from the problem of transcortical sensory aphasia in which comprehension is also impaired. In transcortical sensory aphasia, words and sounds are perceived normally and the patient can repeat them. Repetition is not possible in pure word deafness.

Speech seems muffled, or sounds like a foreign language. Sometimes, patients can actually recognize foreign languages because their prosody is so different from spoken English. For the same reason they may also be able to determine who is speaking, but not what is being said. This suggests a preserved ability to comprehend paralinguistic aspects of speech, including the emotional intent of speech. The ability of patients with pure word deafness to watch other people speak allows them to utilize gesture and facial expression to partially counteract their failed aural speech comprehension.

ADVANCED ISSUES REGARDING THE COMMISSURES

I do not wish to leave you with an overly mechanistic impression of the corpus callosum or its role in clinical neuropsychology. To be frank, we really know very little about the nature of the information it transfers. Is it sensory, abstract, or something else? Is transfer bidirectional or unidirectional, and does the nature of what is conveyed vary depending on the type of cortex connected, or perhaps the context of the stimulus? These remain unanswered questions.

More interhemispheric connections exist than the ones I have just discussed. For example, we know little of the function of the habenular, hippocampal, and posterior commissures. Figure 6.1 showed how the subcortical commissure of the pulvinar and the brachium of the superior colliculus project the most peripheral parts of the retina to visual cortices of both hemispheres. These subcortical commissures as well as other divergent retinal projections are one possible explanation of blindsight, for example.

Different sections of the callosum transfer different modalities. Both the splenium and anterior commissure, for example, participate in transfer of visual patterns, color, and brightness. Anterior to the splenium one finds somesthetic transfer, while the most anterior parts connect the frontal lobes in which subcortical circuits are known to mediate many aspects of human behavior (Cummings, 1993).

MRI scans now are used to verify whether commissurotomy is complete or whether unsevered fibers remain. Detailed study of split-brain patients who do have callosal remnants, the locus and extent of which are known with certainty, are beginning to clarify *what is transferred and how*. For example, semantic knowledge can transfer in the anterior part.

In general, these studies are beginning to reveal the remarkable specificity of *what* is communicated between the hemispheres (Gazzaniga et al., 1989). Gazzaniga's patient VP, for example, is capable of comparing both phonological and orthographic information across hemispheres in making correct judgements about whether words rhyme when they both look alike and sound alike. However, she cannot make correct judgements given other combinations of phonology and orthography (e.g., when words sound alike but look different, sound different but look alike, or both sound and look different). The specificity of this finding is notable given that in previous studies she showed no ability to transfer information between her hemispheres. The point is that such cases, which illustrate the cross-integration of highly circumscribed information, make it necessary to prove even the simplest inference.

Contemporary MRI studies of patients who underwent commissurotomy twenty or more years ago confirm that the callosal syndrome appears only with complete severing of the commissures. Yet naturally occurring lesions such as tumors, trauma, and hemorrhages cause disconnection when a small part of either the anterior or posterior callosum is destroyed. This paradox is unresolved.

Old arguments over Liepmann's conceptualization of apraxia, however, may be nearly settled. The apraxia following callosal lesions appears to be truly due to callosal damage rather than to the supplementary motor area that is often associated with naturally occurring lesions. Clinical cases also support the idea that the left hemisphere is dominant for praxis in both hands, although the robustness of its expression varies among individuals. Verbal apraxia endures longer than visual apraxia and, therefore, how you test patients matters. For example, miming an action to command is more difficult than visual imitation (Graff-Radford et al., 1987).

Your own visual inspection of scans has by now impressed on you that the configuration of the corpus callosum varies considerably from person to person. But does this have any significance?

One study found that the mean callosal area did not differ significantly between normal individuals and epileptics, between left-handed and right-handed individuals, or between men and women. However, the mean callosal area was greater by 18% to 28% in persons with right-hemispheric speech as determined by the Wada test. These individuals contrast to those with either left-hemisphere or bilateral speech representation. This difference is significant and could represent as many as 37 to 54 million additional callosal axons in subjects with right-hemisphere speech dominance (O'Kusky et al., 1988).

Because the number of callosal axons in neonates exceeds that in young adults, these inquiries bear on the topic of non-standard cerebral organization discussed earlier (chapter 3). They suggest that individuals with right-hemispheric speech undergo less physiologic necrosis in the competition for synaptic targets.

In the 1970s, demonstration of consistent asymmetries in the planum temporale led to the demonstration of other neural asymmetries in lateralized structures, and by the 1980s, neuroanatomic interest had turned to individual differences in the midline morphology of the commissures (Witelson, 1992). The human adult corpus callosum varies greatly in shape and size (as measured by width, area, axis length, and perimeter). Gender and functional asymmetries are currently receiving much attention, though all we can say presently is that gender differences in callosal anatomy are not attributable to any measure of overall brain size between the sexes. When considering the factors of sex, age, hand preference, and hand consistency one can assign shared features of callosal morphology to two dichotomous groups: Consistent right-handers and inconsistent right-handers (Cowell et al., 1994) rather than simply considering the writing hand as was done earlier. A sex-related (possibly hormonal) factor acting during gestation may explain a larger anterior half in inconsistent right-hand males and a larger posterior midbody in consistent right-hand females (Habib et al., 1991).

In schizophrenia, one sees developmental abnormalities of both the corpus callosum and those limbic structures with which it is intimate embryologically (i.e., hippocampal formation, fornix, septum pellucidum, and cingulum). We know that individuals with callosal agenesis also show abnormalities in the aforementioned limbic structures, and that neuropathological studies have particularly implicated abnormal neurogenesis in the hippocampal formation and cingulate gyrus in schizophrenia, an extremely common mental illness (prevalence, 1%).

The term *agenesis* is a misnomer given that callosal axons actually are formed; the pathology lies in their failure to cross the midline (Swayze et al., 1990). Compared to 0.1% for callosal agenesis in the general population, the prevalence rate of 1.4% for callosal agenesis in schizophrenia is significant ($p < 0.001$). At present, callosal abnormalities in schizophrenics are associated not with mental retardation but with severe, refractory delusions and hallucinations. If you have imputed a causal relationship between the two, you stand rebuked because there are far more patients with schizophrenia who have normal callosi. Neither are there any reports of patients with surgical commissurotomies who have turned psychotic. Instead, a small subset of schizophrenics appear to have gross developmental anomalies of the callosum and related limbic structures, suggesting that there may be more subtle limbic abnormalities in patients with schizophrenia in general. Histologic dystrophies do exist in schizophrenia, and this seems a fruitful association to pursue.

The last advanced issue I want to address is whether we "really" do have multiple minds in our single heads. Gazzaniga, among others, suggests that conscious awareness is asymmetrically distributed and represented only in the left hemisphere. Evidence for this comes from split-brain patients. In particular, one asks to what extent overt behavior is governed by non-conscious processes.

One of Gazzaniga's patients, JW, was able to name or write about information presented only to the right hemisphere, a capacity not seen in adults who have complete, verified commissurotomies. Further experiments showed that his capacity was not an instance of right-hemispheric expression but that somehow his right hemisphere was able to induce his left one to respond in speech or writing. Moreover, the left hemisphere was not consciously aware that it possessed the information transmitted to it by the right brain (Gazzaniga et al., 1987). This finding is remarkable. Then again, it is hard for those who have never personally examined a split-brain patient to appreciate the visceral resonance that witnessing such a dissociation produces. Split-brain patients are extraordinarily rare but, should you ever have the opportunity to examine one, the interaction may permanently upset your comfortable certainty about mental unity.

Evidence for non-conscious cognitive processes also comes from a variety of circumstances such as blindsight; the capacity of amnesics to learn skills but to have no recollection of their training; learning during anesthesia (Jelicic et al., 1992); the capacity of those with parietal lesions to use information in their extinguished hemifield which they cannot "see"; and a galvanic skin response in prosopagnosia, which indicates that covert facial recognition has occurred at an autonomic level.

Gazzaniga himself is surprised, though he shouldn't be:

The dramatic finding that a left hemisphere response system such as speech can be prepared and capable of functioning without the left hemisphere being aware of the information the speech system possesses is consistent with the view that preconscious processes can be active in the production of behaviors.

These kinds of dissociations seem still more paradoxical given that even patients who have had complete commissurotomies still retain a subjective sense of mental unity. This is true despite the experimental evidence that each disconnected half-brain has separate and isolated experiences.

Based on the observation that commissurotomized patients seldom display signs of confusion or dissociation in their activities outside the neuropsychology laboratory, Canadian psychologist Justine Sergent (1950–1994) offered the provocative viewpoint that perceptual disunity and behavioral unity could coëxist because *subcortical structures* permitted information divided between the disconnected hemispheres to be related and acted on. In other words, she argued that the empirical evidence points to a *mental disconnection at the level of informational content but a coherence at the level of behavior* (Sergent, 1987). Although brainstem areas are intimately involved in the regulation and elaboration of behavior, they are limited, and Sergent suggests that processes involving a many-to-one rather than a one-to-one mapping may be within the functional capacity of subcortical structures that are operative in split-brain patients.

Far less satisfactorily, Gazzaniga (1989) speculates that the left brain includes an "interpreter" that generates hypotheses about an individual's responses. The interpretation is of course unique to the individual because it has access to past experiences and future goals. For example, mood shifts can be induced by experimentally manipulating the disconnected right hemisphere. When one induces a positive mood the left hemisphere interprets positively whatever is happening to it. Similarly, when the right hemisphere triggers a negative mood, the left hemisphere will suddenly interpret negatively a previously neutral situation. The purported interpreter makes up a reason why the mood has changed that sounds plausible to the left hemisphere but that has no real basis. (Some might ask if manipulating the right hemisphere isn't real in the sense that it sustains an actual physiologic change.)

That the left hemisphere contains such an interpreter that comes up with plausible reasons for our behavior and why things are the way they are is not so radical an idea as Gazzaniga seems to think. There is no reason to resort to "interpreters" or other sorts of homunculi. Research on what are called *cognitive errors* and *cognitive dissonance* lay bare the long-standing human tendency to find patterns, associations, and cause-and-effect relationships where none in fact exist (Gilovich, 1991). That is, we seem to have a penchant to explain "why" and an innate tendency to impose order on chance occurrences, perhaps in an effort to bring order to a disordered world.

8   Emotion, Consciousness, and Subjectivity

Emotion permeates every experience. Mental process has both emotional and cognitive content at all stages of its development. But despite the rich phenomenology of both consciousness and emotion, we understand them only superficially. Vestiges of behaviorism's Draconian restrictions against the study of "inner" and "unobservable" states are largely responsible for this circumstance, although Flanagan (1992) enumerates other reasons for our paltry knowledge. I am optimistic that both bottom-up and top-down approaches will be fruitful as they penetrate these issues.

Precisely because our understanding is weak and our approaches to the phenomenology of emotion and consciousness diverse, the contents of this chapter may not seem coherent on first reading. I did not wish to halt describing merely the cerebral localization of emotional symptoms, however, because growing interest in emotion and consciousness makes these topics ones with which students should be familiar, even though initially they may seem more philosophical than practical.

We reviewed in chapter 3 how emotion exerts a constant tone and how it is more than the extreme up and down states by which we customarily label it. We are continually in an emotional state, and that state is ever changing. This chapter considers (1) the clinical manifestations of emotional symptoms whose cerebral localization is known, (2) how the phenomenal dichotomy between reason and emotion does not hold up at the neural level, (3) how emotion influences cognition and how the two are not necessarily congruent, (4) the illusive nature of self-awareness, (5) a distributed system that sustains the attentional matrix and directs its focus to desired targets, and (6) the false dichotomy between first-person and third-person points of view that are usually labeled *subjective* and *objective*, respectively.

The anatomy of emotion is largely, but not exclusively, that of the limbic system and frontal lobes. The central limbic axis is modulated not only by hippocampal and amygdalar inputs, but also by ascending visceral afferents from spinal cord and medulla as well as by circulating molecules (volume transmission). I pointed out earlier that the central nervous system has an emotional core reaching down to the spinal cord. Because the components of this core are reciprocally interactive, they constitute a distributed system (a neural organization that was explicated in chapter 3). It is probably worth repeating here that the primary emotional constituent of the neocortex is the prefrontal lobes; that of mesocortex the cingulate gyrus; that of archicortex, the hippocampal formation; that of basal ganglia the amygdala; that of the diencephalon, the dorsal thalamus and hypothalamus; that of midbrain, the central gray; that of pons and medulla the nuclei of autonomic relays; and that of spinal cord, the intermediolateral cell column nuclei.

The hypothalamus is the suprasegmental integrator of both sympathetic and parasympathetic autonomic divisions. We can say broadly that the hypothalamus is concerned with the expression of emotion whereas cortex is concerned with its experience. The hypothalamus is the center of the limbic system and projects and its efferents in three directions in a way somewhat analogous to that of Papez's division of diencephalic projections (see the box, "Papez's Three Thalamic 'Streams'," in chapter 3).

Papez's "three streams" of *movement* (basal ganglia), *thought* (neocortex), and *feeling* (limbic system) as well as the hippocampo-mammillo-thalamo-cingulate-hippocampal Papez circuit appeared in chapter 3. In chapter 6, I reviewed the salient manifestations of focal lesions involving frontal, temporal, and limbic structures. You should now grasp that all these structures are capable of modulating emotion as part of a larger behavioral expression that contains both objective and subjective elements. In particular, dysfunction of paralimbic and limbic tissue can severely disrupt the synergy among sensation, thought, behavior, and feeling.

EMOTION AND FOCAL LESIONS

Great license is taken with the term *emotional*. Most people's concept of emotion is both heuristic and psychodynamic. The emotional response that follows any disease, such as stroke or cancer, or the emotional exacerbation of symptoms (such as anxiety or the presence of an audience worsening the tremor of Parkinson's disease) is really a general medical issue that is not unique to neuropsychology. Also, some circadian, environmental, and endocrine factors that modulate emotion have not customarily been considered part of neuropsychology's domain. An example is seasonal affective disorder, a periodic depression that depends on the duration of the photoperiod. Shift work, sleep deprivation, and either periodic or episodic hormonal changes in both men and women are further illustrations. Whether officially part of a discipline's domain or not, however, it needs saying that those who hope to arrive at the big picture must consider all such aspects.

To make this discussion manageable, we will first proceed from the assumption that emotion is physically mediated and, second, limit our discussion to those neural-behavioral relationships wherein a physical basis can reasonably be ascertained. These constraints are of course arbitrary, but they do aim to keep us focused on the neurological side of neuropsychology.

Cerebral lesions can alter mood, affect, and emotional tone. These changes may be subtle or dramatic. Emotion requires an appropriate cognitive state as well as arousal that is mediated by the reticular formation, thalamic nuclei, and frontal neocortex. The hypothalamus generates the visceral part of emotion and is itself influenced by limbic entities that in turn receive input from the cortex, particularly the frontal lobes. In short, *emotion is affected by cortical, basal ganglionic, limbic, and hypothalamic structures.*

Not long ago we thought that depression following cerebral lesions was a normal and common-sense reaction to loss. That is, we made up psychodynamic explanations, forgetting a prime axiom that science usually is counterintuitive. Now, we know that mood change is both a direct effect of a lesion as well as one due to interruption of aminergic projections. This fact suggests treatment with antidepressants. Although biogenic amines clearly are involved in emotional arousal, however, the situation is not so straightforward that you can expect currently prescribed antidepressants to produce the same behavioral effects as catecholamine or indolamine agonists. This is because some antidepressants reduce the number of postsynaptic receptors and actually decrease the level of aminergic transmission.

In our eagerness to document external and so-called objective signs of disease, we sometimes forget that some illnesses present solely with a dramatic alteration of feeling or comportment. The examples of acute frontal lesions and herpes simplex encephalitis should come to mind. Less well known is the fact that unprovoked rage can be the main feature of neurologic disease, occurring in a small proportion of mental retardates, and individuals with psychomotor seizures, hemorrhagic leukoëncephalitis, or temporal lobe glioma. Most criminals are neurologically normal, yet neurologists have often been asked to justify the violence of such criminals (Pincus, 1993; Restak, 1993). Although there is evidence that brain damage can unleash violent behavior, it does not explain it.

Well-recognized emotional signs are lability (the unstable transition from one mood to another), forced laughing or crying, violent outbursts, placidity or apathy, hyposexuality or hypersexuality, panic, and the dysphoria that accompanies acute autonomic storms (e.g., tachycardia or bradycardia, bronchospasm and bronchorrhea, hypersalivation, diaphoresis, pallor, gastrointestinal hypermotility [with consequent borborygamy, diarrhea, or nausea], piloerection, and so forth). The lesions responsible for some effects are well localized whereas the anatomic correlations of others remain unsettled.

Neocortical Lesions

Previous analyses of the neurology of emotion tended to assign a unitary character to the emotional processing of each hemisphere. For example, the right hemisphere was said to deal with unpleasant "negative" emotions, whereas the left hemisphere was said to concern itself with pleasant "positive" ones. This overly simple scheme has never been substantiated, although the model did acquire a richer texture once we began to distinguish between emotional feeling, emotional surveillance, the appropriate direction of attention, and the communication of affect (via speech, behavior, or both).

One's emotional state depends on a correct analysis of conditions, but cognitive awareness alone turns out to be insufficient to inform emotion. Patients with frontal lesions, for example, exhibit a classic dissociation between cognitive discrimination and their usual placidity. Cortical lesions influence emotions through (1) inadequate cognitive appraisal, (2) impaired arousal, and (3) disconnection of cognition from limbic-hypothalamic influence.

Lesions of either hemisphere (though more often the right one) uncouple verbal behavior, affective behavior, and the internal mood that one feels. Verbal-behavioral dissociations engendered by emotion-producing lesions are similar to those witnessed in split-brain patients. That is, patients may show vegetative signs, act depressed, and even go so far as to attempt suicide—yet they vigorously deny feeling depressed. Instances such as these are stout caveats against uncritical reliance on verbal reports in the presence of contradictory external signs.

Dissociations of speech and action do not necessarily relieve patients from actually feeling deep concern, or even mental anguish, about their plight, all the while acting euphoric, facetious, or perhaps even gripped by uncontrollable laughter. Conversely, flatness, placidity, and detachment may lead you to conclude erroneously that a patient is clinically depressed when in fact the individual is not.

The orbitofrontal cortex receives inputs from the amygdala and anterior thalamic nuclei, and is also the neocortical terminus for all the multiplex neocortical projections whose cascade begins in idiotypic cortices. *A key member of both limbic system and the paracrine core, the orbitofrontal cortex is the only neocortical projection to the hypothalamus that consists entirely of heteromodal cortex.* It is not surprising, therefore, that focal lesions produce emotional flatness and abandonment of personal and social strictures, as if thoughts can no longer relate personal actions to one's internal experiences.

Right-Hemisphere Effects

Individuals with right-hemisphere lesions may be impaired by apathy, an unrealistic appraisal of emotional priorities, and flawed feeling or affective expression. One reason for altered emotional *expression* is that right-hemisphere lesions dampen arousal more often than do left ones. Right-hemisphere lesions are often associated with euphoria or indifference (e.g., the profound indifference of anosognosia), difficulty comprehending the affect of someone else, or difficulty in expressing one's own affect. Interestingly, such patients' lack of appropriate concern extends beyond their immediate physical illness to include indifference to such matters as financial woes or social conflicts. Bear (1983) suggests that this represents a failure of emotional surveillance to sustain attention, register emotional concern, and initiate an adaptive response to a perceived threat.

What is said constitutes the linguistic content of speech, whereas how it is said conveys its affective content. *Perception* of others' emotional intent is related to the right hemisphere's mediation of prosody, attitude, and the kinetics (gestural aspects and visage) of emotional perception and expression. *Prosody* refers in part to nonverbal aspects of speech such as pitch, tempo, rhythm, and melodiousness. But prosody also conveys affect. The superiority of the right hemisphere to recognize and respond appropriately to the affect contained in prosody has been shown by lesion analysis, dichotic listening, discrimination testing, and the Wada test.

Patients with right-hemisphere lesions also have difficulty interpreting visual stimuli such as facial expression, gestures, cartoons, and the general *mise-en-scène*. We believe this is related somehow to the right hemisphere's talent for recognizing faces and the related observation that tachistoscopic viewing in normal individuals consistently shows a right-hemisphere superiority in discriminating facial emotion. Regional cerebral blood flow also shows increased right hemisphere activation, especially frontal and parietal, when volunteers discriminate facial emotion (Gur et al., 1994).

When it comes to expressing emotion, patients with right-hemisphere lesions have difficulty inflecting neutral sentences, even though they understand what is required of them. They may also have difficulty remembering emotionally charged discourse or stories. The faces of individuals with right-hemisphere damage are less expressive than those of their counterparts who have left-hemisphere injury. (In normal subjects, emotions are said to be expressed more intensely on the left side of the face.)

Patients who fail to apprehend negative nonverbal feedback commonly frustrate their caretakers. Explicit declarations, on the other hand (e.g., saying "Jack, you make me very angry when you pull out your catheter. Don't do that."), can produce the desired results. That is, it helps if you repeatedly remind the language hemisphere about the individual's proclivity to neglect, discount, and overlook social cues. Such patients appear to have both impaired cognition and reduced arousal, a conclusion supported by the demonstration of dampened galvanic skin resistance.

Left-Hemisphere Effects
Patients with left-hemisphere lesions tend to be depressed. Their MMPIs show elevation of the depression scale, whereas those with matched right-hemisphere lesions do not. Differences in emotional reactions between patients with similar lesions on different sides are not entirely due to differences in their perception and expression of affect. What causes patients with left-hemisphere brain damage to be depressed is not certain, although disruption of asymmetrically distributed norepinephrine projections is suspected (Starkstein & Robinson, 1993). Depression is most often seen in patients who have anterior perisylvian lesions and nonfluent aphasias. The severity of their depression in such instances led to the descriptor *catastrophic reaction.*

This description is unfortunately misleading because even patients with severe aphasia are able to intone their utterances affectively, possibly via right-hemispheric pathways that remain intact. Typically, individuals with Wernicke's aphasia can easily communicate anger and exasperation. Some nonfluent aphasics may actually be very fluent when using expletives. They can also communicate by facial expression and gesture.

Galvanic skin resistance measurements show that individuals with left-hemisphere disease are hyperaroused compared to normals; those with right-hemisphere lesions are hypoaroused.

The right-positive and left-negative dichotomy is not universally accepted. In a neurosurgical series of 141 patients with brain tumors, lesions of heteromodal frontal or parietal association cortices, combined with paralimbic lesions, caused a negative mood; lesions in sensorimotor cortices assuaged the negative effects of the heteromodal and paralimbic lesions. The state of a patient's mood was not influenced by the laterality of the lesions (Irle et al., 1994).

Limbic Lesions

Ablation of the amygdala produces placidity, as seen in the Klüver-Bucy syndrome, named after the German psychologist Heinrich Klüver and the American neurosurgeon Paul Bucy, who described a dramatic behavioral syndrome in 1937 after extirpating both temporal lobes in the monkey (Klüver, 1937; Klüver & Bucy, 1939). Such animals (1) lose their powerful and customary aggressive-fear reactions and become surprisingly docile, (2) indiscriminately attempt fornication regardless of the appropriateness of the target, and (3) are unable to discriminate visually the edible from the inedible, putting nearly every object, both animate and inanimate, in their mouths for inspection.

The singular deficit in these diverse manifestations is a failure to *associate emotional drive with an appropriate extrapersonal target*. Drive remains normal; its association with a proper target is what fails. Today, we think that the Klüver-Bucy syndrome is expressed when the amygdala is severed from its cortical inputs (Mesulam, 1985a).

The anatomist Walle Nauta has characterized the amygdala as an "active explorer" of the world, a concept that counteracts the passé, hierarchical view of neocortical dominance by emphasizing the "omnisensory" amygdala's robust modulation of neocortex. The standard model thinks of sensation as projecting inward. The amygdala demonstrates the reverse situation, wherein connections are directed outward, projecting to those parts of the neocortex that receive the final cascade of sensory data *en route* to the limbic system. What projects from the neocortex is "a repeatedly preprocessed multisensory appreciation of the organism's environment" (Nauta & Feirtag, 1986).

In contrast to the placidity of amygdalar lesions, those of the septum lead to irritability and rage. The septum is the classical pleasure center based on animal stimulations. Patients with septal tumors (destructive lesions) may fly into a rage and exhibit general irritability. Patients who receive electrical stimulation of the septum confirm that the sensation is in fact pleasurable or even explicitly sexual. Anterior temporal lobectomy performed for seizures has been reported to increase sexuality.

Hypersexuality in either gender is rare but well documented in neurologic disease. Standard explanation is that the removal of moral and social restraints by orbitofrontal lesions leads to indiscriminate sexual actions. Similarly, the general apathy produced by superior frontal lesions is said to reduce all impulses, including sexual ones. Rarely, a hypersexual frenzy can develop abruptly in encephalitis or gradually in instances of temporal tumors. Presumably, the medial dorsal thalamus, medial forebrain bundle, or septal preoptic region is involved in such instances because these are the limbic structures from which MacLean could evoke erection and orgasm by electrical stimulation.

Although the hypothalamus figures largely in both theories of animal emotion and in the human Papez circuit, patients with lesions restricted to the hypothalamus only show an unexpectedly low incidence of altered social-emotional behavior. It appears that some of the neural circuits whose damage is implicated in well-described emotional symptoms by-pass hypothalamic nuclei (Weddell, 1994).

Type I herpes simplex virus produces a hemorrhagic necrosis of the inferomedial temporal and orbitofrontal lobes. Emotional lability, impulsivity and other disinhibition, distractibility, agitation, and amnesia are frequent and often permanent sequellæ if patients survive. Adults essentially revert, behaviorally speaking, to impulsive and unwieldy children. Limbic encephalitis is also associated with carcinoma and produces a clinical picture similar to that of herpetic encephalitis. Lastly, the neurotropic rabies virus has a predilection for limbic entities and produces profound anxiety and agitation.

Gelastic (laughing) and *dacrystic* (crying) seizures are associated with temporal foci. Auras associated with temporal lobe seizures may be pleasurable, fearful, sexual, or disgusting. Fear is the ictal affect most common in temporal lobe seizures (though it can also be experienced because of cingulate foci). The hippocampus plays a time-limited role in fearful memories evoked by polymodal (contextual), but not unimodal stimuli (Kim & Fanselow, 1992). The amygdala appears to be the structure critical for the experience of fear.

Behavioral manifestations of limbic epilepsy are discussed in chapter 11.

Basal Ganglia Lesions

In the hierarchical model of brain organization, the basal ganglia were considered motor relays. Compelling evidence that their dysfunction can produce either cognitive or emotional symptoms changed this view. MacLean (1990) and others showed that lesions here exclusively produce not motor symptoms, but alterations in behavior that are highly complex and even species-specific. The basal ganglia and thalamus can evoke emotional symptoms because they influence cortical and limbic tone via specific neurotransmitter projections.

Depression is common in both Parkinson's disease and dementia, each of which suffer marked degeneration of basal nuclei and corresponding neurotransmitters. That the depression is not an entirely reactive one is demonstrated by a poor correlation between mood and motor impairment. Not surprisingly, depression in either group fails to respond to L-dopa or cholinergic agonists. Because norepinephrine and serotonin are reduced in Parkinson's disease, nortriptyline or electroconvulsive treatment can be dramatically helpful, however.

A mood disturbance, especially depression, can precede the chorea and dementia of Huntington's disease, a neurological malady characterized by degeneration of the caudate and putamen nuclei. It has been difficult, however, to disentangle firmly the emotional reaction of patients to their inevitable fate from those mental symptoms that can be attributed directly to neuronal loss and the profound chemical depletions of gamma-aminobutyric acid (GABA) and acetylcholine.

Brainstem and Cerebellar Lesions

Bilateral corticobulbar lesions between thalamus and medulla release facial expression from supranuclear control. The result is involuntary (called *forced* or *spasmodic*) laughing and crying, sometimes abruptly shifting from one action to the other. Once started, the emotional display is uncontrollable and must run its course. Laughing, crying, or rage can be triggered by the seemingly most innocuous or inappropriate event.

A lacunar state, multiple sclerosis, motor neuron disease, or other diffuse diseases in their advanced stages most often produce the state known as *pseudobulbar palsy* (so named because what appear to be bulbar, [meaning medullary,] symptoms are produced by supranuclear lesions—i.e., pseudobulbar ones). Patients with pseudobulbar palsy *feel* various emotions, but often their only means of expressing them are through laughing or crying.

We can learn to inhibit, but not excite, subcortical centers that subserve emotional expression. The faciorespiratory coördination of laughter, for example, is believed to involve the medial thalamus, hypothalamus, and subthalamus (Poeck, 1985). But only in response to a limbic stimulus reaching a subcortical nucleus can we smile, laugh, or cry. When facing a photographer, for example, we always smile badly when asked to do so, and even the most experienced actor cannot cry on command.

In chapter 6, I reviewed the mental symptoms associated with cerebellar disease. Because paralimbic projections synapse in the basis pontis and continue via the middle cerebellar peduncle to the cerebellar cortex, it is reasonable to ask whether cerebellar disease can elicit emotional symptoms. There is a paucity of relevant observations, perhaps because clinicians overlook emotional symptoms when dealing with a neural entity that has historically been characterized as solely motor.

Prodromal laughter can apparently be released by lesions as high as the posterolateral thalamus (Ceccaldi & Milandre, 1994). In three cases of stimulus-specific forced laughter, two occurred with diffuse brainstem dysfunction and the third with a left cerebellar hemorrhage (Doorenbos et al., 1993). Directional gaze was the stimulus in the first two patients. In the patient with the cerebellar hemorrhage, cerebellar intention tremor of either hand or foot always invoked forced laughter, without fatigue, and without an experience of amusement on the patient's part.

In situations with diffuse cerebral disease, pathologic crying (Poeck, 1985) is said to be more common than pathologic laughter (Ironside, 1956). When pathologic laughter is caused by a focal lesion, it is usually in the posterior fossa. What little information exists about treatment notes that forced laughing and crying may respond to dopaminergic (L-dopa) or serotonergic (fluoextine) agonists (Allman, 1992).

EMOTION AND CONSCIOUSNESS

Compared to what we know about the neuropsychology of other states, our knowledge of emotion and consciousness is meager and confused. That our thoughts seem *intentional* while feelings seem to happen *passively* to us is a schism that dates back to antiquity. Plato, for example, said that we are prisoners of our feelings and should therefore "hold fast to the sacred cord of reason" lest we become lost. Euripides agreed, declaring that folly occurs only when desire conflicts with reason. Aristotle, on the contrary, argued that emotion has a logic of its own and must be understood in its own terms. He asserted that emotions were not simple animal passions unleashed, but that they were a complex part of our thinking.

There is a similar schism in the way contemporary scientists and the general public view emotion. Scholars concur that emotions are complex states involving perception, affect, cognition, salience, drive, judgement, and action. That is, the nature of emotion is partly rational (de Sousa, 1983; Solomon, 1983; Rorty, 1980). The public, however, is inclined to favor Plato's dichotomy that emotion somehow conflicts with and threatens reason.

For example, In *The March of Folly*, American historian Barbara Tuchman argues that from Troy to Vietnam, leaders have pursued policies contradictory to their self-interest, even after the negative repercussions of those policies have become plain. Their decisions were short-term judgements that had an emotional bias and that history judged to be follies—grand miscalculations, the consequences of which were predicted at the time by minority voices. In asserting that emotion rather than well-reasoned statesmanship steers the ship of state, and that "the rejection of reason is the prime characteristic of folly," Tuchman illustrates the lay belief in the Platonic dichotomy.

We conclude that the Platonic view perceives a strong dichotomy between reason and emotion, while the Aristotelian view sees a weaker one. Ommaya (1994) nicely eliminated the dichotomy altogether by proposing that consciousness is a type of emotion, and that emotion serves as a "cognitive homeostat." Emotion and reason are interdependent because their anatomy is interdependent.

In chapter 1, I asked you to imagine an equilateral triangle with one of neuropsychology's major disciplines (behavior, neuroscience, and psychology) at each vertex. I now ask you similarly to picture a triangular relation between feeling, knowing, and doing to impress on yourself that cognition, emotion, and action are interactive rather than linearly hierarchical. Multiplex models emphasize the dynamic interplay between feeling, knowing, and doing. This interdependence is evident especially when we look at the role of emotion in consciousness, self-awareness, and directed attention.

Psychodynamic models once claimed that emotion is a consequence of cognition. The James-Lang "feeling" model, for example, proposed that emotion is merely one's awareness of visceral sensations. According to this view a nightingale, asked whether it sings because it is happy, would reply that it is happy because it sings. Strictly biological models of emotion, on the other hand, place emotion as the causative antecedent of cognition. Two consequences of this are that emotion can (1) exist in the absence of thinking, and (2) precipitate various ways of thinking. Just as emotion can produce a specific motor behavior (such as smiling, crying, screaming, jumping, or thrashing), it can likewise precipitate *specific patterns of thought* (Niedenthal & Kitayama, 1994).

The conjecture that emotion is specifically encoded and can be experienced in the absence of thought is supported by experiments in split-brain patients (Ledoux et al., 1979). Although the perceptual nature of a stimulus exposed to the right hemisphere is unavailable to the left, its emotional tone somehow gets consciously represented in the left hemisphere. Possibly, the intact anterior commissure subserving interlimbic connections is responsible for interhemispheric judgements observed in such individuals.

The observation that the verbal system of split-brain patients can accurately read the emotional tone precipitated by a stimulus whose nature it cannot know implies generally that individuals cannot always be aware of the origins of their moods, just as they cannot always be aware of the origins of their actions. In other words, the conscious self notices that the person inhabits a particular mood without knowing why. The process of verbal attribution takes over and concocts an explanation that, while perhaps plausible, is nonetheless incorrect. Our thoughts and feelings about something are not necessarily congruent.

Daniel Dennett's analogy likens consciousness to the press releases of the government's spokesperson who is personally out of the decision-making loop. Press secretaries often are the last people in government to know what is actually going on; consciousness is likewise the last to know what is going on in our minds. Being conscious of our own thinking seems to have emerged with the appearance of brain areas capable of the symbolic precursors to language. But language is hardly the only means of self-expression. Our brain can direct the hands and body in piano playing, painting, mime, dance, or other creative acts in which non-linguistic motor outputs express a highly sophisticated self-awareness that is strongly allied to the æsthetic capacity that I argued depends on emotion rather than reason. When experiencing the insight of the lightbulb going off, we first discern a feeling of recognition and coherence, followed by a conscious awareness of understanding ("This is it").

That the conscious realization of an insightful recognition is secondary to the recognition itself is splendidly shown in prosopagnosia, in which in patients are no longer able to distinguish the details of a particular face from the general class of faces and attach it to a memory of who that person is. This is true even if that person is a spouse or someone the patient has known for years. One can show, however, that another facet of their mind does recognize the person to whom the face belongs. When patients with prosopagnosia are shown a picture of someone they knew well before their illness, two contradictory things occur. The cognitive mind says that it does not know who that person is, while a sharp galvanic skin response betrays that recognition has indeed occurred. In other words, recognition is dissociated from conscious awareness of it.

I defined insight as fathoming a relation between different premises, a capacity that depended on the emotional organization of the human brain. Insights generally are accompanied by a feeling of certitude, or "this is it." That a solution toward which we struggle does not always emerge by attacking problems with the intellect is illustrated by the solution of a Kōan, a mental puzzle given to Zen students. To work on a Kōan the student must be eager to solve it and face it without thinking about it. The more one attacks a Kōan with the intellect the more impossible a solution becomes. "Two hands brought together make a sound. What is the sound of one hand clapping?" This is a famous Kōan (Reps, 1994). If you think there is no such sound you are mistaken. Entities such as Kōans force us beyond analysis and also lead to the premise that the cognitive and emotional minds are but two facets of the same mind. We obviously could have several facets (Gardner, 1983).

Having multiple facets of mind could be the human equivalent of the physicist's duality principle, which states that light is simultaneously a wave and a particle and that any experiment designed to demonstrate one property makes it impossible to observe the complimentary one. Our metaphoric concepts (see below) do likewise: In emphasizing one aspect of an object, they hide others. By analogy to the duality principle, our minds are simultaneously analytical and intuitive, appositional and propositional, holistic and sequential. Even though we scurry among these mental facets we seem unable to occupy more than one facet at a time, nor is any but the linguistic facet fully accessible to awareness and what we customarily call reason.

Awareness

Although he started out as a neurologist who later appeared to abandon the brain, Freud based his explanation of mind on the physiology understood in nineteenth-century Vienna. He was correct in pointing out that the mind codes its experience in ways not wholly accessible to awareness. That is, a level of mentation exists that we cannot consciously fathom but which nonetheless has clear and observable effects on both behavior and experience.

It may be difficult to bring yourself to believe that you are more emotional than rational, let alone coming to grips with the assertion that the entity you know as your "self" is not really in charge of your mind or your life. The illusive nature of self awareness, however, is nicely demonstrated by the work of Kornhüber (1965).

The physical brain has no sensory nerves and is not aware of its own physical substance. You can mechanically poke it with a rod or stimulate it with an electrical current or magnetic field. Regardless of the type of physical energy applied, the patient does not say, "I feel you touching my brain now," but instead reports a sensation in a peripheral body part. Physical movements may be similarly elicited by stimulating brain motor points. This immediately tells us that *there is not an identity between the actual neurons being stimulated and the spatial location of the subjective experience that results from it.* Repeated experience from brain surgery on awake individuals confirms that the brain's reference is always external.

People who have their brains stimulated have experiences that they claim they did not cause. Their reason says that the experience comes from them even though it does not feel like it comes from them. Instead of being aware of its own physical substance, the brain creates a reality outside of itself. A helpful analogy may be to think of a hologram, which produces a real three-dimensional image that exists outside of the film and laser beam that produce it.

The illusive nature of self-awareness was first shown by Kornhüber's work on what is called the *readiness potential* (*Bereitschaftspotential*), which shows that there is more to consciousness than what is apparent from what we can introspect or observe. The experimental subject is told to move a finger whenever he or she feels like it. Devices measure precisely when finger movement occurs as well as electrical potentials in the brain before and after the movement. A special clock permits the subject to record the moment of conscious decision to move the finger. Through a method called *reverse analysis*, one finds a buildup of brain activity—the readiness potential—that prepares the action to be performed (figure 8.1). This occurs in the brain almost one second before the subject makes a conscious decision to move the finger. One second is long on the time scale of physiologic events, much longer than the time required for the electrical impulse to traverse the physical nerves between motor output and the finger muscles. In other words, the readiness potential far antedates the subject's *decision* to make a movement.

Others, especially the American physiologist Benjamin Libet (1985), have replicated and extended Kornhüber's work. One conclusion is that we are deluded in believing that each of us is a free agent who may decide to take an action. Such a decision is an interpretation we give to a behavior that has been initiated some-

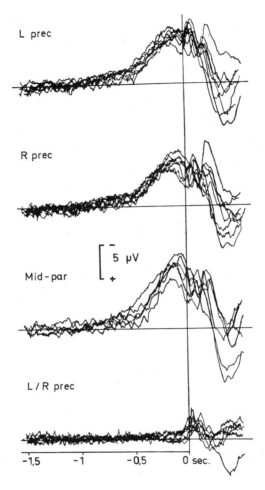

Figure 8.1
Readiness potentials recorded from the scalp in response to voluntarily evoked finger movements. Time zero is the onset of movement. The antecedent potentials are derived by the method of reverse analysis. From Kornhüber (1974), with permission.

place else by another part of ourselves *well before* we are aware of making any decision at all. In other words, the decision has been made before we are aware of the idea even to make a decision. If "we" are not pulling the strings, then who or what is? One answer: A facet inaccessible to introspection.

Kornhüber's experiment can also be performed in the other direction. A stimulation of the skin with a pin prick reaches the brain in ten thousandths (10/1000) of a second; there is more than half a second of readiness potential before the pin prick is consciously perceived. Yet in the subject's own mind there is paradoxically no delay in appreciating the prick relative to the physical stimulation. Libet proposes that the initial signal in the cortex, occurring just ten thousandths of a second after the pinprick, acts as a time marker. After the half second (500/1000) of neuronal buildup necessary to convey a conscious experience, that experience is referred back to the time marker. The subject thus experiences no delay in his or her own mind. Personal experience tells us that the world appears seamless, that the sights, sounds, smells, tastes, and textures of any experience are concurrent. Libet suggests that the unsettling disparity in time between conscious experience and neural events is necessary to maintain subjective synchrony among sensations. My point is that subjective experience has a time base discrepant from the neuronal activity that produces it.

Work such as Kornhüber's and Libet's point to a part of us that is inaccessible to self-awareness but that nevertheless has observable effects on behavior and experience (Kihlstrom, 1987). The implication of their work is consistent with that of split-brain research. For example, the conscious, speaking hemisphere of split-brain patients is surprised at the knowledge and actions of the other hemisphere. This is particularly striking when interhemispheric conflict occurs, as when the left hand undoes a task that the right hand has just completed, or when the left foot goes in one direction while the rest of the body moves off in another. These kinds of mind probes show that we know more than we think we know. And yet we always seem surprised to discover that we know something. In everyday life are we not surprised at our own intuition, creativity, insight, and other manifestations of inner knowledge?

Directed Attention

Mesulam (1981a, 1985b) proposed a network for attention that is lateralized, in dextrals, to the right hemisphere. He proposed that the reticular formation sustains an *attentional matrix*, while three cortical entities provide the *vector force* that focuses attention on appropriate targets. This circuit (figure 8.2) defines a distributed system given that its three cortical entities have robust reciprocal cortico-cortical projections. The reticular system itself sustains complex interactions with entities in brainstem, thalamus, and cortex. Attentional tone and vector can vary independently, producing diverse clinical pictures.

The distributed system of attention includes three *different* representations of extrapersonal space: (1) a sensory map in posterior parietal cortex, (2) a motor map for directing exploration (e.g., scanning, reaching, fixating) in frontal cortex, and (3) a map of the spatial distribution of motivational valence in the limbic system's cingulate cortex.

We previously encountered unilateral neglect (anosognosia) in our earlier discussion of parietal lesions. Profound examples in which the world on the patient's left side ceases to exist are, of course, dramatic and memorable. Neglect due to posterior parietal lesions usually is not so severe, however, and may actually require bilateral simultaneous stimulation to demonstrate.

The frontal aspect of neglect is an underlying disinclination to move toward or within the affected hemispace, a hypokinesia for exploration and manipulation within it. The cingulate component affects the distribution of expectancy for potential events and the correct attribution of salience to actual stimuli on the affected side. That is, impaired emotional vigilance results in less scanning and fixation. In its fullest expression, the patient acts as if nothing could ever be expected to occur in the left hemispace. In Mesulam's words, "the deficit is not one of seeing, hearing, feeling, or moving, but one of looking, listening, touching, and exploring." It encompasses the body schema, extrapersonal space, and interpsychic representations. Damage to any one of the three spatial representations or their thalamic or striatal connections can produce unilateral neglect. The inflection of symptoms depends on which part of the distributed system is damaged.

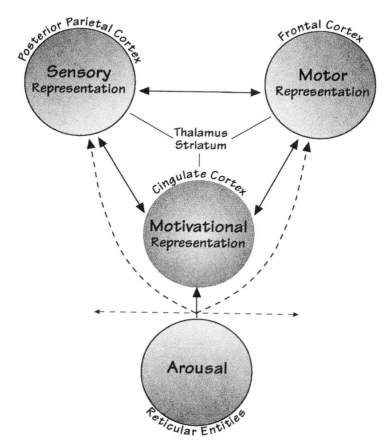

Figure 8.2
A network for spatially distributed attention. See text for details. Based on
Mesulam (1985b), with permission.

Three points relevant to the system's lateralization in the right
hemisphere are that (1) the right hemisphere attends to both sides
of space, but is biased toward the contralateral (left) hemispace, (2)
the left hemisphere attends almost exclusively to the contralateral
right hemispace, and (3) the right hemisphere devotes more synaptic resources to attention than does the left hemisphere. Therefore, left-hemispheric lesions tend not to produce neglect because
the right one is able to attend to both sides. On the other hand,
right-hemispheric lesions cause marked neglect because the left
hemisphere monitors the contralateral space almost exclusively.

We should be suspicious of simple models of attention given that it is far from unitary, involving wakefulness, consciousness, arousal, affect, motivation, salience, memory, and perception (McGlynn & Schacter, 1989). The behavioral relevance of a stimulus may even be affected by lesions as early (hierarchicaly speaking) as unimodal association cortex, which leads to modality-specific deficits of attention. More abstract features are managed by heteromodal association cortices (i.e., prefrontal, posterior parietal, and ventral temporal), areas that receive input from multiple unimodal association cortices, limbic entities, and paralimbic areas.

That attention is filtered at advanced rather than early stages of multiplex processing was shown in an elegant series of cerebral blood flow studies using auditory, visual, and tactile stimuli (Roland, 1982). Although all three senses were stimulated in each trial, subjects were instructed to attend to only one modality during a discrimination task. Even so, both primary and unimodal association cortices for each of the three senses activated, with the activation in the one sense being attended to exceeding that of the ignored modalities. Regardless of the sense in which the subject was instructed to discriminate, the prefrontal heteromodal cortex always activated. Because the idiotypic and homotypic cortices belonging to a given sense continue to activate even when that sense is ignored, the attentional filtering appears to occur at the higher (less differentiated) stage of processing. One can speculate that greater behavioral flexibility results from this arrangement than if the input were filtered at an earlier (more differentiated) stage.

Clinically, individuals with heteromodal parietal lesions (area 7) show multimodal extinction when tested with bilateral simultaneous stimulation, they neglect their internal schematic of left-sided extrapersonal space, and they cannot adequately shift their attention to the left hemispace. Single-unit recordings show that area 7 neurons respond to sensory, motivational, and motor contingencies. The cortical and thalamic input of area 7 is already highly abstract. Reciprocal and monosynaptic projections feed back to those three qualitatively different inputs, just as its outputs to the frontal eye fields, striatum, and superior colliculus have reciprocal projections that come into play during orientation, search, and exploration. Developmentally, attention matures late. Indeed, getting children to "pay attention" is a major part of their socialization.

Those who approach behavior computationally have likened the direction of attention to a searchlight assigned the task of sampling cerebral activity to determine "where the action is" (Crick, 1984). This searchlight purportedly helps when disparate features (such as color and shape) must be co-joined, as when, for example, we distinguish a red ball from an apple (Julesz, 1981). How different attributes can be assigned to a single object is known as the *binding problem*, and the hypothetical attentional searchlight is suggested as a possible solution to it. Recently discovered electrical potentials that oscillate at 40-Hz are said to explain how the brain assembles sense impressions into a single object (Gray et al., 1990; von der Malsburg, 1981).

A feature that some find attractive is that the time scale of the 40-Hz oscillations corresponds to the psychological time scale of attentional shifts from object to object. Neurons stay phase-locked for several hundred milliseconds, long enough to possibly establish and break their temporary functional configurations in roughly the same time frame that an individual's conscious attention moves from one physical object to the next.

Computationalists such as Crick believe that the synchronous firing of neurons in disparate brain regions is a natural solution to the binding problem, because their joint firing on other neurons throughout the nervous system will be extensive. "The content of the cell assembly—the 'meaning' of all the neurons so linked together—can in this way be impressed on the rest of the system...." He further wonders if the oscillating mechanism that purportedly binds disparate aspects necessary for awareness might also link neuronal groups responsible for ideas and thoughts that might not even originate in the senses. (Parenthetically, if you do not adhere to modularity, there is no binding problem.)

Unilateral neglect is an example in which the vector of directed sensory attention is impaired with little, if any, disturbance of attentional tone (Robertson & Marshall, 1993). The confusional states serve as opposite examples in which attentional tone is the primary disturbance.

Objectivity and Subjectivity

A system of mental concepts determines how we think and act. We are not normally aware of our conceptual system; we just think and act along certain lines. Concepts structure what we perceive and how we relate to objects and other people, thus centrally defining everyday reality. If our conceptual system is metaphorically based, then the way we think, what we experience, and what we do must also be metaphoric.

Metaphoric Concepts in Language and Action

I want to present the case that everyday language and actions are permeated with metaphoric concepts based in *physical experience* rather than *abstractions* (Leary, 1990; Lakoff & Johnson, 1980). The premise that metaphor is merely language (something like rhetoric or poetry) perpetuates the view that the world is dispassionately objective, meaning free from human concepts of it. However, concepts are not defined by fixed properties but rather in terms of how we physically interact with objects. Understanding grows out of the entire scope of our experience.

Consider the premise that metaphor is experiential (thus subjective) and visceral (thus emotional), an a-rational transfer of connotations from one thing to another. Metaphor physically encapsulates our relations with the world and, though it is a means of discerning the similar in the dissimilar, it is emphatically not the product of logical analysis.

The objective person claims to comprehend something in terms of its inherent properties, some disembodied ideal. To suggest this is false, let us turn to a most subjective example, namely LOVE. Dictionary writers allude to affection, sexual allure, and the like. Metaphorical comprehension sees love as a JOURNEY, MADNESS, or a BATTLE—things grasped in the course of experiencing it directly. Consider these examples (from Lakoff & Johnson, 1980, passim):

LOVE IS A JOURNEY

Look at *how far we've come* only to *go our separate ways*. It's been a *long, bumpy road* and this relationship *isn't going anywhere*. It's *on the rocks*.

LOVE IS MADNESS

I'm *crazy* about you and *insanely* jealous. You drive me *wild* and make me go *out of my mind*.

Love Is a Battle

She is *besieged* by suitors who *pursue* her *relentlessly*, causing her to *flee* their *advances* and *fend them off*. The *tactics* they use in *fighting* over her are unbelievable.

Trying to pen an objective definition of love reveals the concept to be entirely metaphoric. A metaphor is defined as experiencing one thing in terms of another, as the metaphorical knowledge of love illustrates. Metaphoric understanding is the ability to perceive similarity among seemingly dissimilar objects. As Aristotle put it, "It is from metaphor that we can best get hold of something fresh" (*Rhetoric*, 1410b).

The easiest metaphors to understand are those based on simple spatial directions such as UP. We change our physical orientation during activities such as standing, sleeping, climbing, or diving. Since a physical orientation is central to having a body, orientation is central to our conceptual system. That is, the structure of our spatial concepts emerges from our direct physical experience.

Conscious Is Up; Unconscious Is Down

Wake *up*. I'm *up* already. I'm an early *riser*. I *dropped* off and *fell* asleep. The patient *went under* anesthesia, *sank* into a coma, then *dropped* dead.

Controlling Is Up; Being Controlled Is Down

He's *on top* of the situation, in *high* command, and at the *height* of power in having so many people *under* him. His influence started to *decline*, until he *fell* from power and *landed* as *low man* on the totem pole, back at the *bottom* of the heap.

Good Is Up; Bad Is Down

High quality work made this a *peak* year and put us *over the top*. Things were looking *up* when the market *bottomed out* and hit an all-time *low*. It's been *downhill* ever since.

Rational Is Up; Emotional Is Down

My heart *sank* and I was in the *depth* of despair, unable to *rise* above my emotions. I *pulled myself up* from this sorry state and had a *high-level* intellectual discussion with my therapist, a *high-minded*, *lofty* individual.

The physical bases for these metaphors is that most mammals sleep lying down and stand up when awake. Well-being, control, and things characterized as good are all UP. Because we control our physical environment, animals, and sometimes even other people, and because our ability to reason is assumed to give us this control, CONTROL IS UP implies HUMAN IS UP and therefore RATIONAL IS UP.

Spatial orientations such as up-down, front-back, and center-periphery are the most common ones in our system of concepts but, given the variety of ways we interact with the world, others certainly exist. We make inside-out distinctions between reason and emotion, for example, and generally characterize rationality as up, light, and active, while the emotions are down, deep, and murky—passive, irrational passions over which we have little control. Intellectual functions of the brain are called "higher" while the emotions and habits are "low."

Anthropologists tell us that the major orientations of up-down, in-out, central-peripheral, and active-passive exist in all cultures. But which concepts are most valued varies from place to place. Some cultures prize balance, whereas America seems taken with the extremes of UP or DOWN orientations.

We see that forming metaphoric concepts is like culling tidbits of our experience and then treating them like autonomous entities that we can arrange. Our interactions in space yield *orientational metaphors*. Other experiences give rise to what are called *ontological metaphors*, ways of treating events, actions, emotions, and ideas as reified, self-contained objects. Cultural influence elaborates ontological metaphors. We can elaborate THE MIND IS AN ENTITY into either THE MIND IS A MACHINE or THE MIND IS A BRITTLE OBJECT to get the following:

THE MIND IS A MACHINE

We are *cranking out* a lot of paperwork. You could see his *wheels turning*. Their proposal just *ran out of steam*.

Compare this with the results of a different elaboration:

THE MIND IS A BRITTLE OBJECT

He *cracked* under pressure. It was a *shattering* experience. You *bruised* his ego.

Metaphors emphasize some facets of an object but hide others. The MACHINE metaphor paints the mind as having a source of power, an expected level of efficiency, an optimum production capacity, and an on-off state. However, it hides the vagaries of thought, its ability to deal with fragmentary information, and other abilities resulting from its subjective properties.

By switching metaphors, we alter how we comprehend something and thus alter reality. Words do not change reality, but changing our concepts does alter what we perceive and how we act on those perceptions. Ontological metaphors are so pervasive that they seem natural and self-evident descriptions of mental thought. It never dawns on us that they are metaphors. Ponder the experience implicit in the following:

Understanding Is Seeing; Ideas Are Light

I *see* what you are saying. It was a *brilliant* remark and a *clear* discussion. Your point of *view* gave me the *whole picture*. Their proposal is *murky*, the ideas *opaque*, and their premise is *transparent*.

Emotion Is Physical Contact

The verdict *bowled him over*. I was *struck* by his generosity. His donation *made an impression* on me. That model is a *knockout*. I was *touched* by their kindness.

You can see how different metaphors produce different flavors of a given concept. The intuitive appeal of a concept rests on how well its metaphors fit our actual experience. One factor contributing to the irrationality of the human mind is the conflict among metaphors that arises from *real differences in their physical foundations*.

For example, "That's *up in the air*," and "The matter is *settled*" are each physically consistent with "I *grasp* your meaning." If you can grasp something you can examine and understand it, and things are easier to grasp if they are down rather than flying up in the air. Thus, UNKNOWN IS UP and KNOWN IS DOWN are coherent with UNDERSTANDING IS GRASPING. However, UNKNOWN IS UP is inconsistent with the orientational metaphors GOOD IS UP or FINISHED IS UP (e.g., "Finish up this last piece of pie").

Logic demands that FINISHED be yoked with KNOWN, and UNFINISHED yoked with UNKNOWN. But our experience disagrees. We do not consider the unknown to be good, and the physical experience leading to UNKNOWN IS UP is entirely different from that on which the two incongruent metaphors are based. This shows how the ability to be at odds with ourselves or the ability to hold conflicting beliefs simultaneously is based not on reason, but on physical experience.

Beyond Opposites

We try to make sense of the world by creating dichotomies and by thinking in categories. We split our existence into objective and subjective parts that respectively compartmentalize external demands and inner concerns. But reality is not the same as our thoughts about it, and we often fail to ponder what a burdensome imposition intellectual categories are in diminishing our direct experience. A pervasive distrust of direct experience is evident in stock phrases such as, "Sorry, I wasn't thinking." No one ever says, "Sorry, I wasn't feeling."

We are prone to identify ourselves with the rational, the external, and the objective. This is particularly evident in the psychiatric activity called psycho*analysis*. Evoking the psyche rather than analyzing it moves you away from external concerns so that you can better grasp your depth. It seems obvious that you should understand yourself better than you could ever understand anyone else. But when you actually try to fathom what you do, feel, and believe, then such efforts at understanding take you beyond yourself. This is the definition of transcendence.

Ineffable, noëtic, and *transcendent* are words that point to something behind what the philosopher Kant called "ordinary experience as we know we have it." William James said that the ineffable defied expression: "Its quality must be directly experienced, it cannot be imparted or transferred to others." *Noëtic* refers to knowledge that is directly imparted, an illumination that is accompanied by certitude. *Transcendent* means "to climb over or beyond," and refers to that which we cannot name. These three terms all point to the existence of inner knowledge that words cannot display. This is the experiential view, in contrast to one that is either strictly subjective or strictly objective.

All three views betray a drive for understanding. Objectively, you seek to understand a world of external objects and relations; subjectively, you seek an internal understanding that makes life worth living. The objectivist believes in a world made of objects with inherent properties about which one can utter statements that are absolutely true or false. The objectivist feels secure in the knowledge that science has a method to avoid the subjective limitations of errors and bias that make the human mind unreliable. The subjectivist, by contrast, rejects the impersonal and abstract, perhaps turning to the romanticism that originated to counteract the ascendancy of an impersonal scientific method.

Both the scientific objectivist and the romantic subjectivist see the individual as autonomous, and both try to overcome the individual's existential separation from nature. The scientist tries to rejoin nature by conquering it; the romantic communes with or becomes absorbed by nature. The objective and subjective views evidently define themselves in contrary terms and seem to exist in separate domains. But a third view based in experience stresses interaction: We cannot live in the world without changing it or being changed by it. The meanings of metaphor, for example, are grounded in physical experiences that structure the conceptual system of what we believe and how we act. These actions in turn alter the world.

Because metaphor joins reason and imagination, the conceptual system on which reality is based is in part imaginative. Likewise, creative ideas are partly rational in nature. Objectivity fails to see that our system of concepts is metaphoric, involving an imaginative understanding of one thing in terms of another. Subjectivity fails to see that even our most imaginative flights occur in the context of objective experience gained by living in a physical and cultural world. The elaboration of metaphors, for example, is an imaginative form of rational thinking.

Life cannot be neatly carved up into wholly objective or wholly subjective portions. Fortunately, we do not need to choose, because the middle view based in experience does not need to be absolute. It produces a system rooted in and constantly refreshed by experience (Schore, 1994). Taken alone, neither the objective nor subjective views can fathom that experience is noëtic and that we understand the world only by living in it. What this means is that humans should be valued not only for their knowledge that can be said, but also for that which cannot be said.

Alasdair MacIntyre, the moral philosopher who wrote *Whose Justice, Which Rationality?*, cautioned that those who espouse "objective" viewpoints always think that their own arguments are the most rational, logical, and convincing. "My civilization, my culture, my method, and my values are better than yours," they say.

The American behaviorist B.F. Skinner (1904–1990) offers an example of extreme faith in objectivity. "In every walk of life," he says, "from international affairs to the care of a baby, we shall continue to be inept until a scientific analysis clarifies the advantages of a more effective technology. In the behavioristic view, man can now control his own destiny because he knows what must be done and how to do it." What this really means is that B.F. Skinner "knows what must be done and how to do it" (Skinner, 1974, pp. 243–251). Like everyone who believes in objectivity, he is sure that he knows what is best for the rest of us. (Politicians, consultants, and other experts often claim this.)

The flaw in worshipping objectivity is that it is possible to have an objective view of anything, but only from your own subjective point of view. You cannot have a subjective evaluation of a species other than yourself, for instance. Hence, you cannot know what it is like to be a bat, a whale, or anything other than yourself (Nagel, 1986). Every subjective experience is connected with a single point of view—namely, yours. The error of persons who place reason and objectivity above all else is in trying to develop a view from nowhere, detached from other values. Perhaps we can imagine a view sitting isolated out in space, but the more we think about it the more we see that it is impossible to have a view from nowhere without beginning with a view from somewhere. That somewhere is yourself. It is difficult to imagine what the *objective* character of an experience would be like. In his famous paper, "What is it like to be a bat?", philosopher Thomas Nagel (1974) asks, "After all, what would be left of what it was like to be a bat if one removed the viewpoint of the bat?"

It is a truism that science tells us how the physical universe "really is" even though it simplifies reality by leaving out whatever fails to fit its conceptual framework. Aldous Huxley expressed this well back in 1946: "The scientific picture of the world is inadequate for the simple reason that science deals only with certain aspects of experience in certain contexts ... most others tend to accept the world picture implicit in the theories of science as a complete and exhaustive account of reality."

Here is the flaw of the objective expert who "knows what must be done and how to do it." Factual concepts of human behavior are far less than a complete picture. Objective frameworks promote themselves as being without values while simultaneously asserting an authoritarianism based on expertise, a value judgement in itself. Proposals for value-neutral, "objective" decisions never acknowledge that value choices have already been made (such as behaviorism's decision to reject the "inner" and "unobservable"). We must beware of abstractions that claim to capture the whole picture.

SUGGESTED READINGS

Cytowic RE. 1993 *The Man Who Tasted Shapes*. New York: Putnam

Flanagan O. 1992 *Consciousness Reconsidered*. Cambridge: MIT Press

Lakoff G, Johnson M. 1980 *Metaphors We Live By*. Chicago: University of Chicago Press

Niedenthal PM, Mitayama S. 1994 *The Heart's Eye: Emotional Influences in Perception and Attention*. San Diego: Academic Press

Schore AN. 1994 *Affect Regulation and the Origin of the Self: The Neurobiology of Emotional Development*: Hillsdale, NJ: Lawrence Earlbaum Associates

Searle JR. 1992 *The Rediscovery of the Mind*. Cambridge: MIT Press

Starkstein SE, Robinson RG. 1993 *Depression in Neurologic Disease*. Baltimore: The Johns Hopkins University Press

9 Memory and Amnesia

One invariably speaks jointly of learning and memory, *learning* being the acquisition of new information, and *memory* being its retention and recall at a later time. We employ the term memory in a positive sense; its negative analogue is *amnesia*, which can refer to the failure of both learning (*anterograde amnesia*) and recall (*retrograde amnesia*). What amnesics forget can be highly specific.

Memory is the most tested aspect of intellect, both for historical reasons and because it participates in diverse mental operations. Clinical and research approaches differ in their emphases. Clinical procedures generally aim to detect structural pathology, whereas the researcher is more often interested in the constituent operations of memory, or even elementary concepts of what memory is. Yet each approach informs the other. For example, amnesia often occurs handily in relative isolation from other intellectual failures. This clinical circumstance has helped the researcher delineate memory's functional components and their anatomic foundations.

A physical parallelism to the Rhomberg test might be useful here in addressing the confusion between what is done in testing memory and what specific steps actually mean in this (see Loring & Papanicolaou, 1987). A huge proportion of clinicians erroneously think that the Rhomberg maneuver tests the cerebellum, but it actually tests the integrity of the posterior columns of the spinal cord. (Perhaps patients' wobbliness makes students assume that the cerebellum must be involved.)

Likewise, the "memory" section of the mental status exam traditionally includes naming the presidents, questioning orientation, subtracting serial 7s, measuring digit span, recalling three objects, and inquiring about remote events. Reflection shows that repeating digits is only one type of mnestic function (in a single category, no less), whereas serial 7s is not a test of memory at all. (Perhaps spitting back information makes students assume that mnesis is involved.)

The conceptual distinction between short-term and long-term memory is often blurred between the bedside and the laboratory. Even though patients parrot information back to you, immediate recall of the cowboy (see the box, "The cowboy," in chapter 5) or Wechsler stories or any brief prose passage is conceptually different from what we normally call *short-term memory*. A few lines of prose is simply too much to hold in immediate memory. Learning is usually tested with several trials of paired associates.

Three main facets of clinical assessment are (1) the impression you form after a face-to-face encounter, (2) the numbers generated by formal testing, and (3) the impact that the amnesia has on the patient's day-to-day life.

CURRENT CONCEPTS OF MEMORY

The French psychologist Theodule Ribot (1839–1916) compiled examples of impaired memory in his 1881 book, *Les Maladies de la mémoire*, believing that their analysis could yield general principles of normal memory. Ribot was especially interested in *retrograde amnesia*: The greater loss of recent memories compared to remote ones.

Since that time, the topic of retrograde amnesia has exercised neuropsychologists, and other vexing questions have been added along the way. For example, is forgetting a loss of biologic substance, like the melting of an ice cube, or is it the blocked retrieval of something that physically endures? Some puzzling aspects of memory yield to experiment. Before the turn of the century, for example, the German psychologist Hermann Ebbinghaus (1850–1909) used tests of nonsense syllables to show that memory could be teased apart in the laboratory and that simple factors such as the passage of time, repetition, and the nature of intervening events can influence one's retention.

You already know that instead of impairing cognition across the board (the conceit of mass action), focal lesions tend to produce highly selective effects. The production of an amnesia isolated from other intellectual domains shows the relative functional separation of on-line perception, cognitive analysis, and the ability to store the record that results from engaging these functions. This non-veridical record can be retrieved at a later time. The term *on-line* refers to the observation that someone's moment-to-moment behavior appears quite normal even though they may have a severe amnesia. Later, perhaps even as the encounter unfolds, the observer realizes that the patient cannot follow the thread of events.

The Plastic Nature of Memory

For a long time one heard the truism that we are born with only so many neurons, meaning that the brain's structure is fixed. I was therefore surprised to learn in the 1970s that the nervous system physically changes as a result of experience (Squire et al., 1992). This plasticity still surprises some students, but then the fact that bone is "alive," that it has circulation and a high rate of cell involution and replacement, also goes against some people's preconceived notions. The brain is no exception to the rule that all biologic tissues change. Brains are inherently unstable, evolving phylogenetically and modified ontogenetically by experience. Examples of structural and functional plasticity include drug tolerance, enzyme induction, the sprouting of axon terminals, facilitation, and inhibition.

In many areas of human endeavor, we rediscover the past as we move forward. The concept that the brain physically changes in response to experience is an old idea dating back to William James (1890), who spoke of the physical paths that sensory impressions take. "The only thing they can do, in short, is to deepen old paths or to make new ones." James metaphorically likened memory to a physical path trodden by sensation. This experiential metaphor did seem to conceptualize a way that memory could persist by leaving a trace. The germ of this idea was found to be correct.

The synapse is the actual site of plastic change. The growth of axon spines, alterations in the number and size of active zones, and the corresponding quantity of neurotransmitter released are all modifiable. We have known for more than two decades that long-term potentiation strengthens the synapses of neural configurations corresponding to the knowledge being memorized, yet we still debate whether that change occurs in the cell sending the signal (presynaptic), or in the cell across the synapse that receives it (postsynaptic). Eric Kandel's work with *Aplysia* (popularly called the *sea slug* or *sea hare*) is interesting reading, not only for its demonstration of how neurons can change their functional efficiency but also because it is a charming story of how *Aplysia californica* and Kandel made each other famous. (The Monterey Bay and other aquaria have sea slugs in tidal "petting pools" for your edification; you must make an appointment to see Dr. Kandel at Columbia.) Kandel (1979, 1992) demonstrated that the habituation of the gill withdrawal response is an experience that *physically modifies* the neural pathways that subserve it.

(*Aplysia* is beloved by neurobiologists because of its many-fold simplicity. Its behavior consists of eating, rest, and copulation. It has only 20,000 neurons compared to billions in a rodent, and these are conveniently packaged into a mere ten ganglia. Best of all, neurons reach diameters of 1 mm—more than 1,000 times larger than human neurons. This combination of size and simplicity has emboldened connectionists to make wiring diagrams showing the role that both *individual cells* and what are called *small circuits* play in specific behaviors.)

In chapter 3 we talked about neural migration in the fetal brain and how the final adult pattern of cerebral organization is influenced by physiologic necrosis, competition for synaptic sites, and the elimination of collateral axons. Analogous events ensue regarding memory. So, instead of stopping after the brain matures (relatively speaking) sometime in childhood, synaptic competition continues in the adult, particularly where the terminal fields of different axons overlap. Although some cells may be lost in their competition for synaptic terminals, those that remain increase their terminal arborization and it is here where plasticity is most readily manifest. The pathway used most often eventually becomes dominant in a way suggested by James' metaphor of "deepening old paths."

Memory: Localized or Diffuse?

After the emphasis on localization of function in the preceding chapters, it is frustrating not to be able to answer the apparently

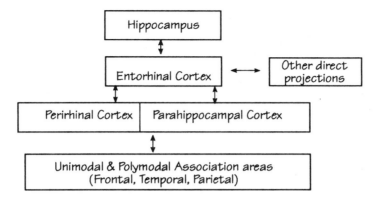

Figure 9.1
The medial temporal lobe memory system. The major gateway to the hippocampus is entorhinal cortex, which receives the bulk of its cascading and reciprocal projections from other cortical areas. The smaller proportion of "direct" entorhinal projections come from orbital frontal, cingulate, insular, and superior temporal cortices. Modified from Squire & Zola-Morgan (1991).

straightforward question, "Where is memory localized?" One often hears that memory resides in the hippocampus. It does not. The hippocampus is essential for forming memories and providing salience so that events will be remembered, but memories are sown throughout the cortex (Fuster, 1995). That is, the hippocampus (and anatomically-related entorhinal, perirhinal, and parahippocampal cortices) binds unrelated events or features that are represented by distinct cortical sites. Engaging this hippocampal formation at the time of learning forms an "index" for the later recollection of the whole event (figure 9.1).

The debate of earlier decades over whether memory is localized or distributed was won by both sides. Memory is widely distributed in the cerebrum, but different aspects of the whole experience—perceptual fragments if you like—are stored in numerous loci. If this sounds like the distributed system, it is. In fact, you might think of memory as the purest type of distributed system because, during recollection, an event is believed to be expressed by activity in the same group of columns that originally perceived it. How can this be?

Thinking modularly, incoming flux splits into multiple streams, each of which concerns a different feature of the environment. A dorsal stream generally aimed at the temporal lobe deals with recognition of "What" is happening, whereas a ventral stream aimed at the parietal lobe is more concerned with "Where" events take place and the spatial relationships among them. Different regions of neocortex are conceived as simultaneously transforming separate perceptual dimensions.

The explanation of memory that is now popular, though not definitively proven, is that an event is somehow stored in the same neural configurations that participate in its perception and understanding. The later stages of cortical processing are particularly emphasized. In vision, for example, the inferior temporal lobe is the terminus for striate projections. For a variety of reasons, it is conceived of as not just a high-order visual analyzer, but also as a repository of memories for these visual processes. So, we can say that memory storage is localized in the sense that a given distributed system represents specific aspects of an event, but memory is also diffuse in the sense that there is no generic memory center, nothing that represents an entire event at a singular locus.

If one thinks linearly, the hippocampus lies at the terminal end of the cortex. Along with the amygdala and orbitofrontal cortex, it is one of the major fields to which diverse cortical areas project. Damage here produces *selective* deficits in perception; memories are affected similarly. Therefore, a lesion in one place can alter the perception of events while a lesion elsewhere can interfere with the memory of those events.

This arrangement recalls Planck's principle of least action in another setting. Earlier (chapter 3), we learned how the limbic system uses the same structures for different functions. Here, memory is registered by the same structure that both analyzes and indexes the experience. This also seems to be a tidy explanation for how we can have so many different kinds of memories—that is, how we are able to remember as many different things as we can perceive. The deduction that analytic and mnestic functions are partly subserved by the same structure generates a dilemma, however. I said that memory causes a measurable change in structure. If memory depends on plasticity, will not the plasticity of cortical neurons destroy the neocortex's analytic capacity? It turns out that only a small percentage of cortical neurons are capable of plastic change, thus voiding our dilemma.

Recall that the Canadian neurosurgeon Wilder Penfield produced "experiential responses" by stimulating discrete points of the temporal lobe. His analysis that these were veridical replays of past events (like a video tape) turned out to be wrong. The brain does not save a record of each and every moment "as it really happened" (a truth that has failed to deter the recovered-memory industry). Replication and extension of Penfield's work by many others shows that electrical stimulation of the temporal lobe does not equate with focal activation of neuronal packets that harbor discrete memories.

For one thing, experiential responses occur mostly when the current spreads away from the point of stimulation (*after discharges*). Surgical removal of the tissue that was stimulated pre-operatively fails to erase the memory that was evoked by its stimulation. Most importantly, limbic structures are involved in experiential responses, possibly because they have widespread reciprocal connections to so many cerebral areas.

Squire's re-analysis (1987, pp. 75–84) of Penfield's work concluded that "these considerations all point to the idea that multiple areas of neocortex, activated through limbic structures, participate in representing the memories and thoughts that give rise to evoked mental experiences." That is, the Penfield studies are best interpreted in terms of widespread parallel distributed processing. No focal memory center exists, but many brain parts each contributes something different to the memory of a singular event.

The amygdala does not participate in the kind of memory (called *explicit* or *declarative*, see below) that depends on the medial temporal lobe system depicted in figure 9.1. Rather, the amygdala plays an important but not exclusive role in *cross-modal associations* and the attachment of affect to neutral stimuli (Squire & Zola-Morgan, 1991). What makes amnesia worse is extending the lesion from hippocampus to include the overlying cortex, not extending it to the amygdala.

The amygdala can be regarded as a neural crossroads since it has direct and extensive connections to all sensory modalities in cortex and thalamus. Sites of amygdalar multisensory convergence themselves project fibers deeper to the hippocampus, possibly thereby associating memories from diverse senses. This bears on the issue that memory is far more than mere recognition. In fact, introspection shows that it is most often a sensory experience of a disparate kind that awakens a singular memory dominated by a particular sense. The issue of what mediates cross-modal associations and their later recall relates to synesthesia (Cytowic, 1989, 1993).

The finding that the amygdala associates a familiar stimuli with emotional valence has been used to reïnterpret the features of the Klüver-Bucy syndrome, attributing them to the destruction of previously formed cross-modal associations. Thus, monkeys with amygdalar lesions were less fearful than normal and unusually willing to interact with novel stimuli, yet their memories were normal as long as the hippocampal formation was unscathed. The converse also was true: All monkeys with lesions of the hippocampal formation or associated cortex had faulty memories, yet their emotional comportment was appropriate as long as the amygdala remained intact.

A further notion currently being tested is that the amygdala not only enables sensory-sensory and sensory-emotional cross-modal associations, but also it may well *enable emotion to influence one's perception of events and subsequent memory of them.* Anatomy shows that sensory cortices not only project to the amygdala, but receive projections back from it. This back-propagation is most dense in heteromodal cortex. Finally, the amygdala is rich in endogenous opiates. Not only is there a gradient of opiate receptors in the back-projections to sensory cortices, but this gradient is highest in the terminal processing areas. The reciprocal amygdalar projections to sensory cortices together with its projections to hypothalamus may explain why, in both animals and humans, emotional experiences are so well remembered.

Lastly, a word about memory as a hologram, an idea originally promoted by Karl Pribram and appropriated by pop magazines. A hologram is a record of the interference pattern made by mixing laser light scattered from an object with mutually coherent reference light. In one commonly used technique, the hologram is a physically stored Fourier transformation of an optical image into spatial frequency. During reconstruction, the inverse transform automatically reproduces an image of the object. If the storage plate breaks in half, each half still contains the whole scene, and so forth toward an infinite regression. The smaller the fragment the less the resolution, of course, because data are lost with each reduction. Nonetheless, each part contains the whole scene. This idea seems attractive in regard to memory because such a distributed storage is resistant to focal disruption, and thus it seems compatible with the notion of mass action.

However, the elements of holographic photography have neither physical nor functional parallels in the brain, and Pribram explored this idea only in metaphoric terms. Despite its aggrandizement by lay popularizers, it is doubtful that it will ever produce deep insights into mammalian memory given its lack of biologic parallels.

Aspects of Memory

The concept that the brain contains multiple memory systems (figure 9.2) is currently a popular idea supported by decades of evidence (Cohen & Eichenbaum, 1993; Perani et al., 1993; Schacter & Tulving, 1994). From the commonly observed dissociation of WAIS and WMS scores, it seems self-evident that the brain dissociates its perception and its intelligence from memory. That memory is

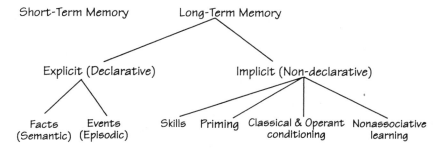

Figure 9.2
Classification of memory. Short-term memory is limited (e.g., a phone number) and decays in seconds if not refreshed. Long-term memory has unlimited capacity and spans minutes to a lifetime. Implicit (nondeclarative) memory refers to a heterogeneous group of abilities that are independent of the medial temporal lobe system and that modify behavior without any conscious recollection of content. Nonassociative learning includes habituation and sensitization. Explicit (declarative) memory is the conscious recall of facts and events that does rely on the medial temporal lobe system.

itself not a unitary faculty should also be evident from observing that amnesic patients who are horribly disabled in their daily living nonetheless perform normally at some learning tasks. Whatever underlies the ability to read a story *faster* with successive repetitions, for example, is disparate from the system that enables recall of that story's *content*. Similarly, facts and events make up the content of conscious recollections, whereas the process by which we learn to do things is qualitatively different and largely unconscious. For example, "What did you learn?" is a difficult question to answer after a tennis or music lesson. Such a question is best answered through performance rather than words.

If my use of different terms—declarative, procedural, episodic, semantic, implicit, explicit, and so forth—for the same concepts seems confusing, it is only because neuropsychologists have not settled on a standard terminology.

Short-Term and Long-Term Memory

This distinction looks at the temporal aspect of memory. I have already said that testing immediate ("Repeat these words"), short-term ("What three things did I ask you to remember?"), and long-term memory ("Where were you last holiday?") in the mental status exam really describes performance rather than being tests that are conceptually based.

Earlier, we considered short-term memory (also called *working* or *primary memory*) to be some kind of buffer that belonged to the back side of the present moment. It is the space where one holds a heard phone number before dialing it. Now we consider working memory to be intrinsic to *each kind of perceptual processing* rather than a single buffer. Repeating digits, therefore, has only to do with the temporary capacity of auditory-verbal phonological encoding.

Working memory has an approximate capacity of seven items, whereas long-term memory is much larger. If rehearsed, the contents of working memory can be held for about two minutes, after which the material is learned and becomes part of the long-term storage. Rehearsal, attention, distraction, and interference are all concerns of short-term memory. If permitted to rehearse and if not distracted, amnesic persons can retain information for many minutes.

Long-term memory depends on structural changes in synaptic connections believed to take place outside the medial temporal lobe. PET studies in patients who are amnesic for episodic events of explicit long-term memory show a common pattern of bilateral metabolic depression in several interconnected structures—namely, hippocampus, thalamus, cingulate cortex, and frontobasal cortex—that suggests a distributed system for long-term episodic memory apart from the medial temporal system (Perani et al., 1993). Protein synthesis seems mandatory for memory consolidation, and material that has entered long-term memory does degrade over years, although that degradation is not uniform over time (i.e., it is non-linear, some memories fading quickly, others enduring). The distinction between short-term and long-term memory applies only to explicit memory.

Declarative and Procedural Memory
Declarative and *procedural* are synonyms for *implicit* and *explicit* memory. This distinction refers to the memory of facts and episodes compared to those for skills. Declarative memory itself is divided into episodic and semantic parts, considered in a moment. These distinctions are made because some kinds of learning are severely impaired in amnesia while other kinds remain normal. That is, amnesic individuals show a dissociation between knowing how and knowing that.

As the name implies, declarative memory is that which one can declare, facts one knows. The *conscious* knowledge of facts is impaired in amnesia. In contrast, procedural memory—the knowledge of how to do something, solve a problem, or reason about a particular thing—is spared, and one is not consciously aware of how, where, or when one acquired the skill. Even if amnesic individuals engage in some task repeatedly, they never gain a sense that it is familiar.

This distinction is often confusing to the clinician and irrelevant to the care of individual patients, yet it surfaces repeatedly like a philosophical debate. The terms originally came from artificial intelligence, but were abandoned by that discipline when it became apparent that any knowledge can be formally represented as either a procedure or a declaration (a moot accomplishment).

What really matters to the clinician is that two qualitatively different kinds of knowledge seem to rely on different cerebral organization. One can say that procedural memory requires the structures subserving the skill to be intact, because the memory presumably resides there (a necessary assumption of the model). If ideas about the cortex sharing perceptual and mnestic function are correct, then a given lesion is unlikely to destroy *all* procedural memories in the same way a hippocampal lesion can obliterate all of declarative memory. The elaborate development of the limbic system in mammals suggests that declarative memory evolved recently as a way to access specialized knowledge across modalities, something that should enhance survival. If you do not understand this idea, reread the chapter 3 section on evolutionary development of the limbic system.

Episodic and Semantic Memory

A conceptual distinction is also made between episodic memory (events) and semantic memory (facts), but somehow this oft-discussed schism seems to miss the essence of what actually happens in memory impairment, because all amnesics have some difficulty with both facts and events.

One view holds that only episodic memory is impaired in amnesia. That is, patients with poor episodic memory (who can't learn new events) nevertheless seem to have good semantic memory (they can tell you lots of old facts). For example, language is considered to be one of the dimensions of semantic memory, yet language usually remains intact in amnesia. The other view says that both episodic and semantic capacity are diminished. Perhaps the distinction is better seen as one of disproportion rather than an either-or choice.

Patients with anterograde amnesia have difficulty acquiring both facts and events. In retrograde amnesia, there is difficulty also remembering both facts and events if they were recently acquired, yet both episodic autobiographical recall and general information is preserved from long ago. The error seems to be in comparing two different time domains: Old facts and new learning. If one compares them in the same time domain, then episodic and semantic talents appear more equal. Semantic memory by its nature is acquired over multiple exposures, whereas episodic events are acquired in one episode, as the name denotes. So semantic memory would always seem to be easier to remember than particular episodes, given any particular level of deficit. Therefore, the question is really a technical one: Is it the case that episodic memory is disproportionately impaired relative to the level of impairment of semantic knowledge? Is the ability for semantic day-to-day learning worse than one thinks it should be given the level of difficulty in learning new events?

This issue is discussed frequently but is a difficult one to settle experimentally. The episodic-semantic distinction may be more useful in frontal lobe lesions, where one often sees a dissociation between performance and knowledge.

Working Memory

I said earlier that *working memory* is another term for *short-term memory*. It is, although the concept of working memory continues to be developed to help clarify exactly what we think goes on in that string of moments that form the immediate past.

Instead of a unitary short-term memory, we now conceive of working memory as an abstract brain system that provides simultaneous storage and processing of diverse information that, in turn, permits cognition such as learning, reasoning, and linguistic comprehension. The triple division of working memory is conceived to contain (1) the central executive, which also controls attention, and two slave subsystems called (2) a visuospatial sketch pad, which manipulates visual images, and (3) the phonological loop, which stores and rehearses speech information (Baddeley, 1992).

The prime function of working memory is considered to be the coördination of mental resources, although functions other than concurrent storage and processing are suspected to exist. Experimental evidence for the existence of a tripartite working memory system is seen in situations requiring concurrent visual and verbal tasks. For example, in the early stages of disease, Alzheimer patients can perform either type of task well, whereas performance on the combined tasks deteriorates markedly compared to elderly controls. This is consistent with the hypothesis of a central executive deficit in Alzheimer's disease.

Evidence for the phonological loop and visuospatial scratch pad also is demonstrated by this analytic approach using dual-task paradigms. This method has disclosed separable visual and spatial components, with different tasks differentially recruiting the two. For example, some imagery tasks rely more on pattern than spatial information or vice versa. Having found ways of separately disrupting spatial and verbal processing, investigators currently are exploring the relative contribution of different subsystems to complex intellectual tasks.

Clinical experiments with the phonological loop concept suggest that short-term phonological memory is crucial in the acquisition of new vocabulary, both in native and foreign tongues. Patients with specific phonological loop deficits typically have difficulty comprehending certain types of complex sentences, although they otherwise have remarkably few signs of cognitive impairment.

In summary, the concept of a hypothetical working memory integrates memory, attention, and perception. Conceptual links between working memory, attention, the control of voluntary action, visual perception, visually directed action, speech perception, and speech production are expected to be derived from this model, although how this will relate to biology remains to be elucidated.

Priming

There is a recently discovered aspect of memory called *priming* that is not episodic, procedural, nor semantic. Instances of priming are unconscious and are believed by those who experience them to be instances of perception rather than memory. The role of priming seems to be, in fact, to enhance identification of objects so that they seem *familiar*.

Priming is said to exist when the appearance of fragments of a previously encountered target (the first few letters, a sketchy outline, tachistoscope presentation) either increases the probability of identification or decreases the latency of identification.

Tulving and Schacter (1990) explain priming by conceiving a "pre-semantic perceptual system that can operate independently of episodic memory." In keeping with ideas of the distributed system they suggest that both priming and object recognition are expressions of "a single perceptual representation system (PRS), which exists separately from but interacts closely with other memory systems."

That this might be so is suggested by the response of those confronted with ambiguous stimuli; they may either respond in a perceptual mode (i.e., try to figure out what the stimulus is) or a mnestic one (they recall it). Priming occurs both verbally and with nonverbal pictures, shapes, and faces. The fact that priming is demonstrated with complex three-dimensional structures, but not with Escher-like impossible objects, suggests that priming of object perception depends on perceiving these objects as structured wholes.

Studies with dyslexics who are able to read irregular words (those that cannot be sounded out on the basis of grapheme-to-phoneme conversion rules) further suggest that the perceptual representation system conceptualized does exist at a presemantic level.

Other properties of priming are (1) its early appearance (priming effects are as large in children as in college students, and do not wane in the elderly), (2) its lack of degradation by drugs, such as alcohol and scopolamine, that impede other categories of memory, and (3) its presence even in the most densely amnesic individuals. Priming is currently a topic of scrutiny. What its clinical implications will be are unknown at present.

Retrograde and Anterograde Amnesia

Most of what is known about *retrograde amnesia* comes from study of head trauma or electroconvulsive therapy. At its simplest, recent memories are more disturbed than ones formed long ago. With time, the gap narrows yet never resolves completely, leaving patients with a span of personal history that is blank. Retrograde amnesia may mar recollection going back years. This suggests an interaction between medial temporal components and more lateral cortical sites.

The existence of retrograde amnesia sheds some light on the question of forgetting, and whether amnesia is a defect of storage or retrieval. A straightforward failure of retrieval would mean that all recollections are equally impaired, not just the ones most recently acquired. The return of apparently forgotten memories with time suggests that biologic substrate was not lost, but that access to it was somehow impeded. This explanation, however, neglects the most obvious fact that amnesia for the time immediately preceding injury is permanent, a fact irreconcilable with a blockage of retrieval. This is an unsettled question.

Anterograde amnesia really refers more to learning than to recalling. It is the inability to learn new information after an acquired lesion. Patient HM, of course, remains the most famous instance of failure to learn new material across all modalities. Aside from head trauma, the other common condition producing both anterograde and retrograde amnesia is herpes simplex encephalitis, which preferentially attacks the temporal lobes. Heretofore, the neuropathology has been considered to always be bilaterally symmetrical, and the consequent neuropsychological profiles accordingly similar across cases. Not until widespread availability of both in vivo imaging and more sophisticated neuropsychological probes in the early 1980s did we appreciate that marked asymmetry could exist in herpetic encephalitis and that such asymmetries disclosed robust dissociations between lateralized processes in both retrograde and anterograde memory.

The case of Esslinger et al. (1993), which had nearly unilateral right-sided damage, suggests that the right temporal lobe (possibly in combination with the basal forebrain and insula) is critical for retrograde memory in all modalities. Additionally, the interruption of specific verbal linkages regarding personal and public events suggests an obligate interaction of both temporal lobes to process autobiographical and contextual aspects of retrograde memory. Their patient is most accurate when she has to retrieve the least amount of unique visual detail. For example, while she recognizes the generic class of dogs, she does not recognize her own dog or his particular breed. Her retrograde amnesia therefore includes not only the expected episodic items, but also non-episodic non-verbal knowledge that is "not bound by time, space, or specific personal experience" (Esslinger et al., p. 149).

In contrast to this patient's total non-verbal anterograde amnesia, new verbal knowledge accrues normally and with appropriate lexical relationships. Another noteworthy dissociation is conscious (anterograde) learning. Though she cannot consciously recognize her examiners, this patient generates consistent and significantly larger galvanic skin responses to certain new faces, indicating that covert learning does take place.

A similarly selective impairment of non-verbal anterograde memory followed right-sided damage to the anterior commissure and fornix (Botez-Marquard & Botez, 1992). Anterograde amnesia for visual stimuli, new visual images, loss of topographic memory, and cessation of dreaming were all affected and dissociated from normal verbal performance.

Lesions in the ventral part of the dorsal thalamus, the mammillothalamic tract, and the rostroventral medullary thalamic lamina also produce an anterograde amnesia that can be predominantly verbal or visual depending on the side of the lesion. Appropriately placed lesions are most commonly found in patients with Korsakoff's psychosis and those with thalamic infarcts. This material-specific anterograde amnesia occurs in the absence of dementia, neglect, or disturbances of arousal or attention (Pepin & Auray-Pepin, 1993).

Though our attention had been fixed on the hippocampal formation for decades after the 1957 report of HM, we now know that the medial temporal lobe system (figure 9.1) plays both a temporary and a narrower role in memory than previously thought. The hippocampal system mediates conscious, explicit (declarative) memory, whereas implicit (nondeclarative) procedural memory is handled by systems in thalamus, diencephalon, and neocortex. While the hippocampal formation has robust, reciprocal projections to neocortical columns, information from neocortex need not even reach the hippocampus in order for *some* memory to consolidate. In monkeys, for example, disconnecting the inferotemporal neocortex from the limbic system severely disrupts memory. By comparison, lesioning the fornix (a major subcortical projection to hippocampal formation) or the mammillary bodies (a major diencephalic projection of the fornix) causes only mild amnesia (Squire & Zola-Morgan, 1991).

Confabulation

Confabulation is a recitation of imaginary experiences, a filling in of gaps in one's knowledge to compensate for perceptual loss or amnesia. Patients with amnesia tend to *confabulate*. Patients' comments are a product of their speech area, and one could possibly reckon amnesia to be the inaccessibility of knowledge to speech. Patients are unable to introspect about activities in a piece of brain that has no access to speech, so confabulation is an attempt to explain what the patient cannot understand. In normal usage, "confabulate" means to chat or talk familiarly together (*con* ["together"] + *fabulari* ["chat"]; *fabula* ["story"]). Although medical usage of the form implies falsification of events, the implausible fabrications do flow smoothly in a chatty, easy way into the texture of the conversation.

Little has been added to the characteristics of confabulation since Weinstein (1955, 1963) and Geschwind (1965a) elucidated them: (1) it does not occur in the absence of a deficit, (2) it is less marked when aphasia is present, (3) it is more likely if there is some general clouding such as dementia or encephalopathy, and (4) it is more likely when association cortex or fibers (either commissural or intrahemispheric) are injured than in solitary damage to primary sensory pathways up to and including unimodal cortex. The less prominent the dementia and a cloudy sensorium are, the more confabulation depends on lesions of association cortex or fibers.

Geschwind's explanation of confabulation is similar to that of release hallucinations. He assumed that the association areas never fail to send a message to the speech area and always send positive messages regarding circumstances. If the primary visual cortex is destroyed, the speech area still remains innervated by visual association cortex. In this case, association cortex, receiving no stimulus from striate cortex, would send the message to the speech area that there is no visual message—that is, everything is black.

The destruction of association cortex or its projections is an unphysiologic state—one in which *no message* reaches the speech area. In this state, the speech area may react to its own spontaneous firing or to random firing from subcortical pathways. A partial disconnection means that the neural signals are inadequate to convey all the information for the "true" stimulus to reach conscious perception. This may lead to errors that are less bizarre than in total isolation of the speech cortex.

Confabulation may be spontaneous. That is, patients may say things that are obviously not true. Knowing full well that none of these events happened, examiners may draw out a confabulated response with leading questions such as, "Do you remember me?", "Didn't we have lunch together?", and "When did you see me last?" Some patients may deliberately make up answers just to please the doctor, which is not confabulation at all. (Patients are shrewd creatures who often tell you what you want to hear if you carelessly pose your questions. Technique matters.)

Confabulation is an interesting quirk of mentation that has no clinical use, yet students and even seasoned examiners may become excited when encountering it. In this regard, confabulation is similar to the eosinophil: Both elicit joy on their recognition by individuals who often can recognize little else.

The Role of Prefrontal and Cerebellar Cortices

That the prefrontal cortex modulates memory was first suggested by lesion analysis in animals and in humans with frontal leukotomies. Unfortunately, lesions tended to be large and variably placed, making satisfactory correlations difficult.

Patients with frontal lesions do not have amnesia in the usual sense, but fail when recall involves context, temporal order, or spatial order. Such tasks include the chronological ordering of events, recency discrimination, frequency-of-occurrence estimations, and recollection of specific autobiographical dates. Also, in addition to failing a variety of metacognitive abilities, patients with frontal lesions are impaired on metamemory judgements (Pepin & Auray-Pepin, 1993). All modality-specific areas project to prefrontal cortex, which is also reciprocally connected to limbic structures.

It is appropriate to consider the role of the cerebellum in memory here, because specific cerebellar nuclei appear to be part of a distributed system involved in cognitive planning, and the most lateral parts of the cerebellar hemispheres may enable prefrontal cortex to execute learned procedures optimally (Appollonio et al., 1993). As reviewed in chapter 3, reciprocal cerebro-cerebellar projections operate via neocortico-ponto-cerebellar and dentato-thalamo-neocortical pathways whose principal projections are to prefrontal neocortex. Patients with cerebellar atrophy perform similarly to controls on implicit memory tasks that, by definition, do not call on conscious resources. In contrast, cerebellar patients do show retrieval deficits when intention and sustained effort is required. Such patients manifest frontal symptoms in their poor planning and execution of a sequence. SPECT studies reveal a dopaminergic link involving cerebellum, basal ganglia, and the frontal lobe (Botez, 1993). Additionally, low cerebrospinal fluid homovanillic acid levels (a dopamine metabolite) are noted in cerebellar atrophy patients.

Modulating Factors

It seems that many neurotransmitters and hormones can influence memory. This knowledge has been gleaned from pharmacological manipulation in animals as well as natural human diseases in which a diminution of given substances has been detected. For example, acetylcholine is lacking in Alzheimer's disease, norepinephrine in Korsakoff's syndrome, and GABA and acetylcholine in Huntington's disease.

At present, norepinephrine, dopamine, serotonin, acetylcholine, GABA, alpha-melanocyte-stimulating hormone, and the pituitary hormones adrenocorticotropic hormone (ACTH), vasopressin, and oxytocin are all firmly implicated as memory modulators. How they act in this role has not yet been precisely determined.

SPECIFIC CLINICAL DISORDERS OF MEMORY

Dementia of the Alzheimer's Type

Loss of memory probably is the most salient feature of Alzheimer's dementia and will eventually be found at some course of the disease in every case. Sometimes, it is the presenting symptom; at other times it follows a decline in other cognitive spheres. Though episodic long-term amnesia (table 9.1) stands out as one of the more salient features of Alzheimer's disease, the memory impairment also includes short-term and semantic failures and some aspects of implicit memory (e.g., word stem completion).

There is a marked death of small neurons in the basal forebrain, particularly the nucleus basalis of Meynert, a structure rich in cholinergic neurons. This relationship was what first suggested that acetylcholine was vital to mnestic integrity. However, basal forebrain degeneration alone does not cause amnesia. The pathol-

Table 9.1
Clinical Amnestic Syndromes

---

1. *Amnesia of sudden onset and short duration*
   Transient global amnesia
   Post-concussive syndrome
   Temporal lobe-limbic seizure
2. *Amnesia of sudden onset, long duration, and incomplete recovery*
   Hippocampal infarctions (posterior cerebral artery territory)
   Hypoxia-ischemia (carbon monoxide poisoning, Stokes-Adams attacks)
   Trauma to medial temporal and diencephalic structures subserving
      memory
   Subarachnoid hemorrhage (? due to diaschesis)
3. *Subacute amnesia with lasting impairment*
   Wernicke-Korsakoff disease
   Herpes simplex hemorrhagic encephalitis
   Basal meningitides
4. *Progressive amnesia*
   Alzheimer's disease and other degenerations that target temporal
      structures
   Third vertricular tumors

---

ogy in Alzheimer's disease imputable to memory is in the entorhinal cortex and subiculum. The clinical features are discussed
in the next chapter.

Transient Global Amnesia

Transient global amnesia is a dramatic, acute, and reversible amnesia that occurs in middle-aged to elderly persons. Patients are
addled and perplexed for hours, and keep asking what is going on.
They are amnesic for current and recent events, but all other cognitive functions remain normal, as do the neurological and general
medical exams.

Recurrences are rare but do happen. Transient global amnesia
is a benign albeit dramatic event, so no intervention is required.
Elaborate or invasive workups are uninformative and unwarranted.
The exact cause is uncertain, but one proposal suggests that transient global amnesia represents a vertebrobasilar transient ischemic
attack, whereas another posits a temporal lobe seizure. Progression

to stroke is rare and definitive evidence of seizure has never been reported.

Korsakoff's Psychosis

Korsakoff's psychosis consists of an anterograde and retrograde amnesia. Confabulation is classically regarded as part of the syndrome although it is not an invariant feature. The memory deficit is distinct from any other disturbance of higher cortical function or, if deficits are found, they are mild.

Patients with Korsakoff's psychosis have a clear sensorium and understand what is required of them. There is no aphasia. The absence of additional cognitive impairments distinguishes Korsakoff's psychosis from a variety of other conditions. Here, a global amnesia is the salient feature.

The pathology centers on the hippocampal formation and dorsomedial thalamus. Earlier, it was thought that the pronounced lesions of the mammillary bodies caused the amnesia, but ideas about this have changed and cases are seen in which either the mammillary bodies or thalamic nuclei remain unscathed. At present, it is not possible to say definitively whether damage to one or both structures is required to produce symptoms. Ablations in monkeys, however, unequivocally show that lesions of the mediodorsal nucleus alone can cause amnesia. Bilateral thalamic infarcts in humans have produced selective deficits instead of global amnesia. The patient of Malamut et al. (1992) who had thalamic infarcts, for example, had anterograde episodic and semantic amnesia, yet priming and remote memory remained intact.

Korsakoff's psychosis occurs from third ventricular tumors, infarctions, or herpes simplex encephalitis. Most often, however, it is caused by thiamine deficiency in chronic alcoholism. In this setting, it is usually part of the *Wernicke-Korsakoff syndrome* and is quite stereotypical.

Wernicke's disease consists of ophthalmoplegia, gait ataxia, and encephalopathy. Features of Korsakoff psychosis have already been described. Once alcohol withdrawal has subsided, the existence of Korsakoff's psychosis may be evident. Peripheral neuropathy is present in more than 80% of cases, and alcoholic cardiac disease is also common.

Both the retrograde and anterograde amnesia may be severe, with patients incapable of recalling the simplest of three objects despite numerous attempts. This is striking given the fact that they can repeat what is requested of them and even explain its significance. Yet memory fails completely.

The symptoms of Wernicke's disease and Korsakoff's psychosis do not represent separate diseases, even though their coöccurrence in the Wernicke-Korsakoff syndrome implies otherwise. Rather, the physical and mental signs are the multifaceted manifestation of a single disease. The syndrome is not due to alcohol toxicity either. Rather, thiamine deficiency is specifically responsible for all symptoms, including the mental confusion during the acute state. However, the persistence of amnesia to some degree and the pathological changes in the diencephalon and midline entities suggest that the amnesia is due to structural loss or lasting functional impairment rather than simple substrate deficiency.

Indeed, the cognitive impairment of patients with Korsakoff's psychosis correlates with their deficient central catecholamine activity. CSF samples from a large cohort show significant reductions in 3–methoxy-4–hydroxy-phenylglycol (MHPG) and homovanillic acid (HVA), the respective primary brain metabolites of norepinephrine and dopamine. Patients with amnesia have more consistently diminished CSF MHPG, and lower levels of CSF HVA correlate with performance on tests of motor learning but not memory impairment (i.e., there is a double dissociation).

Alcoholic Blackouts

The term *alcoholic blackout* refers to a transient amnesia during severe intoxication. This is almost always seen in chronic alcoholics with marked tolerance who are able to consume prodigious amounts of ethanol without dying. Far less often, acutely intoxicated individuals with no tolerance may also fail to recall their drinking spree. Patients in a blackout act normally for many hours and acquaintances notice nothing unusual. The patient may suddenly "come to" in strange or dangerous circumstances, far away from home, having indulged in uncharacteristic acts, and yet have no inkling how this all transpired.

Blackouts are an early and extremely serious prognostic sign of alcoholism. A drinking, drug, and social history should be taken and appropriate advice given to cease drinking permanently. The danger of this sign should not be underestimated.

Concussion

Individuals may have amnesia following a shaking injury to the brain. Previously, much was made of the duration of post-traumatic amnesia as a prognostic sign. It was also thought that patients had to be unconscious (often for hours) for amnesia to occur. These ideas are now known to be overly simplistic and wrong.

There is a noteworthy one-way dissociation between consciousness and amnesia following concussion. It is possible to have amnesia following a shaking of the brain that does not produce loss of consciousness. However, individuals who lose consciousness have an obligatory amnesia. Few practitioners are aware of this dissociation, which is why concussed individuals who did not appear unconscious and yet who complain of forgetfulness are erroneously judged to be malingering. Anterograde learning is more troubling than retrograde amnesia in such persons.

Forgetfulness in the Senium

It was long assumed that mental enfeeblement and forgetfulness were part of normal ageing. This outmoded notion far overstates the case. Though we have all encountered remarkable individuals who remain mentally sharp and productive beyond the eighth decade, it is now becoming clear that some aspects of memory do decline variably in the senium (Albert & Knoefel, 1994).

Considering the elderly as a group, one can say that *learning* (acquisition of new knowledge) declines linearly with increasing age and is not correlated with education, whereas *delayed recall* (forgetting) is stable across age. This selective decline may be clinically useful in that one may suspect organic disease if learning is impaired more than expected or if delayed recall is impaired to any extent. *Cueing* (giving hints) augments a normal elderly person's recall performance to near perfect levels, a feature not seen in Alzheimer's disease.

The definitive basis for progressive decline in learning is not known but may be related to neuronal dropout in hippocampus and parahippocampal gyrus, plus a reduction in neurotransmitter modulation. Consistent with the idea of structural loss is a reduction of hippocampal tissue seen on MRI volumetry that correlates with the severity of forgetfulness. MRI volumetry remains experimental and, like other correlations between imaging and behavior, is fraught with error (cf. Damasio & Damasio, 1989, for a sanguine view).

Turning to the juices of the mnemon, a number of neurochemicals are important to learning and memory, particularly catecholamine-containing ones. As noted earlier in chapter 3 catecholamine-containing neurons are phylogenetically old, numerically sparse, and project extensively throughout the central nervous system. That catecholamine nerve terminals are found both with and without synaptic connections implies both transmitter and modulatory functions. Substantial evidence now indicates that catecholamine systems are impaired in both aged humans and animals (McEntee & Crook, 1990). In fact, treatment with clonidine, an alpha-2–noradrenergic agonist, causes a remarkably similar improvement in mnemonic performance among aged monkeys, young monkeys with neurotoxic depletion of catecholamine in the dorsolateral prefrontal cortex, and humans with Korsakoff's psychosis. Furthermore, clonidine shows an inverse dose-response pattern. That is, the greater the loss of norepinephrine, the lower the amount of drug required for optimal mnemonic improvement.

The three findings that suggest abnormal memory unrelated to expected declines in the senium are (1) a learning performance below that of age-adjusted norms, (2) poor learning that cannot be improved by cueing, and (3) impaired delayed recall (Petersen et al., 1992).

Psychogenic Memory Loss

Psychogenic amnesia is the sudden failure to remember important personal information, and usually follows severe psychosocial stress. Typical stressors involve the threat of physical injury or death, natural disasters, military combat, and rejections and other intolerable interpersonal events. Resolution also is abrupt and usually complete; recurrences are rare. One usually finds a clear precipitating factor—often a situation from which no possible escape other than an illusory one exists. Psychoanalysis long ago suggested that metaphorically "going away" made amnesia and fugue states substitutes for suicide.

Four patterns are typical. *Circumscribed psychogenic amnesia* is most common, and involves forgetting the hours surrounding some terrible event, such as the death of companions in a plane crash one has personally survived. *Selective psychogenic amnesia* involves blockage of selected details of an unpleasant event. *Generalized psychogenic amnesia* encompasses all past life history antedating the precipitant, whereas *continuous psychogenic amnesia* is a global one that advances up to the present moment.

A *fugue* involves amnesia for personal identity plus the key feature of wandering, often far from one's starting point. The individual appears outwardly normal and gives no hint of having lost personal identity. A false identity is given instead. The outwardly normal behavior is contrasted to that of somnambulism or transient global amnesia, in which observers promptly discern that something is wrong. Persons emerge from the fugue having no recall for concurrent events but nonetheless resuming their former identity, or else they emerge with lost identity and amnesia for all past life events.

The European literature suggests that men are more likely than women to experience fugues, that they often have a reputation for lying, history of previous fugues, and depression, and carry psychopathic personality diagnoses. Perhaps this impression has stuck because military sources provided much of the clinical material. The American Psychiatric Association's DSM III manual states that young women are more prone to psychogenic amnesia and has no opinion regarding age and sex ratios for fugues.

Treatment is similar to that for conversion hysteria and may use superficial psychotherapy, hypnosis, narcotic abreaction, or "talk and explanation." The prognosis is good, and often patients speedily recover their memories. Psychogenic amnesia as defined by the DSM manual is distinct from both the "Hollywood amnesia" mentioned earlier and the "recovered memories" of the legal cottage industry that has made *abuse* a household word.

THERAPY FOR AMNESIA

In much the same way that ophthalmologists are interested in blindness but not vision, neuropsychologists often are concerned about amnesia but not remembering. In other words, patients going blind complain that eye doctors have little practical advice to recommend regarding devices or techniques that might help them better use their remaining vision. Likewise, short of saying "Make a list," neuropsychologists fail to suggest how amnesics might compensate for their waning memory.

Amnesia is a severe disruption not only for the individual suffering from it but also for immediate family and coworkers. It disrupts efforts at both physical and mental rehabilitation. Obviously, little can be achieved when patients constantly ask the same questions or are unable to retain the flow of events.

Historically, the muscle-building approach featuring drills, repetitive practice, non-structured list making, or computer-aided exercises has not enhanced practical memory in naturalistic settings. Tasks that emphasize factual organization through mnemonic devices such as imagery or mental "pegboards" likewise fail because they further strain the individual's already limited capacity.

There appears to be some reason for rejecting the widespread pessimism that there is nothing to be done for those who suffer from amnesia (Levin, 1990; Young & Delwaide, 1992). Recent attention has turned from trying to improve scores on laboratory-based memory tasks to seeing what works in a natural environment (Mateer & Sohlberg, 1988). Patients with amnesia need to remember to take their medication, visit the therapist or physician, and do any number of errands much more than they need to remember test material about Anna Thompson of South Boston or the cowboy who got a new suit. In a natural setting, patients are most concerned about their ability to remember future actions they must take (prospective memory) and about attention-based forgetting (remembering why they went into another room, for example). They are far less concerned about forgetting semantic facts or overlearned ones. The kind of things that patients do forget varies from individual to individual, in part depending on each person's unique neuropathology. So, any treatment needs to be tailored to individual needs.

Unfortunately, commonly used formal tests tend to focus on re-call ability rather than prospective memory, and further fail to find out why someone does poorly on a particular test. Mateer and Sohlberg have outlined a triple approach to memory rehabilitation that involves (1) attention training, so that individuals can focus on a particular task, (2) prospective memory training, and (3) memory notebook training. The goal of attention training is to be able to switch between tasks and handle multiple tasks. Pro-spective memory training seeks to extend the interval during which someone can carry out a given task by repetitive rehearsing as the target time approaches. When residual disability impairs daily success in naturalistic settings, then a structured memory notebook may offer some stability.

Unfortunately, clinicians often advise patients to "make lists" but then no more specific instructions, leaving patients and fami-lies to their own devices. Structured and rule-governed notebook training is intensive (giving prospective memory tasks at least three times a day, four days a week), but the results hold promise. Additionally, this kind of training imitates real-life situations.

Systematic training and feedback is necessary to keep the note-book's use from being short-lived (Sohlberg & Mateer, 1989), and notebooks must be tailored for individual needs. Some persons, for example, may need orientation reminders with autobiographical details about where they live, their phone number, and so forth while others have no difficulty with such overlearned information.

Suggested sections for a structured memory notebook include orientation, a memory log recording what the patient has done; a calendar for appointments; a things-to-do section; a transportation section with maps, schedules, and directions for frequently visited places; a feelings log to record emotional events; a name section to deposit identifying information about persons newly met; and a today-at-work section, which helps structure the job environment for those who return to work.

Patients are first trained in *how* to use the memory book and its various sections, and then in *when* and *where* to utilize it. This begins with role playing, advances into the hospital or clinic world, and ultimately moves into the patients's own living situation. Al-though memory notebook advocates make no mention of it, the technique of a structured workbook, as developed by the American depth psychologist Ira Progoff over thirty years, itself exerts powerful associative forces among memory, feeling, noësis, and understanding (Progoff, 1959, 1994).

Lastly, you should be aware that patients looking for hope may turn to pure empiricism, trying anything and everything to see what works, no matter how absurd a purported remedy might appear. Some individuals offering alternative therapies are well-intentioned, others are unscrupulous. One supposed memory aid is aromatherapy, whose legitimacy is based on the common observation that scents often evoke strong memories (even though these memories are episodic). That any scent from chocolate to mothballs to flowers is equally effective on student volunteers taking verbal recall tests indicates that there is nothing unique about whatever expensive olfactory stimuli are being peddled. Any novel stimulus does just as well. And, of course, belief itself is a powerful therapy.

SUGGESTED READINGS

Cohen NJ, Eichenbaum H. 1993 *Memory, Amnesia, and the Hippocampal System*. Cambridge: MIT Press

Dudai Y. 1989 *The Neurobiology of Memory*. New York: Oxford University Press

Fuster JM. 1995 *Memory in the Cerebral Cortex: An Empirical Approach to Neural Networks in the Human and Nonhuman Primate*. Cambridge: MIT Press

Kandell E. 1979 Psychiatry and the single synapse: Impact of psychiatric thought on neurobiologic research. *New England Journal of Medicine* 301:1028–1037

Squire LR. 1987 *Memory and Brain*. New York: Oxford University Press

Squire LR, Butters N. 1993 *Neuropsychology of Memory*, 2d ed. New York: Guilford

10 Dementia: An Example of Diffuse Disease

The terms *diffuse* and *non-focal* distinguish cerebral disorders in which the pathological process is relatively circumscribed. Dementia is my primary example. Diagnosing nonfocal conditions depends mostly on syndromic analysis (see p. 142 to refresh your memory if necessary). That is, you note the temporal course, etiology, demographics, and pattern that its features form. From this, you infer whether any topographic regions are affected and include this inference in the syndromic analysis.

The distinction between focal and nonfocal disorders is not precise. Illnesses caused by reasonably circumscribed pathology can affect remote brain regions (diaschisis), and nonfocal hardly means that the pathology is homogeneous. It may be anatomically widespread even though possibly restricted to a single entity (a disease of myelin, for example, or of one neurotransmitter). This imprecision reflects our struggle to impose intellectual order on what exists.

Dementia is common and a rather prototypical example of diffuse disease, and my purpose is to be representative rather than encyclopedic. Parkinson's disease, multiple sclerosis, closed head trauma, metastatic tumor, and the various stroke syndromes are other examples of diffuse disease, but are not mentioned in detail. One could literally consider systemic and metabolic illnesses to be nonfocal, but this takes the term too far.

Although Alzheimer's disease is presently a very popular topic, I must first provide general information before rattling off the inevitable eponyms. Almost all my comments, however, are relevant to the individual Alzheimer patient. Indeed, many practitioners regard Alzheimer's dementia as the archetypal dementia.

TERMINOLOGY OF DEMENTIA

Dementia (Latin *de* + *mens* = "mind") is an acquired loss of intellect. Aphasia, amnesia, agnosognosia, and similar *isolated* defects are excluded, although these entities may, with time, be among the many symptoms evident in a demented person. Dementia is not a disease but a collection of disorders and, for precision's sake, you need to specify the etiology if possible. Because some dementias are treatable, differential diagnosis is important.

Table 4.1 showed an annual incidence rate of 50 cases of dementia per 100,000 population, regardless of age. The rate is highest in those older than seventy-five years, and dementia is more prevalent in women. Elderly women are three times more likely to develop dementia than men, and women with a history of myocardial infarction are five times more prone to dementia than those without such a history (Aronson et al., 1990). Popular opinion seems to be that dementia is both rampant and widespread, but no more than 5% of persons older than sixty-five years are demented such that they cannot care for themselves. Perhaps up to 10% have mild cognitive impairments that are less disruptive. Several factors lead to overdiagnosing dementia, and Alzheimer's disease (AD) in particular.

First, AD has been singled out as a U.S. Congressional (sic !) *Decade of the Brain* topic, which increases awareness of the disease. Populations in developed countries are getting proportionately older, and the public is increasingly knowledgeable about AD. Second, although pathologic diagnosis is the standard of accuracy, clinicians often must settle for diagnoses of "probable" AD. A mere 55% to 82% of cases are accurately diagnosed clinically (Chui, 1989) when compared to biopsy or postmortem criteria. Because careful thought is not always exercised, the Alzheimer label is liable to be attached to any decline in comportment in the same indiscriminate way that "hardening of the arteries" was thrown about only a decade ago. Though this is neither good science nor an accurate description of what ails the patient, it does show the need people have to label what they do not understand.

Finally, diseases go in and out of fashion just as do other human concerns. Hardening of the arteries has yielded to AD, and neurasthenia to chronic fatigue syndrome and multiple environmental toxicity. Are such concepts social fads, neurotic expressions, or bona fide illnesses? I said earlier that there are more ways of knowing than the scientific method, implying that a good practitioner is holistically minded. Be carefull, however, not to swing uncritically too far with the pendulum. We sometimes do not know what is wrong, but that does not give us license to berate people or call them crazy. Neither should we diagnose disease that isn't there. In some instances, only time yields an answer.

One can classify dementia by pathology, anatomic topography, etiology, or some other way. Table 10.1 classifies dementia according to clinical presentation, whereas table 10.2 shows relative frequencies of some of its etiologies. These distinctions should make it clear that dementia is a syndrome of many causes. It may be the only manifestation of disease, or it may accompany other neurological or general medical signs.

The term *subcortical dementia* was first used to characterize the mental decline that accompanies supranuclear palsy, possibly because the pathology was primarily in brainstem, thalamus, and basal ganglia rather than neocortex. Though pathological change may predominate in one place, *demented patients have pathology in both cortical and subcortical structures*. Thus, the dichotomy is overly simplistic. Unfortunately, the term still is used to refer to the mental symptoms accompanying human immunodeficiency virus (HIV) infection, lacunar state, and Parkinson's, Binswanger's, and Wilson's diseases.

CLINICAL COURSE OF DEMENTIA

Inconsistencies and repetitiousness may be the best way to characterize the insidious onset of most dementias. The clinical course does not follow any set pattern, and you may eventually see every behavioral entity described in previous chapters. Because association cortices bear the brunt of pathology, failures in memory, cognition, and adaptation are the major symptoms. However, it bears noting that dementia affects more than just mentation. *Gait, posture, reflexes, and physical vigor are invariably altered*, sometimes severely so.

The earliest signs may be subtle enough to be dismissed or attributed to psychodynamic causes. General psychomotor retarda-

Table 10.1
Clinical Presentation of Dementia

1. *Dementia as sole manifestation*
   Alzheimer's disease
   Pick's lobar atrophy

2. *Dementia with or without other neurological signs*
   Hydrocephalus
   Multi-infarct, other vascular disorders
   Intra- and extra-axial mass lesions
   Cerebral contusions or lacerations
   Pugilistic dementia
   Marchiafava-Bignami disease

3. *With obligatory neurologic signs*
   Creutzfeldt-Jakob disease
   Myoclonic epilepsy
   Huntington's chorea
   Schilder's disease
   Pediatric disease presenting in adults

4. *Dementia with other medical disease*
   Wernicke-Korsakoff disease
   Subacute combined degeneration
   Folate deficiency
   HIV-associated dementia
   Chronic meningoëncephalitis
   Pulmonary hypoxia and hypercapnia
   Wilson's disease (familial or acquired)
   Myxedema
   Cushing's syndrome
   Pellagra
   Drug intoxication (acute or chronic)
   Multifocal leukoëncephalopathy

Table 10.2
Relative Frequency of Various Dementias

Illness	Frequency (%)
Alzheimer's disease	50
Multi-infarct and other vascular disorders	15
Tumor and infection	10
Pseudo-dementias (treatable)	7
Alcoholic dementia	7
Normal-pressure hydrocephalus	5
Drug intoxication	3
Undiagnosed	3

tion and forgetfulness often herald dementia's onset. Language and memory are involved early, though all intellectual skills eventually suffer as disease progresses. The patient is unable to do familiar tasks and may restrict his or her activities. Deferring to family members when unable to answer questions is characteristic. Word-finding difficulty and repetitious rambling give way to the confusional phase, in which multiple cognitive defects are obvious to everyone.

Irrefutable amnesia, getting lost, having trouble dressing, spatial disorientation, disinhibition and change in comportment, neglect of one's toilette, emotional lability, poor adaptive behavior, and frank paraphasic speech are the collective emergence of parietal, frontal, and temporal lobe signs. The catastrophic reaction mentioned in chapter 6 is the patient's emotional attempt to cope with losing his or her mind. Strict orderliness and compulsion may be one attempt to mitigate against mental chaos; withdrawal may be another; belligerence, verbal tirades, and unfocused anger may be yet a third. One often hears that the premorbid personality becomes exaggerated in degenerative diseases, but enough instances in which milksops become monsters and tyrants turn tame are known to experienced clinicians.

Release of primitive reflexes, rigidity, hyperreflexia, and the frontal gait disorder make their appearance. Bladder and bowel incontinence emerge late in the course. At this point, patients usually are vacant and fail to recognize their family. General physical deterioration and frailty complete the picture. The typical course runs five to fifteen years. Patients end up bedridden, mute, and enfeebled, often in the posture of Yakovlev's cerebral paraplegia in flexion.

REVERSIBLE DEMENTIAS

Because they can be mitigated if detected early, the reversible dementias should rise swiftly to mind in one's differential diagnosis.

Intoxications

The elderly commonly take more than one prescription medication. Coupled with the fact that they metabolize drugs less efficiently than younger persons, polypharmacy is a frequent culprit when an elder's mentation has fizzled. The distinction between whether the patient suffers from dementia or encephalopathy is somewhat academic, because the practical issue is that mental impairment from intoxication is reversible if detected quickly. A distinct danger is that exogenous agents might be lethal.

Common culprits are tranquilizers, sleeping pills, analgesics, steroids, ulcer medications, anticholinergics, antidepressants and other psychoactive drugs, blood pressure medicines, digitalis, and theophylline and other asthma medication. Drug interactions may be synergistic. Exogenous agents capable of producing dementia are the heavy metals, carbon monoxide, and manganese.

The comments I made in chapter 4 about an acute change in mental status are particularly relevant to intoxications. (Review the terminology there as necessary, especially the distinction between encephalopathy and dementia.) Although the mental clouding that results from intoxication can be either acute or chronic, acute changes should make you especially suspicious of exogenous agents. Many in-hospital cases are sadly iatrogenic, the result of polypharmacy, dehydration, or sensory deprivation. By themselves or jointly with electrolyte imbalance, the effects of forgotten standing drug orders are compounded when various physicians and house staff prescribe independently and without reviewing what the patient is already being given. Preparation for diagnostic procedures (enemas, fasting, "on-call" medication) and substances such as contrast media, anesthetics, anticholinergics, and sedatives administered during radiographic, gastrointestinal, cardiac, and similar procedures can trigger an encephalopathy or unmask an incipient dementia.

Iatrogenic intoxications are preventable if one takes care in prescribing and in obtaining an accurate drug history. Patients almost never volunteer that they are taking prescription medication given by someone else and must be specifically asked, especially about sleeping pills. A little forethought would avoid the reflexive response of ordering emergency scans. Searching for a structural cause—especially the muchsought subdural hematoma—in the setting of acute mental change is unproductive and often delays discovering the real cause.

Metabolic Abnormalities

Renal, hepatic, pancreatic, thyroid, parathyroid, adrenal, and pituitary failure all produce an encephalopathy that may be reversible, depending on how well one can address the underlying organ failure. Abnormal values on a multichannel automated blood chemistry profile often make one suspect derangement in one of these organ systems. Jefferson and Marshall (1981) provide a useful review of the mental manifestations of common medical conditions.

Renal Failure

Renal failure is an excellent example of how a metabolic disorder produces diffuse cerebral disease. The common neurological manifestations of renal failure, dialysis, and transplantation are: (1) uremic encephalopathy, (2) dialysis dysequilibrium, (3) dialysis dementia, (4) Wernicke's disease, (5) cerebral hemorrhage, (6) brain tumors, (7) meningitis, (8) central pontine myelinolysis, and (9) peripheral neuropathy.

Uremia is the presence of urinary constituents in the blood and the toxic condition resulting thereby. The earliest sign of *uremic encephalopathy* is a cloudy sensorium (decreased alertness and awareness of the environment) that is followed by variable and fluctuating motor signs (dysarthria, asterixis, gait ataxia, multifocal myoclonus, and seizures). Temporal variability of symptoms and signs, sometimes hourly, is characteristic. One moment patients seem well, but an hour later you must shout and shake them to get any response. Patients initially seem preoccupied or disinterested, and pause for an unnervingly long time before answering. Poor mental control (serial 7s, backward spelling, and the like are hopeless) is evident long before cognitive impairment occurs in encephalopathy, whereas the reverse is true in dementia (i.e., orientation and cognition fail in dementia long before the sensorium clouds). Sleep patterns often are reversed. Forgetfulness, confusion, misidentifications, illusions, and hallucinations ensue.

Surprisingly, the mental state does not correlate with the severity of uremia as measured by clinical chemistry. Rather, some suspect that the rate at which renal failure develops is important, given that profound encephalopathy is common enough in acute renal failure. Though this point is unsettled, it is known that brain calcium increases, oxygen metabolism decreases, and the granular layer of the cerebellar cortex degenerates (see chapters 3 and 6 to review cerebellar contributions to cognitive impairment. Whether granule cell necrosis is causative in uremic dementia or is only an agonal occurrence also remains unresolved.) Accumulation of organic acids and decreased cerebral glycolysis and ATPase activity are suspected to play a role as well.

As in many metabolic encephalopathies, *asterixis* appears once sensorial clouding is apparent. Instruct the patient to extend the wrists and "hold your hands up as if to stop traffic." Note the bilaterally asynchronous, arrhythmic flexion-extension of the wrists and side-to-side finger movements. Asterixis can also be demonstrated in the legs. The EEG shows generalized slowing with periodic high-voltage bursts, and the CSF is full of mononuclear cells (*pleocytosis*) and excess protein (*hyperproteinemia*). Other motor signs mentioned previously may all be present. *Convulsions* usually are a terminal sign.

These symptoms and signs are not necessarily unique to renal failure, and not all instances of renal failure or dialysis lead to dementia. I want to impress the importance of your making syndromic and etiologic diagnoses based on history, observation, and deduction—not on clinical features alone. For example, a large dose of penicillin (especially in those with impaired renal function but also in those with normal kidneys) can cause an encephalopathy of delirium, asterixis, myoclonus, and convulsions that is identical to the uremic type just described. The peripheral and mononeuropathies common in renal failure are outside the scope of this book, but are partly due to the same metabolic derangements that affect the cerebrum.

Hemo- or peritoneal-*dialysis* itself can produce many neurologic derangements—known as *dialysis dysequilibrium*—including headache (70%), vomiting, irritability, agitation, formication, delirium, speech arrest, obtundation, stupor, and coma. The cause is believed to be osmotic fluid gradient shifts that produce intracellular edema in the brain. Reducing the speed and frequency of dialysis helps. Because thiamine is a water-soluble vitamin, *Wernicke's disease* may appear suddenly. Dialysis patients all receive heparin, are more likely to fall than are well individuals, and often have thrombocytopenia: So you can also expect subdural and intracerebral *hemorrhages* and their behavioral accompaniments in this group of patients.

Dialysis dementia is subacute and invariably fatal. Its features are dysphasic speech, dementia, myoclonus, asterixis, facial grimacing, and convulsions. Although elevated concentrations of various substances have been found in brain tissue, the cause of dialysis demntia remains unsettled. Mental and physical signs may emerge and abate over the course of dialysis sessions, but ultimately they are progressive.

Lastly, even life-saving *renal transplantation* has unintended effects that interest the neuropsychologist. Reticulum cell sarcomas and lymphomas occur with increased frequency in transplant patients, probably because of immunosupression (the situation is similar to those with HIV infection). As with any mass lesion, cognitive dysfunction may occur depending on the location and speed of tumor growth. Even infections can produce mass effects in addition to their systemic effects. Fungi (*Candida, Nocardia, Aspergillus*), parasites (*Toxoplasma*), and viruses (cytomegalovirus, papova virus) are all likely in renal transplant patients. *Central pontine myelinolysis* occurs in up to 10% of autopsy series in transplant deaths. It may produce pseudobulbar palsy and obtundation in addition to the motor signs of quadraplegia during life. When initially described in 1959, it was believed to be due to nutritional deficiency; Laureno (1983) persuasively argued that it could be caused by the too-rapid correction of severe hyponatremia

Table 10.3
Childhood Ailments Presenting as Dementia in Adults

1. Neuronal inclusion disease (NID)
2. Alexander's disease
3. Lafora's disease
4. Kufs' disease
5. Cerebrotendinous xanthomatosis (CTX)
6. Polycystic lipomembranous osteodysplasia with sclerosing leukoëncephalopathy (PLO-SL)
7. Adrenoleukodystrophy (ALD)
8. Gangliosidosis 1, type III (GM$_1$-III)
9. Gangliosidosis 2 (GM$_2$)
10. Gaucher's disease, type I
11. Niemann-Pick disease, II-C
12. Mucopolysaccharidosis III-B (MPS) (Sanfilippo's disease)
13. Mitochondrial disorders
    - Mitochondrial encephalopathy with ragged-red fibers (MERRF)
    - Mitochondrial myopathy, encephalopathy, lactic acidosis, and strokelike episodes (MELAS)
14. Metachromatic leukodystrophy (MLD)
15. Wilson's disease
16. Fabry's disease
17. Krabbe's disease (globoid cell leukodystrophy [GCL])

(i.e., an electrolyte manipulation can cause permanent neuropathological lesions). Regardless, autopsy series suggest that the incidence of cerebral pontine myelinolysis is inexplicably high in renal transplant patients.

Inborn Metabolic Disorders

Some inborn disorders of metabolism become symptomatic only during adulthood. These include the many neuronal storage diseases, adrenoleukodystrophy (ALD), metachromatic leukodystrophy (MLD), and hepatolenticular degeneration (Wilson's disease). Wilson's disease and cerebrotendinous xanthomatosis (CTX) are the entities most successfully treated; ALD and mitochondrial disorders are potentially treatable (table 10.3).

The various enzymatic and metabolic deficiencies that cause neurodegenerative disease have long been thought to be difficult to pronounce, impossible to memorize, and rare. They also are considered the proper domain of pediatric neurologists. However, we now know that seventeen so-called pediatric neurodegenerative disorders can manifest anytime from the second to the sixth decade of adulthood. Table 10.2 shows that in 3% of patients who present with dementia, no diagnosis is reached. Because individuals with suspected Alzheimer's disease or any unknown type of dementia almost never are screened for hereditary or acquired errors of metabolism, how rare or common these disorders actually are unknown. It is safe to assume that a proportion of pediatricians know about them, but few general physicians could be aware of their existence, and they are virtually unknown to doctoral neuropsychologists. For this reason, I mention them here with the admonition to consider them in any *atypical dementia*, especially those presenting in young adults. That four of the seventeen disorders are treatable currently makes it morally imperative that more attention be given to disclosing these neurodegenerative disorders.

The details of these disorders are topics for advanced study and may be cogitated when you are experienced enough with the common dementias to recognize an atypical one. Coker (1991) gives an excellent review of the pediatric disorders that present as dementia in adults. Although they should be considered in any atypical dementia beginning in young adulthood, you should remember that the time of onset is highly variable in some. Ceroid lipofuscinosis begins at age thirty, for example, whereas neurologic symptoms may not emerge until the sixth decade in cerebrotendinous xanthomatosis. Table 10.3 lists the metabolic disorders that can present as dementia in adults, and tables 10.4 and 10.5 feature additional diagnostic considerations. Consider the tables as handy reminders, something to which you may refer back later in your career.

The history is paramount as several of these disorders have unique features. According to Coker, the special studies suggested in table 10.5 will permit diagnosis of eleven of the disorders (ALD, GM_1-III, GM_2, Niemann-Pick II-C, MPS III-B, MLD, Wilson's,

Table 10.4
Physical Signs in Metabolic Diseases

Myoclonus:	Kufs, Lafora, mitochondrial, PLO-SL
Organomegaly:	Niemann-Pick II-C, Gaucher's type I, MPS III-B

Dermatologic
   Xanthoma: CTX
   Hyperpigmentation: ALD
   Angiokeratoma: Fabry's

Supranuclear gaze palsy:	CTX, Gaucher's type I, Niemann-Pick II-C
Cataracts:	CTX, Fabry's
Short stature:	MPS III-B, mitochondrial
Extrapyramidal:	GM1-III, NID
Lower motor neuron:	Mitochondrial, GM2, ALD, MLD, GCL
Radiographic leukodystrophy:	Alexander's, PLO-SL, ALD, MLD, GCL
Abnormal skeletal X-rays:	Gaucher's, GM1-III, PLO-SL, MPS III-B

Note: See table 10.3 for explanation of abbreviations. From Coker (1991), with permission.

Fabry's, GLC, CTX, and Gaucher Type I), whereas the remaining six require muscle, liver, fat, rectal, or brain biopsy. Fortunately, the latter six have clinical characteristics that suggest themselves when the less invasive procedures have all turned up negative. Alexander's disease, for example, features progressive macrocephaly and leukodystrophy along with enhancement of the caudate nucleus on CT scanning.

Some of the metabolic dementias resemble Huntington's chorea because of their associated features such as ataxia, dysarthria, psychosis, myoclonus, facial dyskinesia, seizures, agnosia, cortical blindness, and supranuclear gaze palsy.

Rather than a classification of dementias based on their clinical characteristics, such as age of onset, a more logical classification grounded on basic defects probably will emerge in the next decade or two. Increasingly, we recognize that pediatric dementias can present in adulthood and that adult diseases also have metabolic and enzymatic defects (e.g., mitochondrial complex I deficiency in Parkinson's disease).

Table 10.5
Useful Studies for Demented Young Adults

1. Wrist x rays
2. Very long chain fatty acids
3. Sphingomyelinase
4. Glucocerebrosidase
5. GM1 beta-galactosidase
6. Hexosaminidase A
7. Mucopolysaccharide screen
8. Lactic acid-pyruvate
9. Alpha-N-acetyl-glucosaminidase
10. Arylsulfatase A
11. Copper, ceruloplasmin
12. Urinary dolichols
13. Bone marrow for foam cells
14. Alpha-galactosidase
15. Galactocerebroside beta-galactosidase
16. Serum cholestanol

From Coker (1991), with permission.

Substrate Deficiencies

The dementias due to pernicious anemia (vitamin B_{12} deficiency) and folate deficiency are reversible only if detected early. In contrast, pellagra quickly responds to niacin replacement even when dementia has been chronic. (The clinical triad of pellagra is diarrhea, dermatitis, and dementia.)

Wernicke-Korsakoff syndrome in alcoholics is the hallmark of thiamine deficiency, but thiamine deficiency does have other rare causes, such as anorexia nervosa, bulemia, geriatric anorexia (the tea-and-toast syndrome), protracted vomiting during pregnancy, and dialysis. It can be iatrogenic in hospital when you forget to supplement intravenous fluids with multivitamins for a patient who is not eating. It is believed that the amnesia of Korsakoff's psychosis does not respond fully to thiamine replacement because irreversible structural damage may have occurred by the time the patient receives medical attention.

HIV and Infectious Agents

One often thinks of Creutzfeldt-Jakob disease and progressive multifocal leukoëncephalopathy as the sole examples of infectious dementia. However, any central nervous system infection can cause dementia if prolonged and untreated. Examples of bacterial, fungal, protozoal, and viral infections that do so are Whipple's disease, syphilis, cryptococcosis, and HIV (table 10.6). Until the beginning of the antibiotic era, infection was in fact the leading cause of organic mental illness. *General paresis of the insane*, caused by syphilis, was the first disorder to be associated with histologic pathology (Alois Alzheimer's writings on this topic are famous), and penicillin made general paresis the first treatable dementia.

Creutzfeldt-Jakob dementia is rare (one per million), but some of its forms can be easily recognized, such as the extrapyramidal variety that is distinguished by rapid onset, marked rigidity, and a pathognomonic startle response. *Rapid* means that 75% of individuals are dead within one year of onset. Periodic, lateralizing, epileptiform discharges (PLEDS) seen on EEG are helpful, but definitive diagnosis rests on histologic evidence: Finding a spongiform encephalopathy and a transmissible agent called an *unconventional virus*.

I discuss infectious agents with reversible dementias because some infectious agents obviously are treatable, even in their advanced stage (syphilis). It is hoped that more infectious entities will be treatable in the future. As an example of this, consider that the treatment for cryptococcal infection, now seen often in individuals with HIV infection, is fungostatic rather than fungocidal: The fundamental defect of cellular immunity in those with HIV means that cryptococci may not be completely eliminated. On the other hand, the newly available oral fluconazole is far better than the previous standard of intravenous amphotericin-B. As a result, dementia from chronic fungal meningoëncephalitis can now often be averted. Aside from the treatment of opportunistic infections, the effect that specific antiretroviral drugs have on structural CNS changes due to HIV is currently being determined.

Because our knowledge of HIV infection is escalating, I will restrict my comments to what I expect will not become swiftly dated. Tradition holds that textbooks usually are repositories of

Table 10.6
Infectious Dementias

Chronic meningitides

FUNGAL
   Cryptococcus
   Histoplasmosis
   Candida
   Aspergillosis
   Nocardia

PARASITIC
   Toxoplasmosis
   Cysticercosis
   Plasmodia

BACTERIAL
   Mycobacterium
   Treponema
   Brucella

Caused by conventional viruses
   Human immunodeficiency type 1 encephalitis
   Subacute sclerosing panencephalitis
   Rubella panencephalitis
   Progressive multifocal leukoëncephalopathy
   Herpetic encephalitis
   Postencephalitic Parkinsonism with dementia
   Eastern equine encephalitis
   Western equine encephalitis
   St. Louis encephalitides

Caused by unconventional viruses
   Creutzfeldt-Jakob disease
   Kuru

---

that which does not change. Your main challenge is to use the term *AIDS dementia* intelligently, for the oft-overlooked reason that not all cognitive symptoms in HIV-infected individuals are directly due to HIV. I have lost count of the consultation requests for dementia that turned out to be drug intoxications, metabolic delirium, or the compound effects of hospitalization and concurrent illness (physical and spiritual exhaustion). You may be eager to do an in-depth evaluation, but a dispirited and sick patient who has suffered all the indignities that modern medical technology can inflict may be less than enthusiastic. Claiming that dementia is present in such an individual is a pitfall not only in patients with AIDS, but in anyone who is seriously debilitated.

First, you must separate direct CNS consequences of the retrovirus from the nonspecific effects of systemic infection(s) and focal sequelæ of intracranial tumors and infection(s), some of which may produce symptoms by their mass alone. Next, you must factor in the tremendous anxiety and psychosocial stress that accompanies HIV infection. Deciding whether to tell others of one's condition, maintaining income, financing medical care, confronting multifaceted discrimination and legal issues, and seeking whatever emotional support is available are all dire psychosocial considerations not faced in other medical situations. It is true that the retrovirus seems neurotropic but, before you can determine the direct effect the virus has on a given individual's cognition, you must distinguish other factors.

The multiple systemic and intracranial infections that are common in HIV can each cause cognitive symptoms or impair sensory input. The same can be said of the multiple drugs given for prophylaxis against opportunistic infections, for intercurrent diseases, and for antiretroviral therapy. Some straightforward associations are listed in table 10.7 and must be considered as confounds rather than the result of primary dementia.

The Working Group of the American Academy of Neurology AIDS Task Force (1991) proposed a cumbersome nomenclature for the neurologic manifestations of HIV infection. They propose the global term *HIV-1–associated cognitive/motor complex*, which has two subgroups. For severe manifestations they propose *HIV-1–associated dementia complex* and, for mild manifestations, they suggest *HIV-1–associated minor cognitive/motor disorder*. The

Table 10.7
Confounds in HIV Infection that are not Dementia

Visual field defects
CMV, toxoplasmosis, HIV
Headaches, weakness, seizures
Cryptococcosis, toxoplasmosis, lymphoma, PML, *Myocobacterium avium intracellulare*, HIV, and any encephalopathy, myopathy, or neuropathy (including adverse effects of drugs)
Lack of memory, concentration
Depression, encephalopathy, physical exhaustion
Depression, mood swings
Endocrine or electrolyte disturbance, drug side effects
Paresis, paresthesias, and other sensory deficits
Varicella zoster, toxoplasmosis, lymphoma, PML, HIV, and any mass lesion

CMV, cytomegalovirus; HIV, human immunodeficiency virus; PML, progressive multifocal leucoëncephalopathy.

Task Force outlines specific features that qualify for sufficient, probable, and possible diagnoses. Regrettably, academic groups are often years behind frontline clinicians. Because quick revision in nomenclature is certain, I have not bothered to reproduce this scheme here. Consult current journals instead or, better still, become a front-line clinician yourself.

The history of HIV-infected individuals should probe for prior and current psychiatric conditions, including depression, anxiety, memory loss, cognitive decline, suicidal ideation, alcohol dependency, and drug use. Both alcohol and drug abuse can be immunosuppressive. At various stages of illness, but particularly when the disease is first diagnosed or during stepwise regressions, there is somatic preoccupation and heightened vigilance related to fear of death and abandonment. Such situational reactions often resolve, and true cognitive impairment is unlikely until the immune damage is severe. Even then, dementia and depression may coëxist. *In fact depression, rather than true dementia, has thus far been found to be responsible for most self-reported cognitive defects.* Even here, clinically significant depression does not beget significant neuropsychological dysfunction that is objectively measurable (Hinkin et al., 1992).

Neuropsychologists have expended much energy trying to detect subtle mental decline in those infected with HIV who do not manifest obvious symptoms. The reason for this is that neurologic involvement is expected sometime during the course of HIV illness and that histologic lesions, when present, are concentrated in subcortical white matter and nuclei. The extended (seven- to nine-hour) NIMH neuropsychological battery mentioned in chapter 5 actually was designed to detect neuropsychological change early in the course of HIV disease. It has not yet succeeded. Multiple studies have found few, if any, differences between seronegative individuals and asymptomatic HIV-infected ones (Van Gorp et al., 1991; Miller et al., 1991). Most studies have been carried out on cohorts of gay white men who, as a group, are well read and better-educated than the general population. Perhaps this indistinguishability will hold up as HIV continues to infect greater numbers of women and minority races. At present, one can say that asymptomatic infection with HIV-1 does not oblige the presence of any noteworthy neurobehavioral impairment (Selnes et al., 1995).

Similarly, the assumption that there must be subtle mental changes early in the course of HIV infection has led to efforts to determine whether there are any structural changes in the brain that might be identified by MRI scans. At this time, the conclusion of sixteen studies is that atrophy and white matter hyperintensities are seen in controls as well as various subgroups of HIV-infected individuals. Prospective study shows that MRI scans do not distinguish asymptomatic and mildly symptomatic HIV-positive individuals from HIV-negative ones (Doonreif et al., 1992). Postmortem morphometric study reveals that HIV-1–associated cognitive/motor complex is not necessarily related to neuronal loss in the neocortex (Seilhean et al., 1993).

Literature from the first ten years of the HIV epidemic is contradictory because the clinical expression of the disease has changed over that time. Initially, patients were uniformly hospitalized *in extremis* and no antiretroviral therapy existed. Today, outpatient treatment is the rule, patients are much less ill, and survival from the time of seropositive diagnosis is rising. There is every indication that HIV infection is evolving into a chronic disease. Perhaps as individuals live longer and concurrent, opportunistic illnesses no longer dominate the clinical picture, we will be able to ascertain what cognitive effects, if any, are directly attributable to HIV-1.

The multicenter cohort study (Selnes, 1991) showed that dementia, when present, appeared acutely rather than as an insidious decline. Clinical hallmarks were psychomotor retardation, poor concentration, and poor mental control. Histologically, the white matter shows pallor and vacuölation, the pons and basal ganglia are gliotic, and elsewhere are seen microglial nodules and multinucleated giant cells. HIV antigens are present in CSF and tissue, yet neurons are not themselves the target of direct destruction. Rather, infected monocytoid cells and microglia produce neurotoxins. Clinical, imaging, and histologic data all suggest *reversible* dopaminergic dysfunction in demented HIV-infected patients involving N-methyl-D-aspartate (NMDA). Both dopamine agonists and precursors improve motor abnormalities in demented patients, and NMDA receptor blockers may play a useful role in ameliorating dementia (Kieburtz et al., 1991). Antiretroviral therapy has improved central nuclei and cortical abnormalities seen on PET scans and also has improved cognitive function in both adults and children. The reversibility of dementia suggests that neuronal dysfunction exceeds neuronal destruction.

Having said all this, and acknowledging that neuronal damage exists in some individuals infected with HIV, exactly what is AIDS dementia? The best definition I can cite, and one that is unlikely to change, is that it is a clinical dementia in someone infected with HIV in whom other causes of dementia have been eliminated. In other words, I do not believe that there is anything unique about the dementia in individuals who have a clinical diagnosis of AIDS.

Depression

Self-reporting of depression is somewhat unusual in the elderly. Whereas melancholy young persons say that they are blue and depressed, it is an empirical observation that dispirited elders often deny feeling depressed and say instead that they "can't think." The reason that cognitive complaints substitute for self-reporting of depression in the elderly remains a mystery (NIH Consensus Development Panel, 1992).

Depression in the elderly may well present as a pseudodementia. McGlone and colleagues (1990) found that self-assessment and spontaneous complaints of poor memory correlated best with depression, while relatives' ratings correlated well with objective amnesia. Because depression is common, it often should be included in the differential diagnosis of any dementia. If the diagnosis is in doubt, then a clinical trial of antidepressants is reasonable and should always be considered.

The contrary situation—the coöccurrence of major depression in primary dementia—also needs to be considered. How often depression occurs in Alzheimer's disease is hard to say because published series cite a prevalence from 0% to 86%, surely reflecting both the diverse populations surveyed and diverse inclusion criteria for both conditions. Clinical experience shows that in addition to Alzheimer's disease, depression occurs in Parkinson's, Pick's, and Huntington's diseases, as well as in multi-infarct dementia.

Depression can result from transmitter dysfunction. For example, norepinephrine and dopamine have their cells of origin in the pigmented nuclei of the brainstem. These nuclei project widely to various nuclei known to be affected in degenerative dementias. Zubenko and Moossy (1988) showed that demented patients with major depression had associated degeneration of the locus coeruleus and substantia nigra compared to demented patients who were not depressed. These effects are additive. In this series, 39% of patients had both dementia and depression. These findings are noteworthy because the most currently favored hypothesis about endogenous depression relies on single neurotransmitters. That multiple interactions may actually be required is suggested by the fact that antidepressant drugs influence more than one transmitter class.

Formal testing reveals, in a number of studies, that depressed individuals have a pronounced deficit in performance IQ (Sackeim et al., 1992).

Hydrocephalus

Obstructive hydrocephalus at either the foramen of Monro or the third ventricle produces dementia by an unknown mechanism. Normal pressure hydrocephalus (NPH) was discussed in chapter 6.

Only some individuals respond to ventriculoperitoneal shunting, and it is a vexing issue how to select patients who might benefit from this procedure. Most proposals suggest removing some quantity of CSF and measuring whether symptoms temporarily improve.

Daily drainage of the CSF through lumbar puncture for an arbitrary number of consecutive days has been tried. Measuring regional cerebral blood flow by the xenon method before and after CSF removal has also been examined, the hypothesis being that the hydrocephalus causes dementia by altering cerebral perfusion in the frontal areas. The commonly used but still controversial test for NPH is a radionuclide brain scan with twenty-four-hour delayed films. "Hang-up" or persistence of tracer in the cisterns after a day is taken as evidence that CSF flow is impeded. None of these ideas has definitively determined the mechanism by which dementia is produced, and none is accurate in predicting which patients might benefit from surgical shunting. These issues remain clouded since this treatable dementia was first described in 1965.

Vanneste and colleagues (1992a) recently compared clinical and literature series to assess risk-benefit outcomes. They concluded that NPH was, first of all, extremely rare (2.2 individuals/million/year) and overdiagnosed. Overall improvement is poor (15% to 20%) and all too often is perplexedly temporary and short-lived. Complications from shunting are common (up to 30%), and serious (death, stroke, seizures) in 9% of patients (Rosenberg et al., 1993).

PRIMARY DEGENERATIVE DEMENTIAS

Alzheimer's Disease

Leading physicians in the nineteenth century seriously doubted that histology could contribute anything to understanding mental diseases. Alois Alzheimer (1864–1915), a Bavarian clinician-turned-pathologist, demonstrated how unequivocal changes occur in the brains of those suffering not just from the dementia that now bears his name, but from various mental disorders (general paresis, arteriosclerosis, acute delirium). In fact, at a time when most contemporaries believed that dementia was an inevitable part of ageing, Alzheimer shrewdly observed that the pathologies of arteriosclerosis and senility were completely unrelated. If you are not reading this chapter sequentially, go back and review the first four pages, because the general comments there apply to Alzheimer's dementia.

Dementia of the Alzheimer's type is the prototypical example of dementing diseases without associated neurologic or medical findings. Patients usually are in their late fifties or beyond. Because the first patient Alzheimer described in 1907 was only fifty-one years-old, endless confusion ensued over the terms *pre-senile* and *senile dementia*, related to the outmoded sentiment that dementia was a normal part of the senium. The choice to use sixty-five years as the cutoff to label individuals as either pre-senile or senile dements was arbitrary. As mentioned in the opening section, the diagnosis depends on characteristic pathological changes regardless of age of onset; correct antemortem diagnosis of AD occurs less than 80% of the time.

Grossly, the brain shows severe atrophy and may weigh less than 1,000 gm. *Knife edge* describes the thinned gyri, worn away like arrowheads. Definitive diagnosis rests on finding microscopic neurofibrillary tangles (NFT) and senile plaques (SPs) containing an amyloid core in both cortex and central nuclei. The neuropil is thinned, neuron dropout is evident, and granulovacuölar neuronal degeneration is especially prominent in the pyramidal layer of the hippocampus. It is usual to see additional microscopic features such as amyloid angiopathy and Hirano fibers. (To rectify inconsistencies in the neuropathological assessment of AD, the consortium to establish a registry for AD [CERAD] formed to establish a uniform pathologic approach, reduce subjective interpretation, and initiate levels of diagnostic certainty [definite, probable, possible, and normal brain] [Mirra et al., 1991].)

These changes are not homogeneous. Rather, both tangles and plaques each have topologic predilections. SPs in neocortex exceed those in allocortex; the reverse is true for NFTs. Evidence accumulates that it is the NFTs rather than SPs that parallel the duration and severity of AD (Arriagada et al., 1992). Early in the disease, NFTs appear in entorhinal cortex, CA1/subiculum of hippocampal formation, and the amygdala. Tangles then continue to accumulate in a pattern that reflects a hierarchic predisposition of individual topographic regions, heteromodal areas being far more involved than unimodal ones. Clinically, the bias for heteromodal association cortex explains the early emergence of spatial disorientation, poor adaptation, linguistic disturbance, and confusion. Unimodal cortices are nearly spared. For example, Rizzo and colleagues (1992) showed that retinocalcarine pathways are normal in individuals with AD and that these patients' visual impairments (agnosia, contrast sensitivity, stereopsis, color vision defects, field constriction, and reduced acuity) result from involvement of association cortices rather than V1. Metabolic investigations also confirm the preferential involvement of heteromodal cortices (Smith et al., 1992)

The *coup de grâce* in AD occurs in the afferent neurons of entorhinal cortex and the efferent ones of the subiculum; their degeneration functionally disconnects the hippocampus from the rest of the neocortex and is believed to underlie the amnesia that ultimately appears in every case. There is nothing outstanding about the amnesia in AD, and comments from chapter 9 apply. You would do well to review the anatomic relationships of entorhinal cortex, hippocampal formation, and amygdala in your atlas. (Remember this as the ECHFA triad and invent your own mnemonic.) Interested students may also turn to the detailed anatomic study of memory-related structures in AD by Hyman et al., (1990). Their study shows tropism: Specific cytoarchitectural areas and lamina that receive projections from entorhinal cortex, hippocampal formation, and amygdala consistently contain NFTs, whereas other areas, sometimes immediately adjacent, are consistently spared these AD changes. The functional disconnection of these structures from their cortical and subcortical targets would be as devastating as bilateral destruction of the ventromedial temporal lobe. Having consulted your atlas, you will see that what is so remarkable is that the reciprocal connections among these three structures are multiple and overlapping, *yet every single projection is breached* in AD, and not by a gross disruption but by selective pathology in specific neurons and terminal fields that support these reciprocal connections. Figure 10.1 shows this schematically.

If anything general can be said about speech in AD, it is that it is fluent but empty (rambling chatterbox, full of cliché), with semantic paraphasias. Vocabulary becomes constricted and speech becomes concrete, with a mild anomia noted first. Linguistic

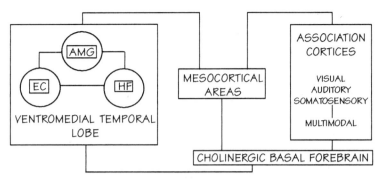

Figure 10.1
Multiple ventromedial temporal lobe connections and their disruption
in Alzheimer's disease. The reciprocal connections among the triplet of
amygdala (AMG), hippocampal formation (HF), and entorhinal cortex (EC)
are paramount. Feedforward and feedback projections connect to meso-
cortical areas (perirhinal cortex, temporal pole, posterior parahippocampal
gyrus) that, in turn, have reciprocal projections with unimodal and multimodal cortices. The cholinergic basal forebrain (nucleus basalis, septum,
diagonal band) is also a link in this multiplex system. In Alzheimer's
dementia, widespread but nonetheless selective pathological processes
accumulate that eventually break every single projection illustrated here.
From Hyman, van Hoesen & Damasio (1990), with permission.

loss is not global, and not all aspects of speech are simultaneously affected. As disease progresses, however, paraphasias become
worse, comprehension suffers, and it is difficult to engage individuals in conversation—either because they are passive and mute, or
because the content of their speech is tangential and irrelevant.
Earlier words and themes intrude into the stream of thought.
Echolalia, logorrhea, grunting, moaning, and repetitive shouting
ensue before the patient becomes akinetic and mute.

Altered personality is integral to AD, although personality
changes per se have been studied less systematically than cognitive ones. Ascertainment of altered personality is through family,
as patients themselves are often unaware that they suffer any brain
disorder. Literature of the last decade agrees that the personality
traits likely to emerge are apathy, irritability, belligerence, anxiety, excitability, depression, and indifference. Petry and colleagues
(1988) compared AD patients to normal retirees and concluded
that the former become more passive, coarse, less spontaneous,

and more rigid as a direct consequence of disease. This profile differs from that observed in cohorts with other neurodegenerative diseases. Also, personality change does not correlate with the level of intellectual impairment (Bózzola et al., 1992).

An explanation consistent with the behavioral-anatomic correlations you have already learned is that indifference and passivity may be related to pathology in the frontal convexity, denial of illness (anosognosia) may be associated with parietal dysfunction, and placidity may be similar to that seen in patients with bilateral medial temporal pathology. I have already pointed out that the nucleus basalis is interposed between neocortex and limbic entities, and that any dysfunction might disconnect the two. Atrophy of the nucleus basalis in AD might explain clinical loss of motivation and enthusiasm.

Psychosis and depression are two accompaniments of AD about whose chemical correlates we know something. Psychosis occurs in up to half of autopsy-confirmed cases and takes the form of delusions and hallucinations (e.g., the patient sees animals in the backyard, hears voices, believes that others are hiding her belongings, or that she must discard all her pots). Psychosis is associated with significantly increased densities of plaques and tangles in the prosubiculum and middle frontal cortex. Norepinephrine is preserved in substantia nigra; serotonin is reduced in prosubiculum and elsewhere. Interestingly, AD patients with psychosis show more rapid mental decline but not an increased rate of mortality; AD patients with major depression show the opposite pattern of accelerated mortality without an increased rate of mental decline (Zubenko et al., 1991). Major depression in AD is associated with selective degeneration of aminergic brainstem nuclei (substantia nigra and locus coeruleus) but not an increase in either plaques or tangles in the cerebrum. Table 10.8 summarizes these differences. The morphometric, chemical, and mortality profiles of AD patients with either depression or psychosis differ greatly. For the sake of future clinical studies, descriptions of Alzheimer patients should include these variables.

An *autosomal dominant familial dementia* with histologic features consistent with AD can begin by age thirty. Other autosomal dominant familial dementias that appear clinically like AD have, at autopsy, been shown through detailed study to be unique hereditary

Table 10.8

Differential Features of Alzheimer's Disease (AD) with Depression or Psychosis

Compared to AD Without Psychosis or Depression	Psychosis	Major Depression
Sex, onset age, duration, brain weight	No change	No change
Mortality	No change	Increased
Rate of mental decline	Increased	No change
Plaques and tangles	Increased plaques in PS, tangles in MF	No change
Degeneration of LC and SN	No change	Increased
Norepinephrine	Increased in SN	Decreased in neocortex and allocortex
Dopamine	No change	Increased in PS
Choline acetyltransferase	No change	Preserved in TH, AM, CN

PS, prosubiculum; MF, medial frontal cortex; SN, substantia nigra; TH, thalamus; AM, amygdala; CN, caudate nucleus; LC, locus coeruleus.
From Zubenko et al., (1991), with permission.

dementias distinct from AD (Sumi et al., 1992). Thus, I emphasize again that the diagnosis of AD rests on histologic confirmation. Knowing this should make you read more skeptically those journal reports whose hypotheses are based on cohorts of "probable" AD.

Pick's Disease

Pick's disease also is called *lobar atrophy*, not because atrophy is confined to the frontal and temporal lobes, but because both gray and white matter are affected. Hence *lobar* is used instead of *cortical*. There are no specifically characteristic signs or symptoms. Although the diagnosis can be suggested by circumscribed atrophy on scans, it most often is discovered at autopsy.

The affected brain parts are dramatically wasted. The white matter is dusky, and the anterior commissure and corpus callosum are atrophied. The caudate, substantia nigra, and other central nuclei are shrunken. The ballooned, surviving neurons contain cytoplasmic Pick bodies (silver-staining inclusions).

Some authors maintain that it is clinically impossible to distinguish Pick's lobar atrophy from other dementias, whereas others insist that the prominent degeneration of limbic and paralimbic cortices produce telling symptoms. This latter camp emphasizes the early emergence of socially inappropriate behavior, such as urinating or undressing in public, inappropriate sexual doings, and an aphasia that progresses to a disjointed jargon. Compared to AD, memory may be relatively preserved. The clinical course is short. Pick's disease is rare, and I have not encountered enough instances to be swayed by either view.

Vascular Dementia

Occlusion of large-diameter vessels, particularly when recurrent, can affect enough brain tissue to render a person demented. Multi-infarct dementia (MID) is rather abrupt in its onset and has a fluctuating and stepwise course, as befits its etiology. Hypertension and atherosclerosis are characteristic. Because hypertension is eminently treatable, some authors conceptualize MID as potentially reversible, or at least preventable. I do not find this semantic distinction useful.

Two other vascular entities—lacunar state and Binswanger's angiopathy—are both subcortical dementias. Infarction of medullary arteries deep in brain parenchyma causes the four classic lacunar syndromes, but lacunæ can occur most anywhere that penetrating arteries roam. It is likely that they do not always produce clinically noticeable deficits (the corollary is that you only find what you are looking for). Medullary arteries usually suffer from lipohyalinosis, which renders them susceptible to thrombosis.

The pathology in Binswanger's disease lies in small vessels, and appears on a background of either systemic vasculitis or persistent hypertension (Olszewski, 1965). Atrophy of white matter is severe, yet the cortex and short U-fibers, which are fed by cortical rather than penetrating arterioles, are spared. A progressive mental decline is characterized by pseudobulbar speech, psychomotor retardation, agitation, irritability, euphoria, and depression with an overarching amnesia that may be difficult to gauge because of

Table 10.9
Mechanisms of Dementia Related to Stroke

1. *Location* of cerebral lesion, specifically regions important for higher functions:
   a. Posterior association areas
   b. Posterior cerebral artery territory, including thalamus and inferomedial temporal lobes
   c. End fields of carotid circulation, superior frontal and parietal convexity
2. *Volume* of lesions, with infarcts exceeding a threshold for brain's ability to compensate
3. *Number* of lesions, with small or large, deep or superficial lesions having:
   a. Additive effects
   b. Multiplicative effects, as in MID
   c. Location-specific effects (disconnection syndromes, Binswanger's disease)
4. *Coöccurrence* of vascular disorders and AD causing:
   a. Additive effects (strokes superimposed on AD)
   b. Multiplicative effects (stroke interacts with AD, aggravating mild AD or unmasking clinically inapparent AD)
   c. Multiple infarcts or Binswanger's disease as a result of amyloid angiopathy associated with AD

From Tatemichi (1990), with permission. AD, Alzheimer's disease; MID, multi-infarct dementia.

inattention. Some pathologically confirmed cases have been diagnosed during life via CT scanning.

Before the advent of CT scanning, Binswanger's disease was considered rare. Now that CT and MRI scans (in conjunction with renewed interest in the entity) are able to detect it as well as lacunæ that might have escaped clinical notice, the relative percentage of vascular dementia will have to be recalculated. One such recent estimate is 23% (Chui et al., 1992).

The terminology that describes the relationship between stroke and dementia is contentious. *MID* is the most commonly accepted term but, as table 10.9 shows, this is only one of several dementias that can result from stroke. As usual, your choice of terms must be careful. Cumulative strokes do not cause the histologic changes specific to AD or any other progressive neural degeneration, yet everyone agrees that stroke can disturb higher functions. It is correct to say that cerebrovascular disease can contribute or cause a syndrome of dementia resembling that of primary degenerative dementia based on location, number, and volume of incidents, and coöccurrence with other pathological processes (Tatemichi, 1990; NINDS-AIREN, 1993).

Parkinson's Disease

Parkinson's disease (PD) is among the ten most common neurological disorders. It affects 1% of the population aged fifty years, and 2% aged seventy-five. Prevalence is one per thousand. Be careful of your terminology: *Parkinson's disease* is the idiopathic "shaking palsy" described in 1817 by the English physician-surgeon James Parkinson (1755–1828), whereas parkinson*ism* describes the clinically similar picture produced by drugs (phenothiazines), toxins (manganese), or infection (postencephalitis).

The clinical triad of PD is bradykinesia, rigidity, and tremor. Because motor signs dominate, most physicians will claim that mentation is unaffected in PD. Jean Marie Charcot, however, took exception with Parkinson's assertion that the mind was unaffected. Today, we know that 20% to 50% of patients will have a frank dementia that waxes as the disease progresses. *Bradyphrenia* describes the mental slowing and hesitation often seen in afflicted individuals. The nature of intellectual impairment is controversial and has not been well described. One can see notable impairments in visuospatial discrimination and difficulty in shifting sets on visual, verbal, or motor tasks. Problems with high-order motor performance are not linked to extrapyramidal deficits. Poor construction, word-list generation, abstraction, and mathematical performance are seen, yet typically conceived cortical deficits such as aphasia or agnosia are not (Huber, 1992).

Depression is common in PD (40% to 60%), and can even be the reason medical attention is first sought: That is, PD may be immediately apparent on examination, but not disruptive enough for anyone to have noticed in normal living. Depression is not an emotional response to disability, but an integral part of the disease.

The pathologic process centers on the dopamine-containing nigrostriatal tract, which has cell bodies in the substantia nigra and axon terminations in the striatum. The signs and symptoms of PD are due to dopamine loss in the striatum and resulting dysfunction brought about by degeneration of the substantia nigra; symptoms improve with restoration of dopaminergic input by supplying dopamine's precursor (L-dopa), by giving dopamine agonists (bromocriptine, pergolide), or by inhibiting dopamine breakdown (selegiline, a selective monoamine oxidase type B inhibitor). Despite symptomatic treatment, nigral cells continue to die and the disease progresses, mean duration of illness until death being eight years. Levodopa remains the backbone of therapy, but it is not the curative acme. Selegiline may retard the natural history of the disease (Klawans, 1990).

Dementia in PD is associated with loss in multiple extranigral populations such as the anterior cingulum, nucleus basalis, and ventral tegmental area (Zweig et al., 1993). PD patients with conspicuous dementia also show pathologic lesions typical of AD in both cortex and nuclei, including the nucleus basalis. The meaning of this has not been elucidated, but is considered to be more complex than a coöccurrence of PD and AD. I should repeat that SPs and NFTs tangles are not unique to AD, but are seen in nearly two

Table 10.10
Conditions with Histologic Neurofibrillary Tangles

Normal aging
Alzheimer's disease
Pick's disease
Parkinson's disease
Down syndrome
Supranuclear palsy
ALS-Parkinson-Dementia syndrome of Guam
Subacute sclerosing panencephalitis
Hereditary cerebellar ataxia
Pugilistic dementia
Vincristine encephalomyelopathy
Infantile neuraxonal dystrophy

dozen neurological diseases (table 10.10). Metabolic imaging shows widespread, but homogenous, cortical glucose hypometabolism in nondemented PD patients; in dements, severe decrease is additionally seen in temporal-parietal regions (Peppard et al., 1992).

The mental state is not necessarily improved by drug therapy. The correlation of bradyphrenia with CSF levels of 3-methoxy-4-hydroxyphenylglycol (MHPG, a norepinephrine metabolite) suggests that mental deterioration may be due more to noradrenergic than dopaminergic involvement. This would be consistent with the frequency of depression in PD.

Formal neuropsychological testing is difficult in PD given that motor symptoms confound all timed tests. Dysphonia (soft speech volume), hesitation, dysarthria, micrographia, reduced vertical gaze (upward worse than downward), and fragmented saccades are conceived of more as motor dysfunction, yet all obviously will impair formal HCF assessment. In a parallel comparison of several types of dementia, Pillon et al. (1991) showed that formal HCF assessment can discriminate among AD, PD, Huntington's chorea, and progressive supranuclear palsy and that, furthermore, each has a specific profile of impairment. Showing that memory and linguistic failure distinguish AD, or that frontal behavior distinguishes supranuclear palsy, however, reinforces my earlier comment that the term *subcortical* dementia really is not useful clinically, because one must further specify its nature. It seems far better, therefore, to state forthrightly the nature of the dementia rather than to apply a label that contributes little to understanding the dementia.

Huntington's Chorea

The combination of dementia and choreoäthetosis known as *Huntington's chorea* is inherited as an autosomal dominant trait and is the most frequent hereditary neurologic disease encountered in tertiary centers. It affects nearly 1 in 10,000 persons.

Changes in personality and mood, especially depression, appear long before motor signs. Impulsiveness, irritability, sexual acting out, and emotional lability are typical. Fifty percent of patients become psychotic late in the disease. The likelihood of suicide is much higher than in the general population. Anterograde memory is especially affected early on, and mental decline progresses until dementia is unmistakable. Death occurs an average of fifteen years after onset.

Wasting of the head of the caudate and putamen is said to be the most distinct pathological sign (easily seen on CT and MRI scans). Most of the small cells in the striatum drop out, and the large ones show no particular pathology. Multiple neurotransmitters are affected. GABA-ergic and cholinergic cells disappear; dopamine receptors decrease in the face of normal dopamine levels; glutamate binding is decreased in the striatum.

Huntington's chorea has been regarded as the prototypical subcortical dementia but, as already stated, this distinction is a superficial one based on gross pathology. PET, for example, shows that cortical dysfunction can be detected even early in the disease. Patients with symptoms lasting less than five years show a 15% decrease in frontal and inferior parietal cortical metabolism; those whose symptoms excede five years in duration have reduced metabolism (by 25% to 30%) in all cortical areas, except temporal, compared to controls (Martin et al., 1992). This illustrates my earlier statement that all demented patients usually exhibit some pathologic change in both cortical and subcortical structures.

A beginning student can easily recognize Huntington's chorea when it is fully developed. The challenge is to diagnose this disease correctly in an adult who exhibits chorea and mental change and in whom there is no family history. The differential diagnosis is often impossible. Some cases are certainly new spontaneous mutations of the Huntington's gene. In an at-risk family, one cannot predict who will be affected until symptoms appear. Onset is usually after age forty, by which time most persons at risk will have already had children. This makes genetic counseling doubly difficult.

Challenging persons at risk with L-dopa to see whether they develop chorea is controversial and yields both false positive and false negative results. It also has ethical implications. The molecular basis of this hereditary disorder is rapidly becoming clearer and diagnosis via recombinant DNA probes is very promising, whereas treatment options are less so.

Pugilistic Dementia

The "punch-drunk" syndrome from multiple boxing knockouts or similar repeated head injuries produces neurofibrillary changes just as in Alzheimer's disease. They are scattered throughout the cortex and brainstem, but are most prominent in the medial temporal lobe. SPs are absent. Cerebellar gliosis, with Purkinje cell dropout, and loss of pigmented cells also are evident. A cavum septum pellucidum usually is present, as is hydrocephalus, although whether the latter is from multiple subarachnoid hemorrhages or is of the ex-vacuo variety is not settled. The corpus callosum is thinned.

Affected individuals are dysarthric, ataxic, rigid, forgetful, and slow. Parkinsonism may be evident. It is incredible that many people see nothing wrong with the "game" of boxing, the object of which is to render one's opponent unconscious. Only recently have several medical organizations condemned this so-called sport as immoral and unjustifiable given that cumulative trauma makes permanent brain injury inevitable.

Pseudodementia

The term *pseodudementia* does not refer to anything specifically but generally to disorders that are treatable if accurately diagnosed. Depression is obviously the main concern, although conversion reaction and bipolar disorder can be mistaken for dementia. Some types of aphasia (transcortical sensory, Wernicke's, jargon) are likewise mistaken for mental disease. Dementia and psychosis are not mutually exclusive. Qualitative differences, mode of onset, clinical course, and ancillary tests usually will sort the situation out.

DIFFERENTIAL DIAGNOSIS

Absolutely nothing can replace a careful history that is taken from both the patient and a relative who has frequent contact with the patient. Symptoms must obviously be interpreted in the individual's own context. At times, information from the patient's employer, colleagues, or neighbors is necessary. The family history should inquire explicitly about dementia, Down's syndrome, Parkinson's disease, and psychiatric illness, as all are associated with an increased incidence of dementia in first-degree relatives. The general physical exam and the neurological exam—with emphasis on higher cortical functions—are most productive when done by someone both interested in and knowledgeable about normal patterns of cognition in the elderly and the typical patterns of loss that constitute the many eponymic diseases outlined above.

The differential diagnosis is essentially pattern analysis, in that certain combinations of symptoms and signs are more or less characteristic. Some types of dementia may be recognized early; others are confirmed only at autopsy. Foremost, one should strive to disclose treatable causes of dementia. Although signs such as rigidity, stooped posture, agraphesthesia, sensory extinction, snout, grasp, and glabellar reflexes appear during the course of AD, they are too infrequent early in the disease course to serve as diagnostic markers that might distinguish AD from normal ageing (Galasko et al., 1990).

The dementias associated with metabolic abnormalities are particularly difficult to disclose, especially by those with no medical training, because the overlap between dementia and encephalopathy is particularly notorious. Reference to the distinguishing guidelines in chapter 4 and to table 4.6 may help.

Assessing the severity of any given dementia is problematic. As with memory, where neuropsychologists' interest has turned from scores attained on standardized tests to remembering in naturalistic settings, we no longer assume that impairment in activities of daily living can be predicted from a test situation. In fact, Teunisse and associates (1991) showed that no single aspect can adequately describe the severity of any instance of dementia. Caretakers themselves experience emotional, social, physical, financial, and spiritual burdens of which the patient can be oblivious. These confounds can make third-party opinions unreliable. For example, caretakers may dress invalids for their own convenience, even though patients might be able to dress themselves if they were permitted the time. Hence, a caretaker's own sense of frustration may lead him or her to overstate the severity of their charge's impairment; denial of infirmity leads to the opposite conclusion. The ability of patients to execute the activities of dailiy living varies dramatically depending on the social surroundings. Clinical as-

Table 10.11
Minimal Workup for Dementia

---

1. Complete blood cell count
2. Electrolytes
3. Metabolic panel
4. Thyroid function
5. Vitamin B_{12} and folate levels
6. Serology for syphilis; depending on history, serology for HIV
7. Urinalysis
8. Sedimentation rate
9. Electrocardiogram
10. Chest x ray

---

sessment of dementia severity, therefore, should state clearly the purpose of the rating, and should be multifaceted, if possible.

Laboratory Tests

Table 10.11 contains the most common first-pass tests used in evaluating dementia. Nothing, however, can replace an adequate history and examination. Together with the ten minimum procedures listed in the table, these should permit you to identify most treatable dementias. The evaluation of dementia is not quick; in fact, one must strive to make repeated evaluations. It is also a mistake to think that dementia can be accurately diagnosed in one sitting. The following are general guidelines based on recent National Institutes of Health consensus conferences. Be mindful that too much testing not only is expensive, uncomfortable, and often unwarranted, but also increases the yield of false positive results, which engenders yet more testing. Both shotgun and cookbook approaches are signs of intellectual laziness.

One of the most overlooked diagnostic maneuvers is to stop all medications that are not lifesaving. Do not hesitate to hospitalize the patient if adequate observation cannot otherwise be obtained, if the patient is agitated, when the onset is acute, or when the history is muddled.

Noncontrast CT and MRI scans are appropriate when focal signs are present, when mental deterioration has recently begun, or when a mass is suspected.

Episodes of altered consciousness, automatisms, wandering, or falls in which individuals injure themselves suggest seizure. Get an EEG.

Lumbar puncture should be done on everyone with HIV infection who shows neurologic signs. Obtain titers for syphilis and cryptococcal antigen. Even if negative, these will be a useful baseline.

Formal neuropsychological testing may be informative when the diagnosis is in doubt or when the affected individual is exceptionally smart or has a sophisticated vocabulary. In this light, a neurolinguistic consultation often is extremely helpful yet usually is overlooked.

Regional cerebral blood flow, PET, evoked potentials, and brain mapping are not for routine use. Brain biopsy is likely to yield a definitive diagnosis in patients with atypical dementias after thorough clinical, metabolic, neuropsychological, and imaging evaluations have failed to yield a cause. Biopsy is not something to undertake lightly. Patients must have a progressive disorder and be well enough to undergo open biopsy; disinterested clinicians must agree on the indication for biopsy; informed consent should be obtained from responsible parties; and appropriate technology (electron microscopy, immunocytochemistry) should be available to examine the specimen. Even though biopsy is helpful in atypical dementias, Hulette and colleagues (1992) showed that demented patients with associated neurologic signs such as hemiparesis, chorea, athetosis, or lower motor neuron signs are unlikely to receive a definitive diagnosis through biopsy.

MRI and CT Investigation of Dementia

The general thrust of imaging studies in dementia has been to untangle primary dementia, vascular dementia, and normal aging, and to further ask if imaging can distinguish demented from nondemented individuals. Methodologically, MRI studies often report small numbers of poorly selected patients and offer limited clinical data. One is vexed trying to deduce from these studies clear general principles about the relevance of white matter signals to a given disease or cognitive state.

The white matter hyperintensities of interest are best seen on T_2-weighted images and are of three kinds: (1) periventricular, (2) circumscribed and small, and (3) larger or irregular. Each can be described more fully. *Periventricular hyperintensities* (PVHs) are curvilinear bands seen at the ventricular horns, sometimes spreading to outline the entire perimeter of the ventricle. The small spherical hyperintensities, called *unidentified bright objects* (UBOs), measure 3 to 5 mm and are seen in the space between the gray-white junction and the juxtaventricular region; they do not encroach on the ventricle or subependyma. *Larger or irregular white matter hyperintensities* are heterogeneous and have a known cause, such as multiple sclerosis plaques, wedge-shaped infarctions that extend to the surface, tumors, and other pathologies. The cause of PVHs and UBOs is not definitely determined.

Distinguishing these white matter signals might seem arbitrary, but post-mortem histology, the correlations of which have only recently begun to appear, suggests that their cause differs. PVHs appear to be associated with demyelination, subependymal gliosis, and increased water content, whereas the hyperintensities in deep white matter are associated with increased water content, gliosis, demyelination, dilated perivascular spaces, and nonparenchymal pathologies. The larger, irregular lesions have pathology specific to their cause. This heterogeneity hampers the assessment of possible clinical associations.

There is no consensus regarding terminology. In 1987, Hachinski proposed the term *leuko-araiosis* (*leuko* = white matter, *araios* = rarefied) as a purely descriptive one that we ought to be able to replace as we arrive at a better understanding of what these white matter signals are. Yet even leukoäraiosis is distinguished from PVHs, vitiating the idea of a global term to signify image-lesions of white matter. My usage of the term *image-lesion* will be to distinguish PVHs, UBOs, and other lesions as indicated above. (*Roentgen-pathology*, a term from an earlier era, would be useful but for the fact that X rays are not used to generate MRIs; *image-lesion* acknowledges a nidus different from surrounding tissue without implying anything about its possible pathology.)

Two opposing viewpoints exist about the meaning of these image-lesions. Unencumbered by either evidence or thought, an ex cathedra group dismisses them as irrelevant by circular logic (because they don't produce clinical effects, they don't produce clinical effects) or else adjures us to accept them as silent strokes (silent, again, because they produce no obvious effects). Because the lesions have signal characteristics different from those of surrounding tissue, the opposing camp puts its faith in structure-function relationships. They believe that image-lesions are probably abnormal, and strive eventually to tease out possible clinical associations.

A scan is not a histologic evaluation—not even an approximation—and major assumptions must be made in the enterprise called *functional neuroimaging*. Attempts at functional neuroimaging immediately followed the appearance of the first scanners twenty-five years ago. Some of these trials have been fruitful, and a minority have been correlated with tissue pathology. In 1975, for example, Hachinski's "ischemic score" conceptually distinguished MID from AD by requiring an abrupt onset, focal signs or symptoms, a fluctuating course and a history of strokes, hypertension, and atherosclerosis. Others proposed adding focal CT lesions as a criteria for MID, but, lo and behold, only 40% of those meeting the Hachinski criteria had lesions apparent on CT or angiography. Subsequent MRI studies showed white matter lesions much more clearly and often were positive in those whose CT scans were negative. By this time, enough histologic studies had been published that showed pathology more widespread than or different from that seen on CT to make it clear that clinico-anatomic associations based on imaging are perilous. Only when done carefully can functional neuroimaging yield results. See the Damasios (1989) and Palca (1990) for such an approach.

The interpretation was first advanced that patients with vascular dementia have white matter lesions, whereas those with AD or Pick's disease do not. Later and better (though not ideal) work showed that white matter lesions cannot distinguish between demented and nondemented patients with a history of stroke, transient ischemic attack (TIA), or reversible ischemic neurologic deficit (RIND) (Hershey et al., 1987).

At present, one can say that there is an overlap in the images of normal aging brains and those with cerebrovascular disease or primary dementia. Efforts to correlate neuropsychological findings with the location of MRI white matter lesions have met with contradictory results, usually because of poor methodology. Aside from selection bias, the following are some other confounds that undermine the effort to discover an imaging protocol that can identify early cases of AD:

• Almost no CT or MRI protocols take into consideration the limitation that one can clinically diagnose antemortem AD with a best-possible accuracy of only 80%.

• Statistical concepts of specificity and sensitivity are ignored in studies that attempt to distinguish normal anatomy from the atrophic brains *expected* in AD. This is true even though not all demented patients have atrophy, and not all patients with atrophy are demented.

• Five percent of AD patients present with mild symptoms that remain stable for years, reducing the likelihood of detecting structural atrophy early on in a subset of demented patients.

• Studies often fail to correct for head size, sex differences, and age differences. Cross-sectional studies suggest that UBOs appear in deep white matter and pons with advancing age (Coffey et al., 1992), although their appearance is not inevitable, given that many octogenarians have no such lesions. This makes it difficult to draw a sharp dividing line between normal and abnormal brains.

• Hypertension and a cerebrovascular history (TIA or stroke) raise the incidence of UBOs in all age groups. UBOs were found twice as often in relatively young hypertensives (mean age, 38.7 years) as in control groups, with no correlation between cognitive performance and the presence of UBOs (Schmidt et al., 1991).

• Hypertension and cerebrovascular risk factors also affect PVHs, which were found in only 7.8% of individuals older than fifty years who had no cerebrovascular symptoms or risk factors. This figure jumped to 78.5% in those who did (Gerard & Weisberg, 1986).

• UBOs are also found in combination with larger, irregular lesions in old, demented patients with stroke (Hershey et al., 1987). Thus, future protocols need to take more care in selecting patients and considering the status of their general health. Without such attention to these and other methodological details, the issues will remain confused.

Turning back to CT, one finds that twenty-five years of data on its utility in diagnosing AD from a heterogeneous group of dements does not clarify the muddle much. The National Institute on Aging has tabulated both sensitivity and specificity for various measures taken by CT compared to pathologic anatomy (DiCarli et al., 1990), and those tables would interest students who wish to pursue this issue. There is considerable overlap when comparing weight, atrophy, and ventricular enlargement in AD and age-matched controls, making these insensitive indicators of whether or not AD is present. Qualitative measures are only slightly better than chance. Even though three-dimensional volumetric measurements are better than planimetry, the skill and resources required to take such measurements render the technique impractical at present. Useful correlations between measures of atrophy and neuropsychological performance also have not been forthcoming.

Our incomplete knowledge of the meaning of white matter changes seen on MRI scans is the result of broad variation in both methodology and assumptions among existing studies. Unfortunately, in both AD patients and controls, neither PVHs nor UBOs bear any relationship to focal neurologic signs. There appears to be a weak association between PVHs and AD, as well as an association with atrophy in nondemented controls. Thus, at best one can say only that the presence of either PVHs or atrophy without PVHs is consistent with AD, whereas the absence of both entities is consistent with normal brain.

After a quarter-century's effort, the promise held by structural imaging in AD and other dementias remains unmet. Though some structural-cognitive associations are true statistically, they are not helpful in individual circumstances. In summary, the meaning of leuko-araiosis in dementia is unclear. It does not correlate with either focal abnormalities or severity of dementia (Mirsen et al., 1991).

The topic of UBOs is germane to closed head trauma, another example of diffuse rather than focal disease. In head trauma as in dementia, however, the clinical correlations of image-lesions continue to be maddingly unclear, largely because of incompatable assumptions and methodologies among the reported studies (Cytowic et al., 1988).

THE NEUROLOGY OF AGING

As Voltaire said, "Everyone complains of his memory; but no one complains of his judgement." Perhaps he was thinking of politicians. This adage reveals that some degree of forgetfulness is normal, or at least socially acceptable if one is not a politician. But it also implies that other facets of intellect fail despite our unwillingness to acknowledge them. Exactly what capacities do fail, and at what point are such failures no longer normal? The neuropsychologist needs to distinguish between true deficits and counterfeit ones that merely reflect age-related decline (Albert & Knoefel, 1994; Huppert et al., 1994).

General Considerations

General opinion holds that many sensory, motor, and cognitive skills start fading at sixty years of age and may be marked by the seventh decade. Obviously, there are exceptions and variation but, in general, all five senses become less acute with time. Visual acuity, the size of the visual field, contrast sensitivity, color vision (blue-green worse than red-yellow), stereopsis, accommodation, upward gaze, smooth pursuit, and saccades all suffer (Cohen & Lessell, 1984). Bilateral high-frequency hearing loss (presbycusis) and impaired speech recognition occur in more than 13% of people older than sixty-five. Sentence identification is worse than single-word recognition. Vibratory discrimination is feeble and often absent in the feet, and touch is modestly weakened in the extremities. Complex sensory discrimination, such as two-point discrimination or stereognosis, is not completely accurate (Kenshalo, 1977). Enfeeblement of taste and smell are less relevant to neuropsychology. I have seen it nowhere in print but have often heard a clinical truism that multiple sensory impairment is the reason the elderly are more prone to an acute change in mental status than are younger persons. In other words, because they do not see well, hear well, or feel well, they are already partially sensorily deprived and easily pushed over the edge into an encephalopathy, dementia, or psychosis.

Swihart and Pirozzolo (1988) point out the cascading effect that basic sensory decline can have on cognition. Common hearing loss, for example, is associated with depression, which in turn impairs cognition and performance—at least on neuropsychological tests. Because we test specific and multiple modalities, neuropsychologists want to know which skills are resistant to ageing and which are not.

The so-called *ageing pattern of the WAIS* is accepted to mean that verbal subtests remain relatively stable while performance subtests decline. This is somewhat simplistic, and it is noteworthy that not all decline is attributable to slower speed alone. A better distinction is between *fluid* and *crystallized knowledge*, the latter being use of familiar knowledge (habit) that does not degrade. Fluid knowledge is required to solve novel tasks in new ways, and this is what declines with age. In short, it *is* difficult to teach an old dog new tricks.

Describing specific failures of memory with ageing is more difficult, and there is a large body of literature on this topic, the nuances of which are perhaps better discussed in class or given full attention in individual reading. The common observation that elderly people recall remote events better than recent ones is borne out by testing. Free, gist, and episodic recall all suffer, as does visual recall, but no simple statement can be offered that is generally valid, let alone apt for an individual case. In the end, the practitioner is likely to rely on a clinical judgement based on the severity of impairment relative to other factors.

Vocabulary is said to be resistant to all kinds of brain damage, which may be why utterances cannot always be taken at face value. This is particularly true in casual conversation, where everyone's exchanges tend to be stereotyped and ritualized (again, the confound of overlearned behavior). The lexicon of the elderly is reasonably preserved; in fact, increased complexity of syntax often is noted. Whether the individual was bright to start and still does the New York Times crossword puzzle in ink also matters. That comprehension declines can be stated more confidently. Concurrent hearing loss may account for inconsistent performance.

Visual reproduction, construction, and manipulation all show minor shakiness and disorganization with ageing that might be suspicious in younger individuals (Howieson et al., 1993). Several authors recommend relaxing scoring criteria, especially normative cutoff levels.

Anatomical Considerations

There are many myths of ageing, but only a few things are biologically inevitable. Three features in the cognitive sphere are inescapable as senescence approaches: (1) a general slowing of both movement and thought, (2) a decreased ability to find new solutions to problems, and (3) a decrease in memory.

The old idea that we lose enormous numbers of neurons from birth onward is now known to overstate the case. Technical artifacts in histologic preparations used for counting neurons in various structures across age groups probably accounts for this misstatement. Haug (1984) shows that some areas, such as striate and parietal cortices, do not lose many neurons during adult life whereas the striatum and prefrontal cortex lose 15% to 20%. In other words, it seems that different brain regions have their own course of ageing and neuronal dropout.

Of course, neuropsychologists want to know what happens in the hippocampus and to the pyramidal cells in CA1. Several sources estimate a 4% dropout per decade. Thus, by age eighty, only 20% to 30% of hippocampal pyramidal cells will have died. In contrast to the amnesia that results from more severe wipeout, perhaps this partial depletion explains what has been called *normal forgetting of senescence* or *age-associated memory impairment* (McEntee & Crook, 1990).

Normal elderly brains do show NFTs in hippocampus and parahippocampal gyrus, further suggesting that hippocampal dysfunction may be the biological basis of senescent forgetfulness. Still, elderly patients show types of forgetting that are *not* encountered in amnesic individuals. Amnesics have no difficulty with object naming, for example, and also have good recall of semantic facts.

Hence, the common failure of forgetting someone's name (attaching a verbal label to a face), commonly witnessed in the senium, must be explained another way (Squire, 1987).

We expect demented individuals to show atrophy on CT and MRI scans, but the converse does not uniformly hold—namely, atrophy does not signify obligate cognitive loss. Shortly after the emergence of CT and MRI technology (after 1973 and 1984, respectively), radiologists were quick to suggest dementia whenever they encountered an image of severe atrophy. Aside from the fact that radiologists are untrained in cognitive matters and so should refrain from giving an opinion regarding mentation, this is another example of the counterintuitive nature of science: No simple relationship between ventricular size or sulcal widening and mental status has held up. From earlier autopsy studies, we know that the brain loses weight and substance—about 150 gm—after sixty years, but astrocytic proliferation distorts the significance of even this simple measure.

NFTs, granulovacuolar degeneration, SPs, and other so-called pathological changes are present in senescent brains that displayed no behavioral pathology in life. In general, the pathological changes seen in Alzheimer's disease, for example, may be similar to those noted in normal senile brains, but their frequency and distribution are different. The functional significance of structural and neurochemical changes remains uncertain.

SUGGESTED READINGS

Albert MI, Knoefel JE. 1994 *Clinical Neurology of Ageing*, 2d ed. New York: Oxford University Press

Caplan LR. 1995 Binswanger's disease—revisited. *Neurology* 45:626–633.

Craik FIM. 1984 Age differences in remembering. In LR Squire, N Butters, eds, *Neuropsychology of Memory*. New York: Guilford Press, pp 3–13

Grant I, Martin A. 1994 *Neuropsychology of HIV Infection*. New York: Oxford University Press

Huber SJ, Cummings JL, eds. 1992 *Parkinson's Disease: Neurobehavioral Aspects*. New York: Oxford

Huppert FA, Brayne C, O'Connor DW. 1994 *Dementia and Normal Ageing*. New York: Cambridge University Press

Katzman R, Rowe JW. 1992 *Principles of Geriatric Neurology* [vol 38, Contemporary Neurology Series]. Philadelphia: FA Davis Company

NINDS-AIREN International Workshop. 1993 Vascular dementia: Diagnostic criteria for research studies. *Neurology* 43:250–260

Victor M, Adams RD. 1989 *The Wernicke-Korskoff Syndrome and Related Neurologic Disorders Due to Alcoholism and Malnutrition*, 2d ed. Philadelphia: FA Davis Company

Whitehouse PJ, ed. 1992 *Dementia* [vol 40, Contemporary Neurology Series]. Philadelphia: FA Davis Company

11　The Epilepsies

All-encompassing classifications of the epilepsies come from the International League Against Epilepsy (ILAE, 1981) or tertiary academic centers whose patients are highly selected and unrepresentative of the broad base of epilepsy in the general population. In fact, only one-third of cases from prospective population-based studies fall into any ILAE category, and many rare syndromes are never encountered (Manford et al., 1992). Predictably, such classifications are not widely used. Accordingly, we will employ conventional terminology in talking about seizures that interest neuropsychologists—namely, those that affect cognition and behavior, those whose manifestations might be mistaken for psychiatric disease, or those that suggest an evaluation for surgery. This is admittedly a small part of the epilepsy gamut. You can turn to any number of specialized texts for details on the physiology, epidemiology, and general medical concerns of various seizure types.

The neuropsychology of the epilepsies encompasses empirical relationships between their phenomenology and (1) type of seizure, (2) localization of the *focus*, (3) effects of anticonvulsant medications, and (4) surgical therapy. Ironically, a very small minority of neuroscientists have any firsthand experience with epilepsy surgery, despite its huge contributions to neuropsychological theory. Even the term *surgery* itself refers to a multitude of operations such as epileptogenic tissue resection, hemispherectomy, or commissurotomy as well as the related procedures of depth-electrode recording, the Wada test, neuroimaging, electrical stimulation, and pre-operative and post-operative experimental protocols. Although we emphasize biological and neurological variables, neuropsychologists also are interested in psychosocial issues, creativity, consciousness, and what epilepsy might tell us about the normal brain.

A moment's thought shows just how much neuropsychology is indebted to epilepsy. Hughlings Jackson conceived that the signs and symptoms of epilepsy arose from clear-cut cortical loci; Penfield's homunculi were a result of electrical stimulation in epileptics undergoing surgery; temporal lobectomy opened up a new view of memory; hemispherectomy engendered the twin concepts of developmental plasticity and critical periods in the acquisition of mental skills; intracarotid injection of amobarbital helped to clarify lateralization of brain function; and commissurotomy expanded our concepts of hemispheric specialization and interaction. In the face of this mother lode, it is startling how peripheral a place epilepsy occupies in medical and doctoral curricula.

In defining a seizure, we say that a sudden and excessive discharge of cerebral neurons (not always cortical ones) results in a disturbance of sensation, a loss of consciousness or mental function, convulsions, or some combination of these. The word *seizure* is a broad term, and one can speak of a sensory seizure, a convulsive (motor) seizure, and a psychic seizure. *Epilepsy* is not any specific disease, but refers to the tendency of an individual to have seizures.

Following stroke, epilepsy is the second most common neurologic disorder. Three to four million Americans have recurrent seizures. Physiologically, a seizure is a sudden, synchronous neuronal discharge. Phenomenally, it is a temporary alteration of behavior. Either way, a seizure has a definable beginning, middle, and end. An awareness of its beginning, or *aura*, indicates that a part of the cortex is discharging enough to cause symptoms but not unconsciousness. Only some seizures have auras.

Although we think of epilepsy as an idiopathic condition, it is important to remember that seizures can sometimes be triggered by identifiable factors such as alcohol, strong emotion, vigorous exercise, flashing lights, loud music, illness, fever, menstruation, lack of sleep, stress, reading, eating, or even thinking about certain things.

TYPES OF SEIZURES

The International Classification of Epilepsy broadly divides seizures into *generalized*, meaning "bilaterally symmetrical," and *partial*, meaning "those having a focal onset." Among generalized seizures, we are interested in the tonic-clonic (grand mal) and absence varieties, whilst among the partial seizures we are interested in the simple partial (sensory and psychic seizures) and complex partial (temporal lobe or psychomotor) varieties.

Generalized Tonic-Clonic Convulsions

We usually regard the grand mal tonic-clonic seizure in terms of its convulsion. However, it is worth noting that some mental change occurs both before and after the convulsion. Apathy, depression, irritability, or other subjective feeling constitutes the *prodrome* that may be sensed for many hours before a convulsion. Approximately half the patients have an *aura*, which is not a sign of impending seizure but the beginning of the seizure itself. Typically perceived auras include contraversive turning of the eyes, head, or body; palpitations; tightness in the chest; butterflies in the stomach; and dysesthesia in a body part.

Consciousness then is lost, and the muscular spasm and apnea of the tonic phase, lasting ten to fifteen seconds, next gives way to the clonic phase of vigorous, rhythmic muscular contractions that last one to two minutes. After five minutes or so of a deep, quiet coma, patients awaken to a state of post-ictal confusion that clears within an hour but for which period individuals have no recall save possibly for the seizure's onset (aura). If undisturbed, patients usually sleep several hours and awake with a throbbing headache.

Grand mal seizures can occur during wakefulness or sleep, singly or repeated as groups of two or three over a short period. Slightly more than 5% of individuals with grand mal convulsions will, at some time, have a salvo of seizures without fully regaining consciousness between them. This is the neurologic emergency of status epilepticus. Although this would not normally be a concern of neuropsychology per se, there does exist a *nonconvulsive* status epilepticus that causes extended confusion (Fagan & Lee, 1990; Guberman et al., 1986). These states are also referred to as *electrographic seizures* because you would not suspect anything was wrong until you saw the continuous generalized ictal discharges on the EEG. The point is that some prolonged states of confusion following seizures are not merely the expected post-ictal state but are in fact manifestations of persistent seizure discharge. Therefore, apparent post-ictal confusion that lasts several hours should raise the suspicion of nonconvulsive status epilepticus. The varieties of nonconvulsive absence status, nonconvulsive temporal lobe status, and nonconvulsive generalized status epilepticus have all been described. Aside from confusion, aphasia may be the sole manifestation of continuous epileptic discharges, even in individuals with no previous history of seizure (Racy et al., 1980).

Absence Seizures

Although the brief blank stare ("absence"), unawareness, and amnesia for the attack was described clinically by Poupart in 1705 (hence the French cognate name), it was not until the 1930s that its defining electrographic three-per-second generalized spike-wave discharge was identified. *Absence seizures* are like turning on a switch in that they begin abruptly without an aura and end abruptly without any post-ictal abnormality.

Onset is in childhood after age four and always before the age of sixteen, though the seizures themselves may persist well into adulthood. Vigorous hyperventilation may precipitate an attack even in individuals who have been asymptomatic since adolescence. Absence seizures are hereditary through a Mendelian dominant gene. Each year, 5,000 to 7,000 new patients are seen in the United States. The estimated prevalence is 120,000 cases. Approximately half of those afflicted have a history of at least one grand mal fit.

In contrast, *absence status* occurs in patients with preëxisting epilepsy and happens at any age. Movements, if present, are focal and subtle, the gross bilateral spasms that mark the onset of status epilepticus being unsustained. Finally, *de novo absence status,* meaning that affected individuals are without a history of epilepsy, occurs in middle-aged patients who often receive high doses of psychotropic drugs (e.g., benzodiazepines, neuroleptics, tricyclics, lithium) in a setting of electrolyte imbalance or metabolic derangement (Thomas et al., 1992). There is already a 2.5% to 4% incidence of seizures as a complication of benzodiazepine withdrawal, and the analysis of Thomas's group suggests that de novo absence status epilepticus may constitute a particular benzodiazepine withdrawal symptom.

The brief staring spell in which all activity abruptly ceases is the hallmark of the simple absence attack. If walking, the patient stands still; if eating, food stops on its way to the mouth; if talking, words stop until the seizure ends, at which point they resume where they were broken off. Only normal breathing continues, after an apneic pause. The gaze is vacant. Action recommences a few seconds later where it left off, as if time had stood still. The majority of absence seizures last less than ten seconds; seldom does their duration approach forty-five seconds. The longer the seizure, the more likely it is for both patient and observer to notice that there has been a break in consciousness.

The old synonym *petit mal* is unfortunate, given that the electrical flux of the whole brain is disrupted during an absence attack. Furthermore, the classic staring spell of the *simple absence* represents less than 10% of all absence seizures.

The contrasting term, *complex absence*, indicates that other phenomena join the fundamental impairment of consciousness. These may include mild clonic movements, increased or decreased postural tone, automatisms, and autonomic manifestations. Clonic movements may be seen in the eyelids as rhythmic blinking, in the corners of the mouth, or in the muscles of the fingers, arms, or shoulders. The movements range from barely perceptible to bilaterally symmetrical myoclonic jerks.

Automatisms are actions that seem purposeful to an uninformed observer but that the patient performs without awareness. The likelihood of automatisms increases with seizure duration.

The two principal ictal automatisms are (1) perseverative, and (2) de novo. In the perseverative kind, patients persist in whatever they were doing at the seizure's onset, such as walking, typing, combing, or handling some object. As the seizure continues, such activities fragment and become increasingly aimless. De novo automatisms, on the other hand, emerge after the seizure begins. Licking, scratching, swallowing, rubbing, fiddling, and wandering are common. It is easy to demonstrate that the environmental context can influence the expression of the automatism. For example, placing a cup in the hand may lead to drinking, placing gum in the mouth may release vigorous chewing movements, or scratching the arm may lead to rubbing of the site. If spoken to, the patient may turn toward the location of the voice and utter a rudimentary sound. Such simple responsiveness unfortunately leads to erroneous conclusions by teachers and parents. A teacher's shout of "Bobby, pay attention!" during the vacant stare may prompt the child to turn toward the voice and dully say, "Huh?" The possibility that the child has a medical problem is thereby replaced with an erroneous opinion that he is merely inattentive.

That automatisms occur more frequently with increasing duration of the absence and are shaped by context suggests that automatisms are reactive, representing a released behavior when the cortex is impaired by generalized spike-wave discharges. Therefore, automatisms are not cortically directed.

Pupillary dilatation, perioral pallor, flushing, piloërection, and salivation are autonomic manifestations that require careful observation and therefore often go unnoticed.

Partial Seizures

Partial, or focal, seizures result from a demonstrable lesion in some part of the cortex, a notion distinct from that underlying generalized seizures, in which the location of origin is unknown. The manifestations of *simple partial seizures* are motor, sensory, or psychic, whereas those of *complex partial seizures* are the elaborate behaviors described by the combination of these elements. The terms *psychomotor epilepsy, temporal lobe epilepsy,* and *limbic epilepsy* are used interchangeably, even though this usage is imprecise.

The usual breakdown of simple seizures is actually too simplistic in that it suggests categories with sharp boundaries. For example, we usually regard simple motor fits (e.g., focal motor, Jacksonian, contraversive, epilepsia partialis continua) as purely motor in their expression. However, scrutiny of partial seizures originating in the frontal lobe reveals such features as vocalization, hyperventilation, elaborate gestural automatisms, and bizarre behavior that is easily mistaken for psychiatric disease or hysteria (Harvey et al., 1993; Saygi et al., 1992).

Because individuals with partial seizures very frequently display a combination of motor, sensory, automatic, and psychic alterations, the preferred term is *complex partial seizure*. Although the focus usually is in the temporal lobe in such combined seizures, the precise behavior that actually occurs depends on the electrical spread among nuclear and cortical entities within the temporal lobe. The term *complex partial* is more apt than *temporal lobe* seizure in describing a *psychomotor seizure*, because a similarly appearing seizure with both psychic and motor elements can also arise from frontal tissue. Therefore, the term *psychomotor* is supposed to be purely descriptive, whereas the terms *complex partial* or *limbic epilepsy* denote a psychomotor seizure the focus of which is in some limbic element of the temporal lobe. Still, custom has it that *temporal lobe epilepsy* (TLE) means a "complex partial seizure." (I suppose the only recourse against this confusing terminology is to be explicit.)

The aura of a complex partial seizure is often an elaborate psychic experience, sometimes constituting the entire seizure. If this is not the case, a period of unresponsiveness follows during which the motor elements emerge. These automatisms last up to five minutes, after which awareness returns gradually. In addition to perseverative and de novo automatisms that are the same as those witnessed in absence seizures, far more sophisticated automatisms also appear. When turning toward a voice, for example, the patient may vocalize sounds, words, or stereotyped (overlearned) phrases. Automatic behavior such as walking, driving a car, or stacking dishes are completed successfully. The strong tendency for action to fragment, which is so characteristic of absences, is not present in the automatisms of partial seizures.

Because electrical spread is rapid, only the first ten to twenty seconds of what the patient says is happening is relevant to locating the focal origin. At their end, more than 80% of complex partial seizures have a post-ictal period lasting between one and two minutes. Post-ictal paraphasias, geographic disorientation, and flat affect most likely reflect some functions of the cortical region containing the focus, not the areas involved in the seizure's spread (Devinsky et al., 1994). The scope of post-ictal signs is extensive and can range from paralysis and other motor signs to sensory manifestations, autonomic signs, and higher cortical deficits that last for hours to days following the ictus.

A tendency toward secondary generalization is true of all types of partial epilepsy, and the complex partial attack may segue into a grand mal fit. It is noteworthy that the incidence of complex partial seizures increases beginning in adolescence, as if recurrent generalized fits were somehow leading to cumulative damage of the temporal lobes (medial temporal sclerosis).

I have already touched on most of the hallucinatory, perceptual, and psychic manifestations of complex partial seizures in discussing symptoms of focal temporal lesions (see chapter 6). Furthermore, I indicated that the limbic structures of the temporal lobe have a low threshold for seizures that remain contained without spilling over to other parts of the brain, and that the most distinctive feature of limbic seizures is a *qualitative alteration of consciousness* (see chapter 8). You can easily review these features in tables 11.1 through 11.3 before proceeding with some of the more advanced bottom-up neuropsychological issues regarding partial seizures.

Emotion in Partial Seizures

Crying, or dacrystic, seizures are rare. Luciano and colleagues (1993) could identify only eleven such patients in the literature in addition to their own seven patients who were studied by video-EEG. Maximal ictal discharges were in the right hemisphere (six anteromesial-temporal, and one mesial-frontal). Weeping patients deny a congruous affect, and their crying appears rather mechanical. For example, one patient's seizures began with a "strange, crazy feeling," followed by violent sobbing, head holding, and rocking of her torso, yet she denied feeling sad or fearful or having any headache during her aura. Another patient began crying while still fully responsive and, when asked why she wept, simply stated, "This is what happens."

Ictal emotion is common (15% of patients with partial epilepsy) yet almost exclusively negative. Fear and anxiety, for example, are the most common ictal feelings. Ictal contentment, euphoria, religious bliss, or other positive experiences are extraordinarily rare. This preponderance of negative ictal emotion curiously contrasts the much more frequent gelastic seizures to dacrystic ones: For example, Sackeim et al. (1982) found that 88% of ictal emotional displays were of laughter, whereas only 6% were of crying. Such

Table 11.1

Localization of Partial Seizures According to the International League Against Epilepsy (1981)

Cortical Region	Clinical Manifestations
Precentral	Contralateral movements according to somatotopy; Jacksonian march; speech arrest, swallowing
Premotor	Contraversive movements; aphasia; automatisms
Orbitofrontal	Olfactory hallucinations; autonomic signs; urinary incontinence; automatisms, psychomotor
Frontopolar	Unconsciousness; adversive and contraversive movements; autonomic signs; axial myoclonic jerks
Opercular	Gustatory hallucinations; autonomic signs; fear; epigastric aura; mastication; salivation; swallowing; speech arrest; facial jerks
Supplementary motor	Psychomotor; focal motor; vocalization; speech arrest; fencing posture; urinary incontinence
Cingulate	Psychomotor; automatisms with sexual features; mood and affect changes; urinary incontinence
Occipital	Visual hallucinations, illusions, and distortions
Parietal	Somatosensory auras; formed visual hallucinations
Temporal	Psychomotor; automatisms; autonomic signs; dyscognitive and affective experience; gustatory, olfactory, and visceral hallucinations; other somatic, visual, and auditory auras; vertigo; speech and motor arrest

behavior that is incongruous with feeling recalls the disinhibited expression of pseudobulbar palsy (see chapter 6) rather than an activation of some specific laughing or crying center. Daly (1958) suggested the useful term *affective automatism*, though that term rarely is employed. The lack of an obvious center suggests that crying, and perhaps other emotive actions, are executed by a distributed system. This is, of course, an obvious phenomenal confirmation of what was implied by anatomical facts of the Papez circuit (see pp. 98–99). Further support for this particular case is the fact that facial movements appropriate to weeping are produced in animals by brainstem stimulation, whereas lacrymation is evoked by limbic stimulation (Weinstein & Bender, 1943; Anand & Dua, 1955).

Table 11.2
Manifestations of Complex Partial Seizures

- Affective (fear and anxiety most common)
- Automatisms (perseverative, do novo, gelastic, dacrystic, procursive, and other seemingly purposeful actions)
- Autoscopy
- Cognitive dissonance (e.g., déjà vu, depersonalization, dreamy states)
- Feeling of a presence
- Epigastric and abdominal sensations, indescribable but recognized as outside normal experience
- Hallucinations (any modality)
- Sensory illusions and distortions of ongoing perceptions (e.g., metamorphopsia, separation of color from its boundary, spatial extension of the form constants, paracusia, *umkehrtsehen*, etc.)
- Synesthesia
- Time dilatation and contraction
- Psychosis
- Forced thinking
- Memory intrusions
- Hypersexuality and hyposexuality
- Autonomic dysregulation
- Contraversive movements
- Speech arrest and ictal aphasia

A preponderant right temporal-frontal focus in dacrystic seizures is consistent with a lateralization of negative emotion to the right hemisphere and is consonant with diverse evidence from other ictal disorders, hemispherectomy, intracarotid amobarbital injection, and infarcts. Though negative emotions such as sorrow, depression, or guilt can be evoked by temporal lobe stimulation (Gloor et al., 1982), crying, or even the urge to weep, hardly ever occurs with temporal stimulation (Halgren et al., 1978). This discrepancy may be due in part to poor observation, but the neurology of mammalian emotion is surely involved too. Both Darwin (1872) and Freud (1916), after all, did point out that "unintentional" laughter and smiling often happen in the face of contrary feelings (fear, anxiety, guilt, doom).

Table 11.3
Comparison of Seizure Types

	Generalized		Partial		
	Grand Mal	Absence	Temporal	Frontal	Parieto-occipital
Aura	50%, always simple	Never	90%, usually complex	60%	100%, esp. somatic or elementary visual
Loss of consciousness	Always; consciousness returns slowly	Always; consciousness returns abruptly	Variable; gradual recomposure when lost	Variable	Variable
Postictal confusion	Always	None	Yes	Yes	Yes
Duration	1–3 min	Most <10 s	> 30s	>30 s	>30 s
Automatism	No	Perseverative and de novo	Perseverative, de novo, and complex	Perseverative, de novo, and complex	Seldom
Affect	No	No	Common	Yes	Seldom

That both laughing and crying often are described as *irrepressible* while the patient remains conscious of these automatisms is another striking example of how forced thinking and behavior originating in limbic structures can overwhelm rational thought and intentional action.

Depression related to epilepsy is another topic that interests neuropsychologists. Whether gauging current mood or lifetime prevalence, patients with either generalized or partial seizures have an increased incidence of depression after the onset of their epilepsy. A preponderance of evidence favors an association of depressed mood with left-sided epileptogenic foci. Two-thirds of patients have symptoms of an interictal depression at some time, whereas fully one-third meet the narrower DSM criteria for major depressive illness (Victoroff et al., 1994). Such a prevalence is more than five times that of the general population.

It is possible that factors other than laterality of focus can modify the experience of epileptic depression. In complex partial seizures with unilateral foci, for example, PET studies have repeatedly confirmed ipsilateral temporal lobe hypometabolism in 60% to 90% of individuals. Regional glucose metabolism in nonepileptics with unipolar depression confirms that a depressed mood and cerebral hypometabolism go hand in hand, although such studies find no correlation with laterality (Drevets & Raichle, 1995).

In epileptics, the degree of hypometabolism varies with the risk of depression, regardless of the side of seizure focus. In terms of state versus trait faculties, no association exists between laterality of hypometabolism and *current* depression, whereas a *history* of depression is clearly associated with left-sided hypometabolism. Therefore, rather than being state-dependent, temporal lobe hypometabolism may be an enduring feature of the neural substrate of depressed mood in epilepsy.

Victoroff's group (1994, p. 162) suggests that depression might be "one price that the epileptic pays for the neural adaptations that inhibit the propagation of seizures." Their analysis of focal glucose hypometabolism further reminds us that the left-right dichotomy oversimplifies a complex issue regarding the neurologic basis of emotion.

Table 11.4
Localization of Partial Seizures by Aura

	Temporal	Frontal	Parieto-occipital
Somatosensory		~16%	~88%
Viscerosensory	~95%		
Experiential	~85%		
Elementary visual			100%
Elementary auditory	0		
Cephalic		0	
Rising warmth		0	
Crying, other affect	0	0	
Vertiginous	Unknown		
Awareness of confusion	Unknown		

Note: See text for further explanations.

The Aura

It is worth emphasizing that the details of the aura, when expertly extracted during the history, provide localizing—and sometimes even lateralizing—information as good as that obtained by EEG and imaging (see Palmini & Gloor [1992] for a particularly well-controlled statistical study of this issue). This clinical correlation with seizure foci has largely been confirmed by electrical stimulation (see table 11.4). As used by Palmini and Gloor, *viscerosensory* refers to unpleasant epigastric, abdominal, thoracic, and pharyngeal sensations, sometimes rising from one body region to another. *Cephalic* sensations refer not to vertigo but to dysesthesias and body schema disturbances of pressure, light-headedness, or alteration of head size (like blowing up a balloon). *Awareness of confusion* is a metacognitive state in which patients are aware that they are "mixed up" and their thoughts disjunctive. For example, a woman may hear voices coming from the wall directing her to kill herself, yet she recognizes the unreality of the voices and even concludes that they are related to her epilepsy (this is also a good example of duality). The remainder of the terms employed by Palmini and Gloor follow conventional usage.

Beginning with the earliest stimulation experiments of Penfield, a number of studies have indicated that experiential responses originate more often from the right temporal lobe. Although they fail to confirm a *general lateralizing* significance for auras (Palmini & Gloor, 1992), strict statistical analyses do find that the complex visual, auditory, and déjà vu hallucinations of experiential responses strongly tend to originate in the right temporal lobe. Palmini and Gloor appropriately defend the diagnostic power of a carefully-taken history. They further advocate encouraging patients to describe their auras in everyday language while vigorously discouraging them from using medical jargon (particularly déjà vu) picked up from examiners. To strictly qualify for déjà vu, patients must be acutely aware that their sense of familiarity is illusory and inappropriate to the context in which they experience it. The recognition of incongruity is essential.

Hormonal Modulation

Two of the brain areas in which circulating sex hormones are concentrated are highly epileptogenic—namely, the amygdala and the hippocampus. Cyclical hormonal variations may alter seizure threshold and, therefore, frequency in women with epilepsy. Also, the laterality of a temporal lobe focus can affect the pulsatile secretion of lutineizing hormone (Drislane et al., 1994). The relationship between epilepsy and hormonal dysfunction is well-known, and polycystic ovaries, hypothalamic amenorrhea (hypogonadotropic hypogonadism), and infertility are but some of the reproductive endocrine disorders that are significantly overrepresented in women with limbic epilepsy. Hormonal treatment may be a useful adjunct to anticonvulsant therapy, particularly if the seizures have a catamenial association (Schachter, 1988).

Reflex Epilepsy

Reflex epilepsy is a curious phenomenon in which certain highly specific physiologic or mental stimuli precipitate a seizure. The precipitating stimuli classically fall into five groups as identified by Forster (1977): (1) visual—flashing or flickering light, specific colors, patterns, eye closure in bright light, (2) auditory—specific music, sounds, voices, (3) somatosensory—either a sudden tap or prolonged touch to a specific body part, (4) reading, and (5) eating. Added to these classic groups should be a sixth category of reflex seizures precipitated by (6) thinking along certain lines or performing certain mental tasks. Because patients rarely think to mention these triggers, you should inquire about reflex activation of their attacks.

Flashing or flickering light is by far the most common stimulus that provokes epilepsy. Strobes, the flicker of television, dappled sunlight through the trees, the light-dark alternation experienced when driving steadily past regularly-spaced telephone poles, and even the waving of one's hand in front of the eyes are well-recognized triggers. The precipitation of generalized grand mal convulsions by intermittent light is associated with the electrographic photoparoxysmal response during photic stimulation (Puglia et al., 1992). Photosensitive patients typically respond to frequencies between 15 and 20 Hz, and intermittent red or green light is said to be most provocative. The prevalence of photosensitive epilepsy is 1 in 4,000, with a higher frequency among women (Jeavons et al., 1986). So-called relaxation devices peddled under the rubric of "brain-wave synchronizers" emit intermittent red light at between 1 and 30 Hz, and have been reported to induce grand mal seizures in individuals with no prior history of epilepsy (Ruuskanen-Uoti & Salmi, 1994).

Seizures precipitated by calculation, measuring, decision making, card and board games, crossword puzzles, knitting, or other spatial tasks are noteworthy in that fits appear to be provoked by activation of the parietal lobe (Goossens et al., 1990). In a manner analogous to using strobe-light stimulation to evoke occipital driving, neuropsychological tests sensitive to parietal function (e.g., block design, puzzle assembly) are effective in eliciting parietal electrographic discharges in some individuals (Wilkins et al., 1982).

Reading epilepsy is characterized by myoclonic jerks of the jaw and throat while reading that culminate in a convulsion. Each myoclonic jerk is linked to a bilaterally synchronous paroxysm on the EEG. More than sixty reports exist, yet whether semantic, lexical, or phonological aspects precipitate the seizure remains unclear. In analyzing a case of reading epilepsy associated with acquired encephalomalacia in Brodmann area 6 (anterior to left central sulcus) and further associated with left frontocentral ictal discharges, Ritaccio and colleagues (1992) conclude that grapheme-to-phoneme transformation rather than linguistic complexity is the critical stimulus. For example, the reading of Latin, unknown foreign text, or other "meaningless" material was equally provocative, indicating that decoding is not essential to precipitate reading epilepsy.

Three-fourths of patients with reflex seizures have more than one effective trigger. As many also have additional seizures that are not reflexively induced. In many patients, the reflex activation goes unrecognized until it is casually mentioned. The rate of spontaneous remission is unknown, the response to medication is only fair to good, and to what extent attacks can be controlled by avoiding specific stimuli is unclear.

Dissociation in Partial Seizures

The so-called temporal lobe personality comprises such traits as humorlessness, religiosity, and hypergraphia (see p. 239). Ever since the seminal quantitative analysis by Bear and Fedio (1977) of *interictal* behavior in those with partial seizures, we have gradually progressed in understanding the array of enigmatic and sometimes dramatic behavior exhibited by such individuals. Instances of depersonalization such as autoscopy, the illusion of supernatural possession, or dual personalities are especially noteworthy and possibly not as rare as commonly was believed. To understand the epileptic dissociative states, it is useful to hold sharply in your mind both a distinction between *ictal* and *interictal* behavior, as well as some anatomical facts about the temporal lobe.

In the medial portion of the temporal lobe that is so often home to epileptogenic foci, one finds (1) the fusiform and parahippocampal gyri, where elaborate sensory associations occur, (2) the amygdala and hippocampus, with their direct projections to hypothalamus and its hormonal, visceral, and motivational forces, and (3) monosynaptic projections between sensory association cortex and limbic entities. Accordingly, ictal manifestations may be (1) sensory, such as hallucinations and illusions, (2) affective, such as impending doom or jealousy, or (3) a combination of sensory and affective elements, as in déjà vu or autoscopy.

I explained earlier (chapters 6 & 8) how limbic entities integrate affect, sensation, and thought, and how the customary relationships among these three elements in the context of one's life experience and future expectations are always perceived as congruous. Seizure foci in temporal limbic entities can disrupt the balance of this integration. Therefore, in addition to subjective experience and overt behavior that we describe as *ictal*, limbic foci can introduce certain *interictal* biases or tendencies that become incorporated into the personality of the epileptic individual over time. The often-cited religiosity or sense of portentousness may be taken as examples of successful personality integration, whereas the emergence of alter-ego personalities or possession by alien forces can be considered experience that is too bizarre and inhuman to integrate. Dissociation from the patient's sphere of everyday experience results.

An obvious question is why some epileptics with temporal foci incorporate subjective experience into their personæ while others dissociate it. Mesulam (1981b) speculates that mental events that originate in the language hemisphere are prone to successful integration into one's sense of self, whereas those originating in the nondominant temporal lobe are unincorporable and therefore dissociate. This speculation agrees with the conjectures of Sir John Eccles, some linguistics, and some split-brain researchers who all surmise that the left hemisphere generates the sense of self.

A link between multiple personality and epilepsy was first proposed in the nineteenth century by French neurologists Jean Martin Charcot (1825–1893) and Pierre Marie (1853–1940). A sense of duality is a common enough aura in epileptics with temporal foci: Twenty percent of patients with partial epilepsy experience dissociation (Devinsky et al., 1989b). The personalities can converse with one another or even alternate á la Jekyll and Hyde: A placid persona alternates with a belligerent hooligan, or a highly-controlled citizen becomes a vindictive criminal (this does *not* mean that individuals are unaware of and not responsible for their actions). Such dissociations may be far more common than suspected. Mesulam (1981b) indicates that in the course of one year, 12 (20%) of 61 patients in whom the possibility of psychomotor epilepsy was raised had dissociations of alter egos or supernatural possession, whereas none of 246 patients with other behavioral neurologic diagnoses did.

Patients freely volunteer the details of their astounding experiences and speak with conviction of being invaded by an alien entity or demon. Far less often, a beneficent spirit is the possessor, but patients nevertheless describe a clear sense of depersonalization, that their actions and thoughts are taken over by external forces. Strong feelings of ictal doom and dread are common. These patients' EEGs are unequivocally abnormal, though convulsions and automatisms are the exception. (This is not surprising as it is well-known that individuals with temporal foci need not exhibit any "abnormal" movements in their psychomotor attacks.)

One can approach the issue conversely by starting not with a seizure but with the psychiatric symptoms of multiple personality disorder (MPD). MPD belongs to the broader category of dissociative disorders that are characterized by a disturbed self-identity with amnesia for the episode. Most MPD patients have normal EEGs, although a high incidence of nonepileptoform abnormalities (sharp transients, intermittent theta, 14- and 6-Hz positive spikes) obviously suggests that some neurophysiological derangement contributes to the expression of multiple personalities in the psychiatric population. Interestingly, patients with partial seizures do not experience a significantly higher incidence of dissociation than individuals with generalized seizures, and they report only slightly more dissociative experiences than do nonepileptic individuals do (Devinsky et al., 1989b). This converse approach indicates that ictal discharges are not the prime mechanism for ego dissociation, although dissociation may constitute one behavioral manifestation of abnormal electrical activity in the temporal lobes. Therefore, the neurologic and psychiatric populations that manifest ego dissociation may actually be quite distinct.

Along this line, intracarotid amobarbital injections in patients with temporal foci suggest that the details of interhemispheric interaction may underlie ego dissociation, because each patient exhibited the second personality during inactivation of the left hemisphere (which, in each, was dominant for language as well as being the site of the epileptogenic focus) (Ahern et al., 1993). This observation confirms the previously cited speculation of Mesulam (1981b), whose patients, incidentally, often switched handedness when the other personality took over. This remarkable event, not witnessed in psychiatric reports of MPD, may indicate some shift in hemispheric dominance that would be consistent with the sudden change in temperament witnessed during amobarbital injection.

Lastly, psychiatric descriptions of MPD note up to fifty distinct alter egos in a given patient, whereas those in the neurologic literature number two or three. As such, it might be more apt to speak of *dual personality* rather than multiple personality. Moreover, rather than differences in age, social status, education, occupation, world view, and other traits of character that so clearly mark the various personalities of the psychiatric examples, those neurologic cases with temporal foci emphasize differences in emotional temperament rather than general personality.

PSYCHOSIS IN EPILEPSY

Influential reports in the 1940s suggested that partial seizures with temporal foci had numerous psychotic elements, whereas later reports did not substantiate any increased risk for psychosis. The matter remains controversial, and the relationship between epilepsy and psychosis refuses to yield to cogent analysis. Much earlier work was poorly controlled and suffered confounds. Trimble (1991) reviews this contradictory history.

When it comes to odd behavior, temporal lobe epilepsy is a bit like the subdural hematoma for which everyone is always scanning. Many psychiatric wards have standing orders for routine EEGs because it is often said that psychotic or otherwise bizarre patients may really have temporal lobe seizures. Focal EEG abnormalities in schizophrenics are rare, however, occurring in only 1% of cases (Goon et al., 1973). Despite this, one still hears the conventional wisdom that approximately 7% of all epileptics have some sort of psychotic episodes. A recent study of 1,611 epileptic outpatients, for example, found that 9.25% had experienced schizophrenic episodes (Mendez et al., 1993).

Part of the confusion can be resolved by first acknowledging that two distinct groups exist, one in which there is a clear proximate relationship between the seizure and a *brief peri-ictal* psychosis and the other, a group of *chronic interictal psychoses*, in which the relationship is one of statistical association. Interictal psychosis generally includes schizophrenia, manic depression, and paranoia. Epilepsy beginning in or lasting through puberty is more likely to be associated with subsequent psychosis.

In addressing the widespread belief that epileptic psychosis is particularly associated with temporal lobe epilepsy, the well-designed study from Runwell Hospital in England (Bruton et al., 1994) found that temporal brain damage occurs no more often in individuals with both epilepsy and psychosis than in those with epilepsy alone. General temporal lobe pathology and medial temporal sclerosis in particular, either unilateral or bilateral, occurred with equal frequency in all the patient groups in that study. Pathologic features in other brain regions, however, can separate patient groups.

Only in the last decade have well-designed imaging and postmortem studies convincingly disclosed structural pathology in the brains of schizophrenics. These include enlarged third or lateral ventricles and reduced area or volume of limbic structures, especially parahippocampal gyrus, hippocampus, and amygdala. Microscopic gliosis and neuronal dropout occurs in hippocampus, nucleus accumbens, and dorsomedial thalamic nuclei. Related to these findings in schizophrenics is the greater incidence of histologic abnormality in medial temporal tissue resected from psychotic individuals with psychomotor seizures than in nonpsychotic epileptics. Three neuropathological features can separate the psychotic epileptics: Enlarged ventricles, periventricular gliosis, and a significant excess of pinpoint perivascular white matter softenings scattered throughout the brain. That is, a diffuse white matter pathology appears to be associated with psychosis.

The Runwell study does not support the belief that TLE particularly predisposes to schizophrenia. Partial seizures were no more common in their institutionalized schizophrenic epileptics than in their most self-sufficient group of epileptics who lived in the community. The absence of a significant increase in temporal lobe pathology in their various patient groups strongly argues against a discrete connection among TLE, temporal lobe pathology, and schizophrenia. Overall, the coincidence of epilepsy followed by psychosis was 4% in their highly selected mental population. Under modern conditions of treatment, therefore, both general and partial seizures are uncommon antecedents of either schizophrenia or psychosis.

Epileptics who later became psychotic were likely to have had their seizure onset at puberty and to have a preponderance of generalized convulsive epilepsy. Degree of, type of, laterality, or bilaterality of mesial temporal sclerosis did not distinguish these patients from other groups. Rather, psychotic epileptics were distinguished by larger ventricles and an excess of focal pathology, including periventricular gliosis and punctate white-matter lesions. In other words, psychotic epileptics have more severe and widespread brain damage than nonpsychotic epileptics, their brain lesions resembling both the structural abnormalities and the acquired pathology that has been well described in schizophrenics during the last decade.

The Runwell study concludes that psychoses associated with epilepsy are not the result of the classic epileptic pathology of the temporal lobe nor of complex partial epilepsy, but that "psychosis might arise from a degenerative or regenerative change in the brain, a pathologic response whose nature might be found by using neurotransmitter or neuroreceptor techniques beyond those of classical neuropathology" (Stevens, 1992).

SURGERY FOR EPILEPSY

The first cortical resections for refractory epilepsy were performed at Queen Square in 1886 by the English surgeon Victor Horsley (1857–1916), who reported his three patients in a paper simply titled "Brain Surgery" (Horsley, 1886). He was only twenty-nine years old and operated at a time when brain surgery was confined to trauma and the injury site was determined by external signs. It was also a time when brain operations usually were fatal and speed was vital. Horsley's ability to identify epileptogenic cortex that was visually indistinguishable from the rest of the exposed brain depended on John Hughlings Jackson's concept of localization. Horsley had earlier analyzed the motor responses of cerebral cortex, internal capsule, and spinal cord of higher primates in minute detail via faradic stimulation.

Following advances in electrophysiology after the 1940s that permitted sophisticated localization of seizure foci, epilepsy surgery centers began to appear in North American and Europe. Today, more than a hundred epilepsy centers worldwide perform 10,000 procedures annually (Engel & Shewmon, 1993). The number of procedures more than tripled between 1986 and 1993 compared to the previous six-year interval. Anterior temporal lobe resection is the most commonly performed epilepsy operation, followed by other cortical resections. Increasingly, operations such as amygdalohippocampectomy, lesionectomy, hemispherectomy, multilobar resections, and corpus callosotomy are being performed.

There are 100,000 potential candidates for epilepsy surgery in the United States alone. This demand apparently is not being adequately met because only 10,000 procedures are performed worldwide. One reason for this is that many people believe epilepsy surgery is a last resort, a drastic measure to be taken when all drug therapies have failed and when the patient is disabled by nearly constant seizures. Ever since Horsley's operation more than a century ago, we seem unduly influenced by the notion of intractability. Proper referral actually depends more on recognizing that a particular epilepsy is remediable by surgery than on waiting until hopelessness is established. In short, early surgical intervention in instances of surgically remediable epilepsy offers the best chance of completely assuaging disabling seizures and their psychosocial consequences (Engel, 1993). The goal is to define an excisable cortical area of abnormal excitability and functional deficit.

The most common constellation of findings that prompts referral is known as *mesial temporal lobe epilepsy* (MTLE). This name indicates a partial complex seizure whose focus is in the medial temporal lobe and whose clinical manifestations additionally indicate the presence of hippocampal sclerosis (Weiser et al., 1993). Table 11.5 enumerates the features of this syndrome.

Medial temporal sclerosis in Sommer's sector of the hippocampus was first proposed as a possible cause of partial seizures by none other than Sommer himself (1880). However, we have never resolved the question of whether hippocampal sclerosis is the cause or the result of seizures. Neither do we fully understand the reason for progressive physical and cognitive deterioration in many of these individuals. We do know that repeated seizures are associated with progressive neuronal dropout in hippocampal sectors CA3 and CA1. Perhaps this cell loss explains the reduced glucose uptake surrounding the epileptic focus seen on PET studies.

Typically, the seizures of MTLE appear in youth and initially respond to medication. They may even remit, an improvement

Table 11.5
The Mesial Temporal Lobe Epilepsy Syndrome

History
1. Complicated febrile convulsions
2. Family history of epilepsy
3. Onset between ages five and ten years
4. Isolated auras common
5. Secondarily generalized seizures are usually infrequent
6. Seizure remission for several years until adolescence
7. Seizures become medically intractable
8. Interictal behavioral disturbance (mostly commonly depression)

Clinical seizure
1. Aura usually present—commonly epigastric rising, other autonomic or psychic symptoms (with emotion), olfactory or gustatory sensation
2. Complex partial seizure—begins with arrest and staring; oro-alimentary automatisms, complex automatisms, and posturing of the contralateral upper extremity
3. Postictal phase—disorientation, retrograde amnesia, and dysphasia if seizures begin in the language hemisphere

Neurologic examination
1. Usually normal, but may reveal recent memory deficit

EEG
1. Unilateral or bilateral independent anterior temporal spikes
2. Intermittent or continuous rhythmic slowing in one mesial temporal area
3. Ictal scalp activity seen only with complex partial symptoms; ictal onset recorded in depth eletrode, most often high-amplitude rhythmic spikes or sharp waves
4. Propagation to contralateral side slow (>5 s, sometimes minutes) or never occurs

Focal functional deficits
1. Temporal lobe hypometabolism on interictal FDG-PET, often involving ipsilateral thalamus and basal ganglia
2. Temporal lobe hypoperfusion on interictal SPECT and characteristic pattern of ictal SPECT hyper- and hypo-perfusion
3. Material-specific amnesia on neuropsychological testing and on intra-carotid sodium amobarbital injection
4. Mesial temporal EEG slowing and attenuation apparent via scalp or sphenoidal electrodes, but more evident with depth electrodes; exacerbated by intravenous thiopental test

Structural imaging
1. MRI may slow small hippocampus, small temporal lobe, or an enlarged temporal horn on one side

Table 11.5 (Continued)

Pathophysiology

1. Hippocampal sclerosis (>30% cell loss with specific patterns)
2. Sprouting of mossy fibers by dentate granule cell
3. Selective loss of somatostatin and NPY–containing hilar neurons
4. Hamartomas and heterotopias occur as "dual pathology"
5. Microdysgenesis common
6. Seizures may originate in sclerotic hippocampus, but epileptogenic region often encompasses a newly larger area

Discomfirming Features

1. History of severe head trauma, encephalitis, or other proximate antecedents
2. Focal motor or sensory symptoms, either post-ictal or seizure onset
3. Interictal focal deficits
4. Marked cognitive impairment on neuropsychological testing
5. Bilaterally synchronous, generalized, or focal extratemporal EEG spikes
6. Diffuse or extratemporal focal EEG slowing
7. MRI cerebral lesion other than hippocampal sclerosis

FDG, flurodeoxyglucose; PET, positron emission tomography; SPECT, single photon emission computed tomography; MRI, magnetic resonance imaging. From Engel (1993).

that often leads to discontinuation of medical therapy. Unfortunately, this happy state does not persist, because disabling complex partial seizures return during adolescence and become unresponsive to all medication. At this point, referral for epilepsy surgery is indicated. Yet the earlier remission is a counteracting force that persuades both physician and patient to attempt further pharmacological manipulation. Patient and physician are unaware that once the first-choice drugs of carbamazepine and phenytoin have failed to control these seizures, all antiepileptic drugs are nearly certain to fail. This important period of psychosocial development is the worst possible time for adolescents to be disabled by their seizures.

Good evidence indicates that anterior temporal lobe resections eliminate disabling seizures in approximately 75% of these adolescents. Even two-thirds of adults older than forty-five years obtain satisfactory seizure control (McLachlan et al., 1992), although surgery in later years cannot eliminate the psychosocial pathology that has already taken hold.

Other procedures that generally are regarded as successful are large hemispheric resections for Sturge-Weber syndrome and pediatric hemimegancephaly; corpus callosotomy for drop attacks such as those seen in the Lennox-Gastaut syndrome; and lesionectomies, meaning very limited resections, often restricted to the lesion itself, in seizures due to structural lesions in the cortex. It is important to remember that not all structural lesions are epileptogenic, which is why presurgical evaluation includes a panoply of diagnostic procedures such as ictal EEG, video-EEG, functional imaging (fMRI, PET, SPECT), neuropsychological testing, intracarotid amobarbital injection, and various types of invasive electrophysiology (electrocorticography, depth electrodes, strip electrodes, grid electrodes, and intraöperative electrical stimulation mapping).

A new operation with initially promising results that await long-term verification is multilobar cortical resection in infants and young children who have secondary generalized cryptogenic seizures. Thus far, selected candidates have been those children with rapid neurologic deterioration (Chugani et al., 1990).

Another counteractive force presently limiting the availability of epilepsy surgery to those who would benefit from it is the reluctance of third-party payers to cover the considerable expense of presurgical evaluation. In earlier times, patients without tumors were selected for surgery based on only the clinical exam and the interictal scalp EEG. Then we developed more complicated procedures, in the hope of delineating the focus more precisely. How much this has altered patient outcome is still debated, and we still do not have a firm consensus regarding the optimal use of all the complicated tests at our disposal. For example, the amobarbital test was once considered indispensable in presurgical evaluation until we realized that a third of hemispheres fail the memory test in temporal and frontal epilepsy, as do more than half of hemispheres with generalized epilepsy. Hence, the Wada test is sensitive to, but not specific for, memory disturbance (Dasheiff et al., 1993). The exact anatomy involved in memory varies by individual, as does the distribution of amobarbital. Better correlations between behavior and an anesthetized brain region are obtained by methods such as adding a radioactive tracer, which shows medial temporal structures irrigated in only 28% of amobarbital injections (Hart et al., 1993).

Partly in response to the problems just cited, researchers have sought highly predictive algorithms to replace some invasive procedures, such as the use of intracranial electrodes, which often are employed for presurgical evaluation (Sperling et al., 1992; Engel et al., 1990). Algorithmic selection of surgical candidates does have merit, as approximately 80% of patients so chosen remain seizure-free beyond one year following temporal lobectomy.

PSYCHOSOCIAL ISSUES

Epileptics are deprived of their coping skills at the very moment they need them most. With no consciousness, there is no coping. This helplessness makes even the vague possibility of a seizure a cause for fear. Though it has long been claimed that social stigmas are a major contributor to psychosocial morbidity among epileptics, the few studies that address this question surprisingly show that the effect of discrimination is not high (Caveness & Gallup, 1980; Scrambler, 1987).

It appears that much greater morbidity results from patients being seriously frightened by the imagined consequences of their seizures. These almost always include the fear of death and fear of brain damage. It is perhaps understandable that individuals who hold such fears are afraid to express them, lest they be confirmed. Epileptics do not just have some vague apprehension that their condition might cause serious trouble; they are terrified that they *will die* from their next seizure and that epileptics as a group frequently do die during their attacks. They also believe that death from sudden accidents is likely, that they are likely to swallow their tongue and suffocate, that turning blue during a seizure portends imminent death, and that seizures cause cumulative brain damage that robs their intelligence and leaves them confused (Mittan, 1986).

Given this snake pit, some experts warn never to make a diagnosis of epilepsy without incontrovertible evidence. The single most important source of information is a detailed history that describes what has been experienced by the patient and observed by others. Lack of any clinical response to conventional medications and a persistently normal EEG call a seizure diagnosis into question and may be sufficient reason to consider ambulatory or video-EEG monitoring.

Proactive measures can mitigate unfounded fears. Probing questions into commonly held fears and positive feedback do help. Epileptics abide many social and personal stresses that exacerbate or can even cause psychopathology. In regard to my earlier comments about increasing frequency of attacks as a result of emotional stresses, there is considerable efficacy in education that increases patient understanding of the seizures, decreases a patient's fear of them, and mitigates hazardous, misinformed practices of self-management.

Although it has long been suspected that cognition deteriorates in epilepsy, the literature is inconclusive. Adverse effects of anticonvulsant drugs, particularly phenobarbital, complicate the picture. Despite an avalanche of studies on the cognitive effects of anticonvulsants, we remain confused ourselves. Poor methodology regarding parameters such as intrinsic differences among patient groups, failure to assign drugs randomly, and nonnormal distribution of outcome measures are common confounds. Below-normal performance is reported in visual-motor coördination, general intelligence, attention, memory, and psychomotor speed, though it is difficult to tell whether the person or the medication is the cause.

SUGGESTED READINGS

Aicardi J. 1994 *Epilepsy in Children*, 2d ed. New York: Raven Press

Engel J, ed. 1993 *Surgical Treatment of the Epilepsies*, 2d ed. New York: Raven Press

Hauser WA, Hesdorfer DC. 1989 *Epilepsy: Frequency, Causes and Consequences.* New York: Demos Publications (also available as catalogue No. 141EFC from the Epilepsy Foundation of America, Landover, MD)

Laskowitz DT et al. 1995 The syndrome of frontal lobe epilepsy: Characteristics and surgical management. *Neurology* 45:780–787

Loring DW, Meador KJ, Lee GP, King DW. 1992 *Amobarbital Effects and Lateralized Brain Function. The Wada Test.* New York: Springer Verlag

Trimble MR. 1991 *The Psychoses of Epilepsy.* New York: Raven Press

12 Spatial Knowledge

I considered titling this chapter "Visuospatial Perception," as is common in enumerating neuropsychological categories, until I pondered our customary emphasis on vision when speaking of spatial configuration. The psychology of spatial cognition has long been dominated by the study of visual input, whereas phenomenal experience shows spatial perception to be the superordinate category. In semantic evolution, spatial adjectives are among the first to extend their domain of meaning to other modalities (Williams, 1976). For example, the fundamentally spatial adjectives of *high* and *low* become metaphoric when applied to auditory pitch.

Vision, hearing, touch, and smell can be spatially extended (Klüver, 1966; Siegel & Jarvik, 1975; Sacks, 1992). We distinguish *near* from *far* in the spatial territory of the immediate limb axis as opposed to teleception. Additional concepts regarding proprioception, body schema, vestibular orientation, and auditory scene analysis betray the belief that our self occupies a segment of Euclidean space. (See figure 12.1 [as well, perhaps, as Edna St. Vincent Millay's sonnet, "Euclid alone has looked on Beauty bare"].) Our thinking about objects (qua representation) and Euclidean space (qua attention) is not entirely clear, so in this chapter I will elucidate a model that is more hypothetical than I prefer but that at least is based on clinical observations rather than abstractions.

A number of clinical defects involving spatial knowledge appear qualitatively similar on the surface but have a disparate neurology underneath. For example, an inability to identify an object's formal characteristics (agnosia) dissociates from the inability to represent it or localize it in space. Because we are not absolutely certain whether humans possess an Aristotelian common sensibility of "configuration," we are left with one list describing specific performance deficits and another list of lesion sites. Table 12.1 will

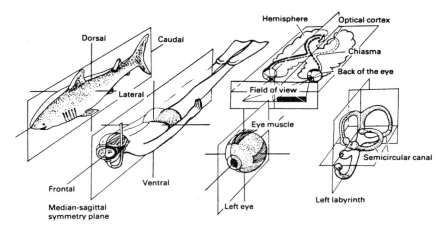

Figure 12.1
Euclidean coördinates in human sensation hark back to the bilateral symmetry that exists in all vertebrates. Not only is the body organized in this frame of reference, but so are the brain and special senses, including the rotational axes of the semicircular canals.

refresh your memory as to some general anatomic correlations of spatial ability.

For more than a century, we have spoken about imperception and "mindblindness," and puzzled over what unifies the behavior with the list of lesions given in the table (Benton, 1993). Perhaps what organizes elements into spatial configurations that form a conceptually whole entity is no more clear than the organizing principle behind color recognition. Color agnosia, achromatopsia, color anomia, color amnesia, and similar descriptions are but a collection of sensory, perceptual, associative, or linguistic disabilities each of which has its own neurologic ground.

It may be that gestalt psychology has provided us with some fruitful ideas.

THE LEGACY OF GESTALT PSYCHOLOGY

The German word *Gestalt* can be translated as "configuration," though it literally means "form" and refers to a perceptual object whose structure comprises a unified whole incapable of being expressed simply in terms of its parts. An example is a melody, as

Table 12.1
General Correlations of Spatial Ability

Distributed
Right-hemisphere network for directed attention = reticular (arousal) plus three separate representations in frontal, parietal, and cingulate cortices for movement, spatial maps, and direction of attention to emotional targets.
Unimodal Visual Association Cortex
Loss of motion, spatial orientation, stereopsis, depth
Unimodal Auditory Association Cortex
Acoustic spatial discrimination
Unimodal Somesthetic Association Cortex
Asomatognosia, right-left confusion
Unimodal Motor Association Cortex
Scanning and exploring contralateral hemispace
Heteromodal Premotor Cortex
Difficulty directing attention to targets
Heteromodal (temporal-parietal-occipital) Association Cortex
On either side: Unilateral neglect (anosognosia, r > 1 parietal)
Language hemisphere: Constructional apraxia, finger agnosia
Non-language hemisphere: Dressing and constructional apraxia, loss of geographic knowledge, spatial misalignment of the body in Euclidean space

distinct from the notes that make it up. Indeed, my *New Cassell's German Dictionary* warns, "In psychological contexts 'Gestalt' should not be translated. National Socialism further perverted its meaning to 'ideal type,' 'usage' and 'concept'."

The central tenet of Gestalt psychology is that the whole is different from the sum of its parts (Kubovy & Pomerantz, 1981; Palmer & Rock, 1994) The Czech psychologist Max Wertheimer (1880–1943) published a paper on apparent motion in 1912 that often is cited as the birth of Gestalt psychology. An illusion of apparent motion occurs when stationary images such as the frames of a movie are viewed in rapid sequence. According to Wertheimer, the movement of the whole is qualitatively different from perceiving the static images of its component frames.

The very idea that humans perceive not the summation of bits of experience but rather the entire configuration of which the bits are part went against the prevailing school of structuralism, which held a Descartian view that complex perceptions could be dissected into elementary parts that are individually comprehensible. A square, they said, was "nothing but" the experience of a particular pattern of retinal points being stimulated, and a melody was "nothing but" the experience of a sequence of tones.

(Up-to-date students will recognize this same reductionist argument in those who today maintain that consciousness is "nothing but" neurons oscillating at 40 Hz. This view insists that a final and wholly physical theory of mind is not only possible, but inevitable. This reduction also denies the existence of subjective qualia that cannot be accounted for in purely objective terms, something "it is like" for a person to smell a rose or feel pain, for example.)

Gestaltists explained perceiving a square or a melody in terms of emergent properties, overall qualities of an experience that are not inherent in its components. Emergent properties are common enough in the physical world. Wetness, for example, is an emergent property of H_2O molecules, and salt has properties not possessed by its constituent elements of sodium and chlorine.

One of the Gestaltists' enduring contributions was pointing out that object perception could not be achieved solely by the image cast on the retina, because light rays coming from different parts of an object are no more related to one another than are rays coming from two different objects. Far from being obvious, their conclusion that the nervous system had to organize sensory elements such as those caused by light rays falling on retinas or sound waves pushing on tympanic membranes was rather controversial at the time. The idea that a retinal image is passively transmitted to the visual cortex for analysis has a long history, and was probably reinforced by the superficial resemblance of the eye to a camera (figure 12.2).

Gestalt psychology proposed an organization based on grouping or configuration, elements being perceptually grouped if they were similar, proximate, formed a closed contour, or moved in the same direction (figure 12.3). Two other Gestalt concepts are *figure-ground*, which distinguishes the object (figure) from the surface behind it (ground), and *induced motion*, which states that objects are perceived in a frame of reference that is determined by surrounding familiar structures. A common example is the illusion

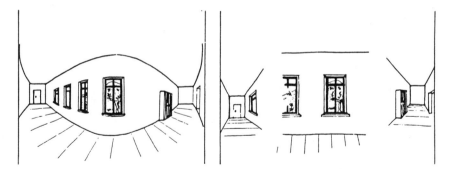

Figure 12.2
The correction of "reality" into Euclidean geometry. (*Left*) The perspective of a double corridor as it is actually cast on the retina depends on the optical geometry of foveation. (*Right*) How our expectation of orthogonal coördinates leads us to interpret the scene.

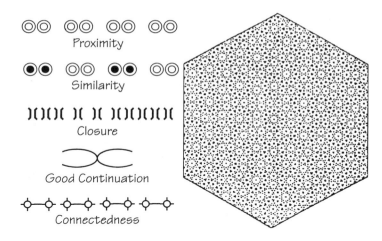

Figure 12.3
(*Left*) Gestalt laws of grouping. (*Right*) Rivalrous grouping of the elements within the hexagon cause a dynamic shifting of the pattern that is perceived.

that your own stationary train is moving when, in fact, the neighboring vehicle is.

The idea that an object's *surround*—what borders it spatially—rather than some direct physical property per se determines how we perceive its color, shape, location, or some other quality is related to one of the most fundamental problems in perception: Given that the environment changes constantly, how does the brain acquire knowledge about certain unchanging physical characteristics within it? Acquiring knowledge of constant features in an ever-changing surround means that the brain cannot passively analyze the flux that reaches it, as that flux is infinite and the brain's resources are not. Although the property of constancy is hardly unique to vision, constancy is best known with respect to color. The *retinex theory* of the American optical scientist Edwin Land (1909–1991) is the accepted explanation of the hoary puzzle of color constancy (Land, 1977; Thompson et al., 1992).

We do not recognize the "color" of certain wavelengths that stimulate the eye, as is so often heard. If we did, the colors of objects would continually change as the illumination changed (this is the problem of color constancy). Rather, we recognize the permanent properties of colored surfaces under different illumination. What remains constant as the lighting changes is an object's lightness, its patterns of light and dark in relation to everything else in the scene. The lightness of an object depends not on the flux of energy reaching the eye, but on everything else in the spatial surround. Land elegantly demonstrated that an object's color depends on its three relative lightnesses; because they are constant, color stays constant, whatever the illumination.

The nervous system constructs one stable aspect of the physical environment in terms of color—namely, the reflectance—from another continually changing aspect—namely, the total energy from different wavelengths reaching the eye. The end result of all the operations it performs on this incoming information is constructing the color of a surface from the spatial surround. Color is a property of brains; it is not a physical property of the world.

A moment's reflection reveals that even mental concepts have spatial qualities, though perhaps they are somewhat difficult to define formally. The Gestaltists claimed that everyday problems contain certain configurational demands that are readily grasped, a

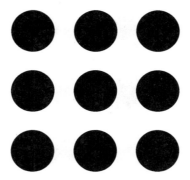

Figure 12.4
Without lifting your pen from the paper, connect the dots using only four
straight lines. (See figure 12.13 for solution.)

feature that inhibited random solutions to a problem (figure 12.4).
The chief obstacle to insight, they believed, was becoming fixated
on implicit assumptions without realizing it. Once the fixation on
one hypothesis or configuration was abandoned, the premise of
a problem could be dramatically reorganized and accompanied by
a self-evident solution (see figure 12.13 for solution to the problem presented in figure 12.4). Aside from examples such as that in
figure 12.4, it is common experience that once you see something a
certain way you cannot revert to not seeing that particular configuration. This shift in how you see a problem is related to the
shifting patterns experienced when faced with rivalrous groupings
(see figure 12.3).

The Gestaltists even found that individuals prefer harmonious
cognitive relations. If Alex likes Bob and thinks that Bob likes
Chuck, then cognitive relations are balanced if Alex also likes
Chuck and unbalanced if he does not. This example also illustrates
the concept of *Prägnanz*, the tendency to achieve the "best fit" or
simplest organization in the sense that psychological organization
converges on the most regular and symmetric perception consistent with sensory data. Figure 12.5 shows *Prägnanz* predicting
how individuals perceive partially hidden figures. *Prägnanz* states
that when stimuli are ambiguous, the perception will be as "good"
(meaning simple, regular, or symmetrical) as prevailing conditions
allow.

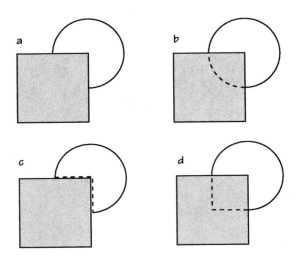

Figure 12.5
An illustration of *Prägnanz*. The partly hidden background figure in *a* is ambiguous. Among all its possible shapes, observers will perceive simple ones (*b*) rather than complex ones (*c, d*).

Gestalt principles of grouping have withstood the test of time, but their idea of isomorphism has not, although a superficial parallel does exist in today's neural networks. Gestaltists initially proposed that subjective experience and its underlying neural events had similar structures. They even pointed to Planck's principle of least energy to support this conjecture. Just as soap bubbles always assume the least energy state of a sphere, Gestaltists reasoned by analogy that the "electric fields" of the brain sought a minimum energy state. This process supposedly explained *Prägnanz*. The parallel in current neural network theory is that activation of a subset of network units propagates through the network until an equilibrium state of minimal energy is reached.

The Gestaltist legacy is impressive, judging by the ideas to which we still refer: Grouping, figure-ground organization, frames of reference, figural goodness, and apparent motion. To the consternation of their contemporaries, Gestaltists' theories often were expressed qualitatively by demonstration (just like Land's retinex demonstrations), and their basic tenet was *prima facie* antithetical to the approach that claimed that whole entities could be understood by reducing them to a set of parts. This paradox, now nearly a century old, still has the potential to make us learn something new if we look at cognition in ways to which we are not accustomed. I raise the point because the psychology and neurology of spatial knowledge is still difficult to express clearly.

GEOGRAPHIC KNOWLEDGE

Geographic knowledge is presumed to be an example of spatial aptitude that depends on the right parietal region. When we ambulate through our own homes, give directions to a stranger, mentally envision which shops we can visit during our lunch-break and what the most efficient sequence would be, or rely on other mental representations of large-scale space, we are said to be using topographic knowledge or a *cognitive map*.

The terms of navigation are largely unfamiliar in neuropsychology. "Map" refers to a large-scale spatial representation. "Placekeeping" is any method of knowing one's current position and orientation on a map. This can be accomplished either by using a "landmark" (identifying a location predicted by the map) or by "reckoning" (monitoring movements to *deduce* changes in position and direction; hence the term *"ded* reckoning," now often spelled as "dead reckoning"). A "compass" orients a navigator with respect to a fixed frame of external reference. Although an accurate map and either careful ded reckoning or landmark recognition are the only obligate tools for navigation, a compass does permit one to follow a steady heading. A compass requires the additional tools of a "sextant" and a "clock," however, neither of which are thought to be meaningfully operative in humans. A talent for distance and angular estimations has been described in humans (Benton et al., 1974), but how these fit in the larger picture is unclear.

We know little of the possible neural counterparts to the above navigational entities. Almost nothing is known about mental placekeeping and how we maintain our orientation relative to Euclidean space. The Pulawat islanders use a colorfully abstract and imaginative system during their protracted canoe voyages (Gladwin, 1970), but this does little to explain how the rest of us make it from home to the office every day. There is also no firm evidence that humans possess a mental compass, though we know that many birds can detect and use the earth's magnetic field as well as skylight polarization (Waldvogel, 1990). (Parenthetically, avian neurology is fascinating in itself. See, for example, the classic work of Stanley Cobb [1960, 1969].) Some intriguing experiments devised to see whether humans can utilize magnetic orientation have been attempted (Baker, 1981), but many scientists find the premise implausible, and no one has tried to replicate this work.

The properties of cognitive maps should not be misunderstood to resemble those of cartographic maps. They are not read and memorized, but are learned by engaging the Euclidean world. Whereas visual knowledge or perception has a single viewpoint, cognitive maps are acquired by personal experience gained from multiple viewpoints.

Two different representations of large-scale space are (1) vector maps and (2) network maps (Byrne, 1982). Vector maps code horizontal distances whereas network maps encode only topological relations. A network map represents nodes along a string, each node marking a physical location and sometimes containing instructions for a directional turn. Underground railway maps such as those of the Paris Metro or the London Tube are good visual examples of network maps (although anyone who has used one to guide walking on the streets above knows that, although the topology is accurate, the vector distance is not).

Network maps are far more common than vector maps, the skill and development of which appear to emerge later. The skills are clearly distinct. To test network maps you might ask, "Tell me all the turns, and whether they are left or right ones, that you would make to get from here to the park." A typical probe for vector map integrity would be, "Point toward the cathedral," or "Is it farther as the crow flies from here to the train station or from here to the park?" When viewed from above, vector maps are isomorphic to the real world.

Psychology has paid more attention to the static aspect of spatial knowledge as a repository of fact rather than to the dynamic aspects of keeping one's bearings. Until more is known of the dynamics of spatial knowledge, it is difficult to know what symptoms to look for. From the preceding information, however, we can predict that certain dissociations should occur in clinical settings.

At the simplest level, topographic knowledge should dissociate from other visual skills requiring spatial knowledge and vice versa. That is, one should encounter patients who cannot follow and describe familiar routes or learn new ones, but who have no difficulty in other visual-spatial realms. Failures of object recognition, visual memory, and imagery, for example, should dissociate from an inability to navigate and should be apparent in everyday performance. Someone with retained networking might describe the steps taken to reach his destination, yet have no idea about the vector of his starting direction (the congenitally blind person approximates this shortcoming). Conversely, someone with retained vector mapping can accurately relate the distance and direction of his starting point but will be unable to retrace his steps or describe how he got to his destination.

Topographic ability is sharply distinct from purely perceptual abilities such as pointing, line bisection, or depth judgement. Patients with defective spatial localization rarely get lost or lose their topographic knowledge, and the two seldom are impaired together. Hemianopic patients seldom get lost either, because they scan effectively with their intact hemifield. Another dissociation concerns constructional apraxia: Those with constructional apraxia usually have no topographic disability, whereas patients who get lost usually do fail at constructions. Constructional apraxia and unilateral neglect often are asymmetrically associated with deficiencies of topographic knowledge.

A rarely noted condition called *environmental agnosia* (Landis et al., 1986) entails a loss of topographic familiarity in that individuals do not recognize familiar surroundings despite intact verbal memory, cognition and perception. You can think of it as a geographical *jamais vu*. Prosopagnosia is often present. Patients can accurately see and describe the surrounding landscape even though they recognize nothing in it. Posteromedial lesions on either side are reported. The deficit is said to be a disruption between memory and perception, an inability to match the perceived environment with the stored memory but, as you will see below, it may be that all agnosics have impaired perception when examined carefully. The presumption that perception would be normal in agnosics has historically biased examiners against scrupulously testing it.

What evidence there is suggests a double dissociation between network and vector maps. There is some clinical support for the premise that those spatial neighborhoods that we cannot see from a single viewpoint, but that we learn instead by locomoting through them, can be treated as a unitary concept distinct from verbally acquired geographic knowledge. Gender differences also exist that persist throughout the lifespan. Normative experiments (Beatty & Tröster, 1987; Beatty, 1989) indicate that males more accurately locate places on maps than do females, and that males perform more accurately on measures of egocentric and allocentric spatial orientation. However, both males and females learn locations of unfamiliar places at a similar rate, whether such learning is intentional or incidental. Age, education, and gender are stable and noninteracting factors in geographic knowledge, though age is the most potent because of the experience gained in living in a landscape. Geographic knowledge does not decay with age.

There are also potential confounds in assessing topographic knowledge. Patients with posterior right-hemisphere lesions have defective judgement for direction and distance. Yet where the lesion is for localizing points in space depends on whether the task is wholly visual and whether stimuli are to be localized within "grasping distance" of the limb axis, require a verbal judgement, or whether the coördinates are relative to the patient's body or to Euclidean references. Some failures of topographic knowledge are actually shortcomings of either memory or representation. Sometimes, derelictions in following familiar routes or in learning new ones are problems with perception or attention. Once past these confounds, we can talk about true topographic knowledge.

BODY SCHEMA DISTURBANCES

In chapter 3, I referred to Yakovlev's tripartite scheme that aligned movement either in reference to the egocentric body axis or to allocentric Euclidean space. The very concept of body schema arose as an effort to explain certain clinical observations by assuming the existence of these two spatial frameworks against which perceptual and motor judgements were directed. Electrical stimulation experiments such as those of Kornhüber and followers showed that our consciousness is not referred to the brain site being stimulated, but is directed spatially outward to a peripheral body part.

Despite its common use, there is no standard definition of the term *body schema*. The three most common connotations are conscious awareness of the body, unconscious bodily representations, and wholly visual bodily representations. Some have dismissed the term as being merely a label denoting self-referential actions and perceptions, including the notion that one occupies a domain of Euclidean space. Other neuropsychologists have used it to mean only verbal labeling of fingers and toes, others to refer to anosognosia or denial of a diseased part. In his distributed system for attention, Mesulam would use the term expansively to include not only a patient who denied the existence of half of space but one also who acted as if nothing could ever be expected to happen in the left half of space. Despite the term's inexactness, we can still justify distinguishing between action and cognition related to the body versus action and cognition related to Euclidean space, because these two categories do dissociate.

Finger Agnosia

Josef Gerstmann (1924) used the term *finger agnosia* to describe an inability to identify either one's own fingers or those belonging to another. From a limited clinical sample, he inferred a causative lesion in the angular gyrus of the left hemisphere. Bilateral finger agnosia became the index symptom of the foursome known collectively as the *Gerstmann syndrome*, which includes also acalculia, agraphia, and right-left disorientation. Neurologists would normally be disinterested in testing for knowledge of one's digits were this odd constellation of signs not alleged to have inestimable localizing value.

Over the years, we learned that finger agnosia neither has unique localizing value nor does it represent a singular cognitive skill. For example, lesions in the left posterior thalamus or parietal-temporal cortex produce it, and it often is seen in conjunction with aphasia or dementia (Benton, 1992b). First, you have to specify what tasks are used to assess the capacity and, second, you must decide whether finger agnosia is present or absent depending on whether the stimulus is verbal, visual, or tactile and whether the required response is verbal, gestural, self-referential, or directed toward the examiner. The syndrome is heterogeneous, meaning that it may be manifested in several ways. Furthermore, it differs from tactile localization of a given finger, a skill that relies on contralateral parietal integrity.

Impaired finger recognition is mildly correlated with constructional apraxia and dysphasia. With which hemisphere finger agnosia is associated in brain-damaged patients depends on whether the disability is demonstrated verbally or gesturally, and whether aphasia is present.

The fact that children between three and five years-old find it increasingly difficult to localize fingers depending on whether the task is visual, tactile, or schematic (representational) suggests different age-related cognitive demands as well as a requirement for representational thinking. Even children at age twelve cannot localize as well as adults can finger *pairs* that are simultaneously stimulated.

Knowledge of Right Versus Left

The concept of right-left confusion is even broader than that of finger agnosia in that it refers to naming of body parts, responding to verbal commands, or imitating gestures. Any meaningful assessment of cognition in terms of right-left orientation requires a clear statement of what is being tested given that verbal labeling, vision, and a somesthetic discrimination whose sensory basis is not obvious are all involved. Commands involving crossing the midline are said to be more difficult to execute than are unilateral tasks.

Right-left confusion has customarily been identified in individuals with left-hemisphere lesions and aphasia. However, as with finger agnosia, the hemisphere that contributes to right-left disorientation appears to depend on what aspect is being tested— namely, commands relative to one's own body, body parts of the confronting examiner, imitation of lateral movements, or crossed movements. Furthermore, combined tasks involving more than one operation or those involving reversals relative to the confronting examiner probably reflect the conceptual difficulty of the task instead of some linguistic or spatial aspect of it (Benton,

1993). Whether manifest by verbal or nonverbal performance, most instances of right-left disorientation seem associated with left-hemisphere lesions.

CONSTRUCTIONAL PRAXIS

It has long been claimed that a right-hemispheric dominance exists for configurational analysis and a left-hemispheric dominance for categorization that is performed by verbal labeling. The ability to make two- or three-dimensional objects by line drawings, block designs, or matchstick constructions is a useful probe for cerebral lesions because these cognitive tasks call on processes of the occipital, parietal, and frontal cortices.

I commented on constructional apraxia in chapter 5. Patients who show constructional apraxia are assumed to have a parietal lesion until proven otherwise. The nature of the errors that they make depends on the side of the lesion. As a general rule, individuals with right hemisphere lesions tend to lose a test object's gestalt, whereas those with left-hemisphere lesions lose its internal details.

The heteromodal association cortex of the parietal lobe is believed to be responsible for the integration of vision and movement, but there is no customary locus for a superordinate skill that we might call *spatial conception*. The inferior parietal lobule (Brodmann areas 39 and 40) is believed to be important, given that this is where vision, sound, and somesthesis converge.

VISUAL AGNOSIA

Visual agnosia is customarily defined as the inability to recognize objects even though basic visual perception is unimpaired. An agnosic patient may be able to describe verbally the characteristic form and function of a chair, for example, or even be able to draw a chair from a real model, a photograph, or line art. Despite this obvious drawing skill and retained verbal knowledge, the patient still cannot "see" that the chair is a chair. The loss of knowledge is specific, because patients can readily identify an object by its characteristic sound, texture, or other qualities. Although such dis-

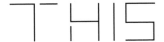

Figure 12.6
Tracing strategies used by visual agnosics show their utter dependence on local contour. Their perception is easily thwarted by discontinuities such as line breaks, cross-hatching, or even stray marks. An agnosic individual consistently read this stimulus as *7415* rather than the word THIS. From Landis et al. (1982), with permission.

orders are rare, we expect that they can tell us much about the normal brain.

Ever since the time of Lissauer (1890) we have split visual agnosias into (1) apperceptive and (2) associative types. *Apperceptive agnosia* is said to stem from an impairment of visual perception that is above the level of an elementary deficit (such as a hemianopia). Patients cannot recognize objects because they cannot see them normally. Individuals without obvious perceptual deficits are called *associative agnosics* in that a presumably normal percept is "stripped of its meaning" (this oft-used term is Teuber's). Note the significant assumption here that the underlying cause lies outside the modality-specific processing of the stimulus.

Visual agnosics frequently are noted to exploit tracing strategies that use both head and hand movements to "outline" what the eyes see. Some patients can read entire pages this way. When prevented from making such movements, patients fail the task under study. Such tracing strategies actually betray the agnosic's slavish dependence on *local continuity* in order to perceive. For example, an agnosic individual consistently read the stimulus shown in figure 12.6 as *7415* rather than the word *"THIS"* (Landis et al., 1982). That agnosics resort to tracing strategies to gain some spatial or kinesthetic sense of an unknown object is consistent with the Gestalt principle of continuity.

That apperceptive agnosics are thwarted by dots or discontinuity in a line that they attempt to trace reveals the necessity of grouping together elements of the very local contour into superordinate sets of contours, regions, or surfaces. The Gestaltists categorized grouping by proximity, similarity, good continuity, and motion. Items can be grouped in more than one way, as figure 12.3 showed.

For example, grouping based on motion can be independent from the set based on spatial configuration. This seems reasonable given that the ventral visual pathway projecting from occipital to temporal lobe deals with static form and color (the "what" system), whereas the dorsal visual pathway in the posterior parietal lobe deals with motion, stereopsis, and spatial location (the "where" system). An obvious question is whether the attentional impairment in the visual agnosias is that of location or object or both.

Can we assume that an individual's ability to copy a stimulus means that he or she can see it "accurately"? Levine (1978) showed that individuals with impaired vision can make accurate drawings using strategies such as feature-by-feature matching or verbal mediation. In her literature review, Farah (1990) argues that we have failed to get past the obvious surface feature of recognition, and have not really examined perception in agnosics carefully. Authors have routinely overstated the perceptual abilities of associative agnosics and, in those cases where perception has been studied carefully, it is found wanting. *It seems that perception may be faulty in all visual agnosias when it is tested carefully.*

If visual perception turns out to be impaired in associative agnosics, is there any reason still to distinguish between apperceptive and associative agnosia? Yes, Farah argues, although the distinction is no longer the dichotomy proposed by Lissauer of agnosia with and without impaired perception, but a distinction between agnosias with different *kinds* of visual impairments. Although the scope of the agnosic deficit varies from person to person and calls upon slightly different perceptual abilities, all agnosias have to do with the overreaching spatial configuration.

Farah (1990) has reviewed a century of literature on visual agnosia, much of it conflicting. The following sections closely follow her monograph.

Simultanagnosia

The term *simultanagnosia* was originally coined by Wolpert (1924) and referred to patients who could accurately perceive individual details of a complex scene but who could not synthesize its overall meaning. Responsible lesions were bilateral and posterior, and spared the striate cortex. Two types of simultanagnosia were

distinguished by their site of presumed causative lesion. Dorsal simultanagnosia followed bilateral parietal-occipital lesions, whereas
ventral simultanagnosia followed left inferior occipital-temporal
ones.

Dorsal Simultanagnosia

Dorsal simultanagnosia is considered a visual attention deficit in
which only one stimulus at a time is perceived—and even that
may spontaneously slip from attention so that the object is "lost"
or suddenly "disappears." Patients act blind even though they have
full visual fields, groping as if in the dark, or walking into furniture
despite the fact that you can demonstrate clearly that their impairment results from visual inattention rather than blindness.
The nature of the attentional limitation is of both the region of
visual space that can be attended to and of the number of objects
that can be attended to. Although it currently is impossible to determine whether the limit of attention is based on the size of the
spatial region or on the foveal spatial location, it seems clear that
the limiting factor is *spatial*.

Dorsal simultanagnosics have difficulty *localizing objects in
space*, even when they can recognize them. In other words, patients cannot reach or point to a visual stimulus that they see, nor
can they describe its location relative to another object. That patients have no difficulty in localizing per se is shown by having
them locate auditory stimuli, or named or touched body parts;
they do this with notable precision.

Dorsal simultanagnosics clearly show that attention is directed
to visual objects rather than points in space. But what is an object?
The century of cases reviewed by Farah suggest that an object is
not an attribute determined by size or visual complexity, but a
flexible configuration subject to voluntary determination. Given
a rectangle made up of six dots, for example, or some other geometric form sketched from discontinuous lines, a patient can
perceive either the entire rectangle or a single dot. However, the
patient cannot count the dots, because once he or she starts to do
so, the dots are seen as single elements and therefore are perceived
only one at a time. In other words, says Farah, "The organization of
the dots into a rectangle did not increase the patient's attentional
capacity to more than one object; rather, it allowed the patient to

view the set of dots as a single object." The same thing is seen in patients with prosopagnosia. They may recognize a face as a face per se but, once they focus on a detail, the relation of that detail to the whole is immediately lost, and so they cannot say *whose* face they are seeing. Attentional processes in simultanagnosia are sensitive to and disrupted by these shifts in what the visual system takes to be an object.

Ventral Simultanagnosia

Individuals with ventral simultanagnosia differ from the dorsal population in that they can see multiple objects but cannot recognize multiple objects. Even when able to describe single elements of a picture sequentially they lack any understanding of the scene as a whole. They cannot grasp the fundamental gestalt. Support of Gestalt ideas is seen in Luria's observation (1959) that two forms can be recognized by simultanagnosics if they are connected, or grouped, by a line drawn between them.

Rizzo and Hurtig (1987) showed that even stationary objects disappeared from the view of ventral simultanagnosics. In their terms, patients were "looking but not seeing." Object disappearance is not related to any disorder of ocular motility, as might be suggested by the searching eye movements that these patients make. Such movements do not cause viewed objects to disappear suddenly. Rather, the movements are the result of the objects' spontaneous disappearance.

In "looking but not seeing," subjects have enough sensory input to permit accurate oculomotor driving and the maintenance of fixation, but they have insufficient data to maintain a conscious experience of the viewed stimulus. That is, they continue to look, but do not see. Three discrete contributions to this situation are (1) abnormal visual perception, (2) cognition, and (3) efferent oculomotor control. In other words, representations that are held in fixation may go unattended, yet may still (beneath the level of conscious experience) drive eye movements.

Vis à vis original reports that striate cortex is spared in simultanagnosia, unit recording in primates demonstrates firing changes in extrastriate but not striate cells when attention changes but fixation is kept steady (Moran & Desimone, 1985). The hypothetical mechanism that modifies the extraction and awareness of

Comparison of Visual Agnosias

Associative agnosia: Shape perceived normally, multiple objects perceived. However, impaired perception is revealed by (1) copying and matching performance that is slavish and effortful, (2) the visual nature of errors, (3) the influence of the stimuli's visual quality on recognition, (4) subjects' own introspection that their vision is abnormal, and (5) experimental protocols involving closure, feature integration, and decisions regarding possible-impossible figures.

Apperceptive agnosia: Depends on very local contour, with recognition readily thwarted by the slightest discontinuity. Shape perception completely vitiated, and guesses are based on color, size, or texture. Conscious modulation is not observed. Movement helps shape perception. Lesions are bilateral and posterior.

Dorsal simultanagnosia: Whole shapes are perceived, even when composed of dots or broken lines. Only a single gestalt is comprehended at a time, though what is apprehended can be consciously modulated (e.g., individual dots arranged in a rectangle or the rectangle alone). Patients can recognize whatever they can see; the trouble is visually perceiving an object's spatial location. Motion impedes shape recognition. Lesions are bilateral and posterior.

Ventral simultanagnosia: Recognition rather than perception is piecemeal (one item at a time)—that is, patients can see but not recognize multiple objects. No understanding of the gestalt. Conscious modulation possible (e.g., familiarity, willful deployment of attention). When carefully tested, perception is found to be impaired. Lesion is a left inferior temporal–occipital one.

---

visual features to which we attend out of all the incoming visual flux is located outside the striate cortex.

The nearby box lists some comparative features of the visual agnosias.

Prosopagnosia

We briefly touched on the topic of prosopagnosia in chapter 6. Prosopagnosics who have difficulty recognizing familiar faces also have difficulty recognizing examples within a class. Thus, a bird-watcher complains that all the birds look the same, a jockey can no longer individuate race horses, a farmer cannot distinguish his cows, and a gardener cannot tell one plant from another. Even distinguishing makes of automobiles, clothing articles, food categories, and public monuments have been reported (see Farah, 1990, pp. 73–74, for references).

Recognition difficulties beyond faces may be the rule rather than the exception in prosopagnosia. When past authors have bothered to test prosopagnosics for the ability to recognize nonface stimuli, it has been cursory. Consistent with these observations is the conclusion that prosopagnosics do not perceive faces normally—in fact, they may not perceive anything normally. This can be demonstrated by covert measures such as galvanic skin resistance (Tranel & Damasio, 1985) or evoked potentials (Renault et al., 1989). Electrophysiology is not necessary to show this, however, as one can disclose it equally well with simpler measures such as reaction time or trials to learning criteria (De Haan et al., 1987). These techniques indicate some degree of covert recognition, but do not conclusively prove a dissociation between conscious and unconscious recognition.

The findings of single-unit recording in monkeys are relevant to prosopagnosia because they provide a different type of evidence regarding the kinds of things that prosopagnosics find difficult to recognize—faces, animals, plants, buildings, and monuments. A population of neurons in the temporal lobe responds selectively to faces, and more than three-fourths of these cells reliably respond more to certain faces than others (Bayless et al., 1985). Cells in the superior temporal sulcus of the macaque have additional properties during facial recognition that remind us of human performance. For example, they respond to pictures of faces under different conditions of illumination, changes of expression, or removal of a feature. Also like normal humans, the cells do not respond to a face whose features have been photographically rearranged. Unlike humans, however, the cells in the macaque can respond to upside-down faces (Desimone et al., 1984).

Much of the earlier confusion regarding the locus of the causative lesion(s) has abated. Clinical studies concur that all prosopagnosics have right anteroinferior or occipital-temporal lesions (the latter is inferred by their left superior quadrantanopia). Those cases that have come to autopsy have had homologous left-sided lesions. The consensus from autopsy, imaging, and clinical methods indicate that bilateral occipital-temporal lesions are necessary to produce prosopagnosia (Damasio et al., 1982; Bruce et al., 1992). Although the most critical circuits responsible for face processing lie posteriorly, pre- and post-operative comparisons in individuals undergoing lobectomy imply that at least four other brain regions (frontal and temporal, on each side) participate equally in perceiving both facial identity and affect (Braun et al., 1994). The possible existence of a more diffuse distributed system for facial perception is discussed in the next section.

A THEORY OF VISUAL AGNOSIA

What kind of spatial coding is heavily required by faces, less demanded by animals, plants, makes of cars, or types of monuments, and even less necessary for the recognition of other kinds of visual stimuli?

Farah (1990) answers this question by demonstrating how all types of agnosia can be explained with only two hypothetical components of recognition. Based on her extensive literature review in which certain combinations of impairments are not observed in otherwise pairwise dissociations of faces, objects, and written words (see her Table 1, pp. 129–132) she proposes the following:

Recalling the Gestaltists, she suggests that some objects are first recognized as a single entity whereas others are recognized only after being decomposed into simpler parts that themselves are apprehended without further decomposition. The remarkable fact, gleaned from primate unit recording, that face-selective cells do not respond to individual facial components or to the complete set of features if presented in an altered spatial arrangement, but only to whole faces, suggests that faces are recognized in a single gestalt rather than being decomposed into subsets of elements. Items such as pencil points, doorknobs, or keyboard keycaps are contrasting examples of representations whose objects are explicitly represented as parts. The most extreme example of objects that are decomposed into smaller units are the individual letters of printed words.

Farah proposes a hierarchy of clinical impairments derived from only two components of recognition: (1) the ability first to represent a part or single gestalt (such as a face that undergoes no further decomposition and thus constitutes a whole object), and (2)

Table 12.2
Five Predicted Patterns Resulting from Combination of Two Hypothetical Processes in the Visual Agnosias

Process 1: Representation of a part (an object that decomposes no further)
Process 2: Rapid encoding of multiple parts

1. Representation mildly impaired = prosopagnosia (*bilateral lesions*)

2. Representation severely impaired—agnosia for all objects except those with the simplest of parts = object agnosia with prosopagnosia but without alexia (*bilateral or unilateral right temporo-occipital lesions*)

3. Normal representation but impaired multiple encoding = alexia (*left posterior lesion*)

4. As in 3, but worse = agnosia with alexia but without prosopagnosia (*left posterior lesion*)

5. Both processes impaired = agnosia with alexia and prosopagnosia (*bilateral lesions*)

the ability to encode multiple parts rapidly, as for objects that decompose into numerous subsets. This hierarchy explains the agnosias as an impairment in representing parts, or encoding multiple parts, or as some combination of the two. Table 12.2 shows this scheme, accounting for all possible stepwise combinations in the ability to recognize faces, objects, or printed words. A review of ninety-nine case reports validates the five predicted patterns enumerated in the table.

Given the confusion that has reigned over the agnosias and spatial localization, Farah's scheme has the merit of being a classification based on clinical observation rather than one driven by theory. It is also predictive. For example, it imposes two intriguing constraints: Object agnosia cannot exist without either prosopagnosia or alexia, and no instance of prosopagnosia with alexia can exist without some degree of object agnosia.

We will have to see how this plan holds up over time. Lissauer proposed his apperceptive-associative dichotomy based on a priori theories of object recognition rather than on clinical observation, yet Farah's review of the past century's literature on visual agnosia shows that perception may not be normal in any instance of visual agnosia. Failure to inquire into visual impairment in agnosia was a result of the prevailing theoretical idea that impaired vision was

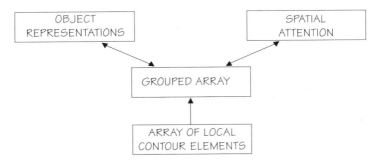

Figure 12.7
The hypothetical grouped array, a scheme for organizing higher vision into either spatial loci or recognizable objects. See text for details. From Farah (1990), with permission.

not the cause of impaired recognition. In other words, progress had been impeded by bringing the wrong theories into research too early.

In summary, *higher vision appears to begin with spatial grouping* of local elements into larger-scale contours, regions, surfaces, and textures. Such grouping appears to depend on the occipital lobes and to be a wholly stimulus-driven process. Witness the "apperceptive" agnosics' dependence on whether lines are discontinuous, curved, or straight, whether they have superimposed hatchings, whether the stimulus is moving, and so forth. Recall how the stimulus in figure 12.6 was perceived as the banal number *7415* rather than the familiar word *THIS*.

With the exception of motion, separate local contours must be grouped into higher-order geometric spatial representations before any further visual processing happens. (This exception holds because local elements can be unified by common motion independently of any unification based on their static properties.) The schematic in figure 12.7 shows how a particular clustering of the grouped array yields either (1) a recognizable "object," or (2) a region of "space" to which one attends. One might say that the *spatial unit* and the *object unit* "look at" the grouped array in a different way when selecting subsets on which to operate. It may help to think of these hypotheticals as follows: The spatial unit = attention, whereas the object unit = representation or recognition.

The spatial unit responds to either top-down forces (i.e., you consciously decide to focus your attention on one part of the array) or to some activity in the grouped array (e.g., the onset of movement, a change in luminance). The object unit's narrow channel capacity prevents it from recognizing all objects simultaneously; it recasts a subset of the array into abstract features consistent with the surfaces, regions, contours, textures, and so forth that cohere to a single object. Both units must cope with satisfying multiple constraints, (e.g., conflicting gestalts) or top-down restrictions, (e.g., familiarity) that can influence the pattern seen.

Figure 12.7 indicates that three sources can determine which portions of the grouped array will be active: (1) a bottom-up influence from stimuli, (2) a top-down influence from spatial attention, and (3) a top-down influence from representation that activates subsets of the array corresponding to objects. The parallel operation of the spatial and object units explains some features of dorsal and ventral simultanagnosics—namely, the effect of spatial attention on the ability to recognize objects in ventral patients and the effect of object recognition on the allocation of attention in dorsal patients.

The piecemeal recognition of a single object among many possible ones that is typical of ventral simultanagnosics is explained first by supposing a spatial cue that prompts individuals to allocate attention to the object's location in space and, second, by supposing that whatever object is at that location gets encoded first. The encoding of a single object evidently exhausts these patients' recognition capacity.

In parsing the grouped array, the object unit of the dorsal simultanagnosic activates segments corresponding to objects, whereas spatial attention is engaged in concurrent spatial regions. Because the underlying impairment in dorsal simultanagnosia is presumed to be one of disengaging attention (Baynes et al., 1986), patients' attention stays "glued" to that one region. The top-down activation from their intact object unit assures that that region almost always corresponds to a whole object. Note the fidelity to Gestalt ideas in that attention in this scheme is spatially based rather than object-based.

The breadth of recognition impairments in visual agnosia suggests that a distributed system likely underlies visual representation and recognition. It is further likely that such a system operates on stimulus properties rather than semantic categories. (Although it is claimed that visual agnosics cannot identify a specific example from a class [Damasio et al., 1982] agnosic errors are, in fact, not bound by semantic categories.) A target face might engender activity in a large population of neurons, many of which could also be active during representations of different faces or other kinds of objects. In analyzing how stimuli are matched against the stored knowledge (memory) of how objects are expected to appear, network approaches indicate that a degradation of stored knowledge is inseparable from a degradation of perception as seen in agnosia. This is what one would expect if recognition occurs when stimulus activation settles into a stable (least-energy) state, determined by the stored patterns of connection strengths. Interestingly enough, this aspect of neural networks recapitulates the Gestalt concept of *Prägnanz* (McClelland et al., 1986).

AUDITORY SCENE ANALYSIS

The study of sound in the context of cognition has generally been limited to speech. Auditory agnosia, the inability to comprehend auditory inputs, has provided some insights into cognition, and the amusias have suggested several theories of auditory perception. Still, the field of auditory cognition is in its infancy, and terminology is not yet standard (McAdams & Bigand, 1993). Sound source determination has only recently been acknowledged as an important element in auditory cognition.

Sound source determination, or *auditory scene analysis*, yields knowledge of the environment, including spatial knowledge. Unlike vision or proprioception, audition does not directly transduce the source sound. Mechanical transduction by the middle ear provides a time-frequency code of the acoustic field, and the central components of audition perform something like a spectral analysis. Perceptual regularities govern the temporal (sequential) and spectral (simultaneous) organization of sensory information necessary for auditory perception. The existence of harmonics, for example, exposes the fundamental nonlinearity of the ear, which transforms the purely sinusoidal vibration of the original source into a more intricate periodic wave the Fourier analysis of which reveals it to contain frequency multiples of the original stimulus.

Although one could argue that peripheral audition is purely perceptual (even though evidence accrues against this), central audition clearly requires attention, memory, and the transformations that we customarily label *cognitive* in making use of information gained about the auditory scene. Analytical hearing implies well-focused selective attention that is aimed solely by central processes. Furthermore, central descending pathways actually modulate the centripetal ones from the periphery and determine what we are to hear in the first place.

Although the auditory organ (the external ear or its analog) varies dramatically from fish to mammal, the labyrinthine architecture is nearly identical throughout the phylogenetic range of vertebrates (Buser & Imbert, 1992, p. 124). Its afferent architecture is almost as complicated as that of the retina, though it differs in being markedly divergent (3,000 inner hair cells support 20,000 output fibers to the central nervous system). Your atlas will provide illustrations of the parallel and recursive auditory pathways.

The *localization* of sound identifies its origin in Euclidean space, whereas *lateralization* distinguishes right from left. Auditory psychophysics tells us that the accuracy of human localization is frequency-dependent and nonmonotonic, maximal errors occurring between 2 kHz and 4 kHz. The complex folds of the external ear play a role in localizing sounds, as do movements of the head. (Animals can additionally move their ears; the horse pinna, for example, has seventeen muscles.) Mostly, however, localization is accomplished largely through auditory means.

It seems that lateralization in sound space begins to be coded at the level of the olivary complex, whereas sound localizing relies on two distinct mechanisms. At low frequencies, one detects phase differences between the sound waves reaching the two cochleas, but at high frequencies one relies on interaural intensity differences. The latter is achieved by binaural cells that respond to the stimulation of both cochleas. Some binaural cells are excited by binaural inputs, whereas other cells are excited by inputs from one ear and inhibited by inputs from the other ear. Usually, the contralateral ear is inhibitory.

Auditory projections are *tonotopic* in the medial accessory and superior olivæ, the trapezoid body, and the inferior colliculus. Although the inferior colliculus has conventionally been considered the main integrative auditory structure, all these structures have a role in localizing sound. It is somewhat surprising to learn that the *superior* colliculus, conventionally known for visual integration, is an additional midbrain site that contains a topography of acoustic space. In addition to its well-known visual projections, the superior colliculus receives auditory and somatic inputs in its middle and deep layers (Buser & Imbert, 1992, p. 283). Figure 12.8 illustrates some tonotopic and retinotopic projections.

In contrast to the strict tonotopic organization found in the auditory inferior colliculus, each "auditory" cell in the *superior* colliculus has a spatial receptive field to which it responds. Some cells are frontal or hemispheric in their orientation, and still others are omnidirectional. Whatever its auditory spatial field, a given cell has an optimum response in both azimuth and elevation. The spatial orientation and most responsive area of these spatial cells are independent of the intensity of the sound stimulus.

In all mammals the auditory cortex is subsylvian. In the macaque, for example, auditory cortex occupies the dorsal part of the superior temporal gyrus. As recourse to your atlas shows, the same holds for humans with the addition that auditory cortex encroaches the posterior parietal operculum. Therefore, it is not strictly correct to say that auditory cortex in humans is completely subsylvian or that it involves only the temporal lobes (Galaburda et al., 1978).

Coëxisting direct and crossed auditory projections assure that each cochlea is universally represented bilaterally in auditory cortex. A tonotopic representation projects sound frequencies in a regular and serially ordered way to the auditory cortex. The cochlea also has a point-by-point representation in auditory cortex as well as multiple maps. That is, many serial maps coëxist within the auditory cortical areas. Our knowledge of multiple sound representations is premature compared to analogous knowledge about multiple visual representations. Figure 12.8 conveys this comparative shortcoming.

The auditory system constantly receives a variety of sounds with different intensities and temporal disparities while also coping with reverberation and echoes. From this chaos, a spatial sound field is somehow synthesized and comprehended. Sometimes, we are surprised when we actually discover how part of this is accomplished. For example, although speech contains many high frequencies, it is the envelope of speech sounds that we exploit for localization, a succession of brief variations of temporal disparity, rather than the individual frequency components of speech.

We have yet to appreciate fully the sophistication of the auditory system. One of its distinctive features, for example, is its descending efferent projections that can modulate many lower pathways from the cochlear nucleus to the receptor hair cells. Moreover, the descending connections are registered with the ascending tonotopicity. The ability of these connections to influence the initial auditory inputs to the central nervous system is another example of how the brain is an active explorer rather than an acquiescent blob. Together with the previously mentioned gustofacial reflex (p. 91), these examples of how even lower-brainstem processes can "decide" about incoming stimuli reflect my point that our hoary distinction between sensing and understanding needs overhauling. For a long time, our conception of this distinction has played a powerful role not only in how we conceive of the nervous system, but also in how we interpret data.

The olivocochlear bundle is the best studied of the descending projections in which efferent fibers from the superior olive directly influence both the inner and outer cochlear hair cells. Other descending pathways include corticothalamic neurons projecting to various divisions of the medial geniculate, auditory cortex projections to the inferior and superior colliculi, and projections from the inferior colliculus to the cochlear and olivary nuclei. All in all, the receptor hair cells of the inner ear can be influenced from levels ranging from the reticular formation to as high as the thalamus and cortex (Buser & Imbert, 1992, p. 323).

Lastly, there is tentative evidence that audition has distinct "What" and "Where" systems in a manner analogous to vision. Part of the anterior cochlear nucleus and the superior olive may form the anteriorly placed spatial auditory detector (the "Where" component), whereas a dorsal system consisting of the posterior and dorsal cochlear nuclei, inferior colliculus, medial geniculate, and auditory

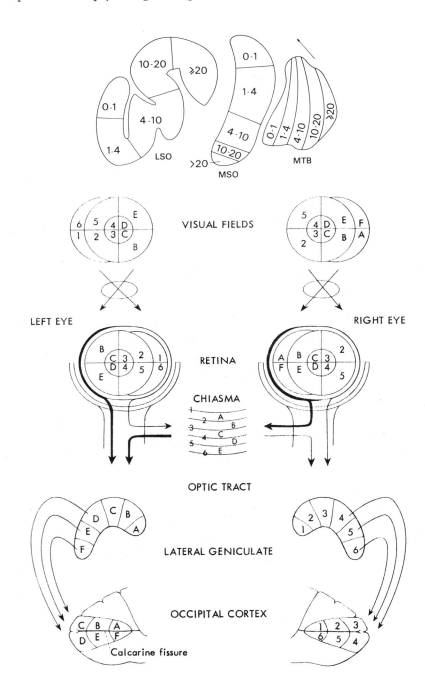

cortex may be sufficient to decode or recognize acoustic patterns (the "What am I hearing?" component).

FORM CONSTANTS REVISITED

If I asked, "How many of you are fond of smoke and explosions?" I suspect that few would raise their hands. If I asked instead, "How many of you enjoy fireworks?" the affirmative response might be unanimous.

Why do we enjoy fireworks so much? Millions of pounds of entertaining explosives go up all over the world, and millions of people turn out to watch them. What are they, these colored lights, moving flashes, and bangs? They are not real things in nature or representations of anything else, nor do they remind us of anything at an intellectual level. They are as abstract as Mondrian or Jackson Pollock—and yet they provoke a strong emotional reaction, inducing millions to watch and walk away satisfied. Onlookers exclaim, "That was wonderful!" without being able to say exactly what "that" was. No other form of abstract visual expression is as popular.

It may be that the form constants can help explain the satisfying appeal of something as unnatural as fireworks. I touched on form constants earlier (pp. 240–243) in the context of release hallucinations, synesthesia, and kindred subjective experiences that, at first glance, seem ineffable. It is often frustrating to those who would understand the neurology of such phenomena that subjects tend to be overwhelmed and awed by the "indescribableness" of their experiences.

The spatial connotations of the term *form constant* give the false impression that what is perceived is stationary and invariant, when in fact the elements are highly unstable, continually reorganizing

Figure 12.8
(*Top*) The boundaries of different frequency ranges (in kHz) in the superior olivary complex. LSO, MSO, lateral and medial olivary nuclei; MTB, medial trapezoid body. From Buser & Imbert (1992), with permission. Similar tonotopic arrangements exist in the colliculus, geniculate, and auditory cortex, although our knowledge of auditory space is premature compared to what we know of visual space and retinotopic projections, some of which are pictured (*bottom*).

themselves in an incessant interplay of concentric, rotational, pulsating, and oscillating movements during which one pattern suddenly replaces another. This kaleidoscopic transition occurs at the approximate rate of ten movements per second (Siegel & Jarvik, 1975). These spatial and kinetic properties are readily seen in synesthesia, number forms, and the auras that herald migraine and seizure. They have less commonly been noticed in sensory deprivation, intoxications, febrile delirium, insulin hypoglycemia, and hypnogogic states, probably for lack of looking.

What synesthetes experience often is projected outside themselves in peri-personal space, rather than being in the mind's eye. Subject DS (Cytowic, 1989) provides an example of spatial extension in vision. On hearing music, this college teacher also see objects—falling gold balls, shooting lines, metallic waves like oscilloscope tracings—"floating on a screen" six inches from her nose. Her favorite music, she explains, "makes the lines move upward."

A spatial extension of touch is described by the trimodal taste-smell-touch synesthete MW (Cytowic, 1989), who describes the tactile shape felt when tasting mint by the analogy of "rubbing cool, glass columns." When pressed to elaborate his sensations, he explains, "I can reach my hand out and rub it along the back side of a curve. I can't feel where the top and bottom end, so it's like a column. It's cool to the touch, as if it were made of stone or glass. What is so wonderful about it, though, is its absolute smoothness. Perfectly smooth. I can't feel any pits or indentations in the surface, so it must not be made of granite or stone. Therefore, it must be made of glass." Hence, MW reasons that the sensory attributes of curved plus cool plus smooth "are like" rubbing a cool glass column. This is a third-person verbal description of a first-person sensory experience.

Even MW's ordinary sense of taste has a spatial quality. He often remarked on tasting flavors in different locations in his mouth and head in a manner that professional chefs, for example, never acknowledged. A spatial extension of taste also appears in the few reports of synesthetically colored taste (Downey, 1911).

The elementary quality of such experiences, in contrast to a pictorial or verbal elaboration, is the essence of the form constants. Once he got his subjects past their awe and their urge to *interpret* their experience, Klüver identified four types of basic hallucinatory constants: Lattices and chessboard figures, cobwebs, tunnels and cones, and spirals. Movement constants of rotation, pulsation, and concentric organization further describe the spatial and temporal *flow* of the experience, whereas variations in color, brightness, symmetry, and replication provide finer gradation. The geometrizing described by Klüver extends past the basic form constants in that the configurations multiply and reiterate themselves. (The term to describe this, *pareidola*, literally means "an image within an image" [Hamilton, 1974].) The self-organization of self-similar structures that differ chiefly in scale are, of course, now familiar from the study of fractals. The configurations of the form constants are not just *visual* phenomena, but *sensory form constants* that can become apparent in any spatially extended sense (see figures 6.5 and 6.6).

What is so striking about the fortification spectrum of migraine, for example, or the geometrizing of synesthesia and number forms is the orientation of their constituent parts. Initially, we believed these spatial and dynamic configurations reflected some anatomic structure such as the cortical columns; later, we tried mapping it to some prototypical mental function. Recently, we have returned to anatomy in asking whether the activation of neuronal pools that respond to different orientations is responsible for perceiving these configurations (Lance, 1986, 1993). The study of nonlinear dynamics tells us that self-organizing systems are far from equilibrium, a property that may underlie their capacity to change radically and unpredictably. Regarding the brain, this property might underlie the kaleidoscopic and scintillating transformations that individuals report as part of these unusual experiences.

At present, we are still not sure what the physical correlates of the form constants are, although we do think that their existence points to some fundamental aspect of perception. This inkling seems to be reinforced by the elementary quality of the perceptions themselves. The distinction between *elementary* and *elaborated* percepts is most readily illustrated in epileptic synesthesia, which occurs in 4% of limbic seizures. That is, seizures in the hippocampus produce synesthesia in persons who are otherwise not synesthetic. An example is the sensory amalgamation of flashing, moving lights, geometrizing, a taste, a feeling of heat rising, and a high-pitched whine. Seizures that remain confined to the hippocampus produce an experience that is elementary—a taste, for example, is described as "bitter," "metallic," or merely "unpleasant." Only when seizures spread to the cortex of the temporal lobe does the perception become more specific and elaborated— "rusty iron," "oysters," or "an artichoke."

In mapping his own scintillating migranous scotoma, Lashly (1941) observed that its configuration remained constant as it expanded, as if some steady centrifugal force were pushing it outward. He noted a scintillation rate of ten flashes per second and calculated its pace of cortical spread at 3 mm/min. The spreading depression of Leão (1944) later confirmed these features, as has the contemporary technology of magnetoëncephalography in showing a slow wave of excitation and inhibition during migraine (Welsch, 1987).

Number Forms

The association of color, movement, and spatial configuration with concepts involving serial order was noted more than a century ago (Suarez de Mendoza, 1890), but one hears little of this today in psychology (see those collected by the mathematicians Bowers and Bowers, 1961). The British polymath Sir Francis Galton (1822–1911) remarked on number forms in 1907:

The pattern or "Form" in which the numerals are seen is by no means the same in different persons, but assumes the most grotesque variety of shapes, which run in all sorts of angles, bends, curves, and zigzags.... The drawings, however, fail in giving the idea of the apparent size to those who see them; they usually occupy a wider range than the mental eye can take in at a single glance, and compel it to wander. Sometimes they are nearly panoramic.

These forms ... are stated in all cases to have been in existence, so far as the earlier numbers in the Form are concerned, as long back as the memory extends; they come "into view quite independently" of the will, and their shape and position ... are nearly invariable (Galton, 1907, pp. 80–81).

As in the form constants, there is also a dynamic quality to number forms. One student complained to her mathematics teacher, "I'm having difficulty because the digits *keep going up to their places* (Bowers & Bowers, 1961, pp. 244–247). Like synesthetes, those who possess number forms express amazement that not everyone "sees" numbers as they do or that anyone should find such forms odd (figures 12.9 through 12.11). As my subject MP

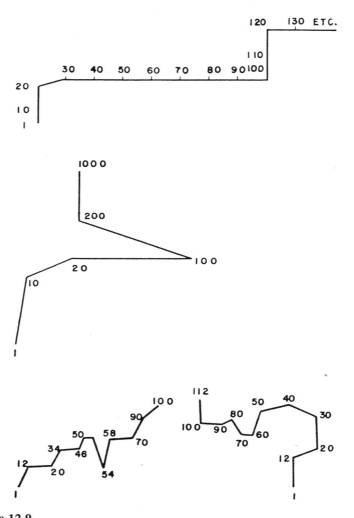

Figure 12.9
Number forms collected by Galton (1907). Note the greater psychophysical space often given to the more frequently used integers. The elements of a number form almost never occupy equal spaces. Elements often are colored, and sometimes have a kinetic quality.

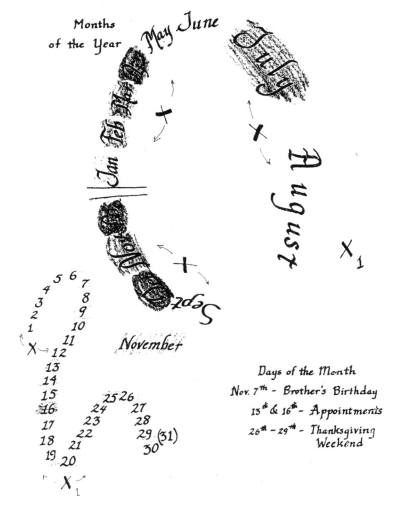

Figure 12.10
(*Top*) Number form for the months of the year, each month being a different color (shown in this black-and-white reproduction by varying shades of gray). As Galton noted, "there are many varieties as to the topmost month; it is by no means always January." (*Bottom*) Each month has its own form for the days belonging to it. Here, November's integers take on the brown coloration of the parent month, whereas special dates and appointments are "marked" with an additional color overlay. From Cytowic (1989), with permission.

remarked, "It never occurred to me that it might be unnatural to visualize the whole alphabet (or numbers)," and subject CS states, "My entire life, everything, has a *place* that goes all around my body" (Cytowic, 1989). Bowers and Bowers (1961) estimate that 3% of the population experiences unique configurations for serial items.

Forms for the alphabet, days of the week, and the months of the year are more common than forms for serial concepts such as ancestry, education, clothing sizes, salaries, weight, time, or temperature (Cytowic, 1989, pp. 191–225). These configurations serve as a mental Filofax or daily planner. The presence of inverted or otherwise oddly oriented forms internested within other forms (see figure 12.11) would seem to require inordinate mental gymnastics to utilize the configuration as a "convenient" mnemonic organizer. Yet the opposite is asserted: "How else could I think? How would I know where anything is or when I'm supposed to do something?" (op. cit., my subject DB).

The forms are vivid, though not always externally projected, and are spoken of in the present tense. Their three-dimensional configurations and their positions in Euclidean space relative to the body remain stable, though the point of view (perspective) may change relative to the individual's age, or the season of year, or as the individual mentally "walks about" within them. In other words, although the perspective may change, the relationships between the elements of the form remain constant. The contents of the form are perceived not so much by their graphic representations as by their shape, spacing, or color. For example, "I know it's 2 because it's white" (op. cit., subject SdeM). The elements usually do not occupy equal spaces. For my subject MP, 6 and numbers containing 6 represent the highest order of magnitude as 6 is physically highest in her spatial representation.

Klüver (1966/1928, passim) described numerous instances of individuals perceiving the form constants by touch as well as sight. "This quickly rotating spiral is moving back and forth in the visual field. At the same time ... one of my legs assumes spiral form ... one has the impression of somatic and optic unity." In another case, "The subject states that he saw fretwork before his eyes, that his arms, hands, and fingers turned into fretwork and that he became identical with the fretwork."

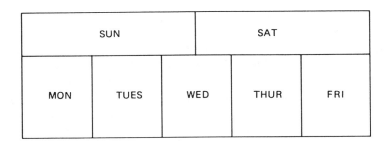
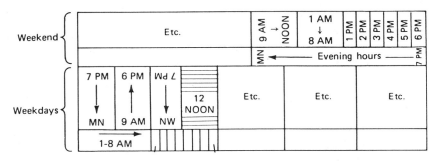
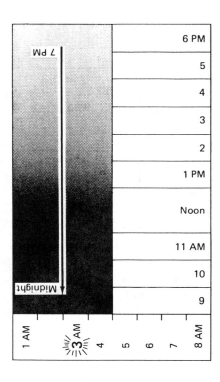

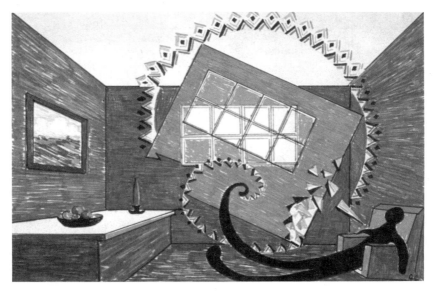

Figure 12.12
Visual-haptic fusion in migraine. This patient experiences the scintillating fortification spectrum, spatial tiltings, and a haptic spiral configuration in the legs. From Sacks (1992), with permission.

A visual and haptic fusion is not uncommon in migraine auras (Sacks, 1992) in which visual gratings also are felt as nets or cobwebs on the body. Even the fractallike "mosaic vision" mentioned by migraneurs is a misnomer because the spatial extension, iteration, and kaleidoscopic transformations extend to touch as well as sight (figure 12.12).

Figure 12.11
Spatial forms for days of the week and time of day. (*Top*) Days of the week. Weekdays are equally spaced; Saturday and Sunday receive more psychophysical space. (*Middle*) Time of day. Close inspection shows that each day of the week contains an upside-down "time cell." Noon and 6 PM are more spacious than other hours, which are spatially equal. The evening hours from 7 PM to midnight are on a fluid continuum, without distinct borders. The relative orientation of time differs for weekend days and weekdays. The subject (DB) performs a mental inversion when she looks at the time cell in detail. From Cytowic (1989), with permission.

The Sensation of Movement

I seem to have yoked our discussions of spatial knowledge and knowledge of movement, but this is all right. *Akinetopsia*, the inability to (visually) perceive motion, is extraordinarily rare, although admittedly examiners do not often seek out the defect. Since the time of the British neurologist George Riddoch (1888–1947), it has been noted that patients with scotoma can often detect movement in their otherwise blind fields (Riddoch, 1917). Amazingly, only one unimpeachable case report of akinetopsia exists (Zihl et al., 1983). This patient lost all knowledge of her visual world when it moved:

She had difficulty, for example, in pouring tea or coffee into a cup because the fluid appeared to be frozen, like a glacier. In addition, she could not stop pouring at the right time since she was unable to perceive the movement in the cup (or a pot) when the fluid rose. Furthermore the patient complained of difficulties in following a dialogue because she could not see the movements of . . . the mouth of the speaker. In a room where more than two people were walking she felt very insecure and unwell, and usually left the room immediately, because "people were suddenly here or there but I have not seen them moving." She could not cross the street because of her inability to judge the speed of a car, but she could identify the car itself without difficulty. "When I'm looking at the car first, it seems far away. But then, when I want to cross the road, suddenly the car is very near." She gradually learned to "estimate" the distance of moving vehicles by means of the sound becoming louder.

Akinetopsia speaks of selective visual motion perception, but the topics we have discussed should make it clear that the perception of motion per se is possible via other modalities (e.g., through sound and touch in Zihl's patient). The complementary observation is found in Riddoch's report, which is based not on the loss of visual motion perception but on its presence in an otherwise blind field (a similar preservation of motion detection exists in blindsight).

Akinetopsia, number forms, and the form constants of synesthesia, migraine and seizure auras, intoxications, and so forth reveal an elementary quality of movement that is nearly as difficult to elucidate as is space. As Klüver experienced in one of his own intoxications (1966/1928), "Sparks having the appearance of *ex-*

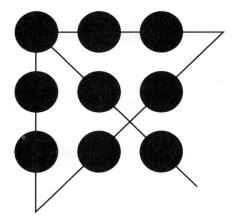

Figure 12.13
Solution of the Gestalt puzzle given in figure 12.4. Once we loosen ourselves from the assumption that a border exists beyond which the connecting lines cannot extend, we see the problem in a new configuration
and can try a novel solution. The Gestalt principles of grouping were said
to prevent random solutions to everyday problems.

ploding shells turn into strange flowers ... gold rain *falling* verti-
cally ... *rotating* jewels *revolving* around a center ... feeling there
is *motion per se.*"

Above all, the form constants are abstract, independent of personal experience, and free of context. They are just configuration,
pulsation, flicker, drift, rotation, perspective .... Do fireworks remind you of anything? When we watch them do we not get a
feeling a salience, as if we recognize something? I suggest that the
"that" of "That was great!" is an ineffable experience of recognition. I do not consider it out of line to suggest that the appeal of
a fireworks display lies in its astonishing similarity to an exter-
nalized catalogue of form constants.

Just as the simultanagnosias turned out to be independent of
striate cortex, so we can guess that the spatial and kinetic aspects
of the form constants must also rely on brain areas outside of idiotypic motor and sensory cortices. (We know, for example, that
electrical stimulation of primary visual cortex causes only simple
flashes and phosphenes, never configurations.) It is likely that
knowledge of space and movement are served by a distributed

system the main entities of which lie outside primary idiotypic motor or sensory cortices, a system that has strong attentional and limbic contributions but the exact reaches of which are yet to be determined. I include limbic entities in the network because people report not only a noëtic sense of certitude but an affect (usually pleasure or satisfaction) that accompanies these experiences.

The selective impairment of visual motion perception in akinetopsia is caused by lesions in unimodal visual association cortex, but the cerebral basis of the other entities I have enumerated is far from certain. What is certain is that our concepts about brain organization must be sufficiently broad to accommodate new observations as we notice them. The occasional bizarreness of these observations invites easy dismissal in light of our prevailing doctrines and treasured ideas about the brain. We would do well to remember history and the nature of science. Concepts that some of us now think of as clear, coherent, and final are unlikely to appear to posterity to have any of those attributes.

SUGGESTED READINGS

Farah MJ. 1990 *Visual Agnosia: Disorders of Object Recognition and What They Tell Us about Normal Vision.* Cambridge: MIT Press

McAdams S, Bigand E, eds. 1993 *Thinking in Sound: The Cognitive Psychology of Human Audition.* New York: Oxford University Press

Zeki S. 1993 *A Vision of the Brain.* Cambridge: Blackwell Science

13 Language

Not long ago, the aphasias were considered exotic disorders of little consequence to the clinician. Indeed, to take any notice of them implied a penchant for philosophical musings. The bewildering array of classifications that newcomers encounter has much to do with aphasia's chaotic history and is probably responsible for most students' initial fear of the subject. Classifying language disturbances according to anatomy is backwards from how you approach a patient who has become acutely aphasic (table 13.1). Clinically, you start by assessing what that patient can and cannot do. Six features that are usually sufficient to diagnose an aphasia are (1) spontaneous speech, (2) speech comprehension, (3) repetition, (4) naming to confrontation, (5) reading aloud with comprehension, and (6) writing (table 13.2). Table 13.3 lists how these variables fare among the different aphasia syndromes.

Aphasia is a disorder of *language* resulting from brain damage. The vocal apparatus functions, but verbal output is linguistically incorrect; likewise, hearing and vision are normal while language comprehension is impaired. In most people, the language-dominant hemisphere is the left one: Aphasias associated with right-hemisphere lesions occur less than once in a hundred cases among right-handed individuals. Even among left-handers, at least sixty percent of aphasias are caused by lesions in the left hemisphere.

The aphasias constituted the earliest demonstration that selective brain damage could affect one class of learned behavior while sparing other classes. Language is not easy to define, but the concept embraces gesture, prosody, semantics (meaning), and syntax (grammar) (Ross et al., 1981). An impaired ability to communicate by writing (agraphia) is found to some degree in nearly all instances of aphasia. Rarely does it exist in isolation.

Table 13.1
Anatomical Classification of Aphasias

Perisylvian Aphasia Syndromes
  Broca's aphasia
  Wernicke's aphasia
  Conduction aphasia

Borderzone Aphasia Syndromes
  Transcortical motor aphasia
  Transcortical sensory aphasia
  Mixed transcortical aphasia
  Frontal aphasias

Subcortical Aphasia Syndromes
  Aphasias from thalamic, striatal, pallidal, and similar lesions
  Aphasias resulting from white matter lesions
  Aphasia of Marie's quadrilateral space

Nonlocalizing Aphasia Syndromes
  Anomic aphasia
  Global aphasia

THE NEUROLOGIC MODEL

Carl Wernicke's 1874 paper, "The Symptom Complex of Aphasia," carried the subtitle, "A Psychological Study on an Anatomical Basis." The American neurologist Norman Geschwind (1926–1984) continued Wernicke's approach in emphasizing the anatomical underpinnings of behavior, though his now-classic formulation (1965b) was informed by additional anatomic and physiological observations. At the time, his coherent scheme of progressive linguistic transformations in serial brain areas explained all clinical aphasia syndromes.

As useful and predictive as was Geschwind's proposal in 1965, however, we understood it to be mistaken twenty-some years later. Electrical stimulation studies showed that the anatomical constraints on language are not as absolute as Geschwind thought, and metabolic imaging and cognitive analysis showed that, contrary to Geschwind's claims, visual words are not converted into auditory representations before their semantic meaning can be accessed. It is worth recounting these developments.

Table 13.2
Clinical Evaluation of Langauge

1. Spontaneous speech
    Rate (fluent = 100–200 wpm; non-fluent < 50 wpm)
    Prosody (rhythm, timber, inflection, melodiousness)
    Articulation
    Content—substantive and meaningful or empty and circumlocuitous?
    Paraphasias—semantic, phonemic, neologisms
    Phrase length (normal = 6–8 words per phrase)

2. Speech comprehension
    Simple and multistep pointing commands (e.g., ceiling, wall, floor,
       door)
    Potential confound: Apraxia

3. Repetition
    Digits, words, phrases, sentences, conditionals
    Echolalia present?

4. Naming to confrontation
    Objects, object parts
    Body parts
    Colors
    Does phonemic or contextual cueing help?

5. Reading
    Reading aloud not equivalent to comprehension
    Comprehension of what is read (either aloud or silently)

6. Writing
    Name or other overlearned data
    Words and phrases to dictation
    Self-directed answer in response to a specific (not open-ended) question

Note: None of these are all-or-nothing deficits in aphasia.

Geschwind noted that the shop-worn distinction between so-called expressive and receptive aphasia was misleading, and urged its abandonment. It was common to assume that patients whose speech was effortful had expressive aphasia and an obligate lesion in Broca's area, whereas those whose comprehension was poor had a receptive aphasia and a corresponding lesion in Wernicke's area. All forms of aphasia, we now believe, have a linguistically incorrect disturbance of speech output.

Geschwind preferred the dualism of *fluent* and *non-fluent* speech. Fluent aphasics produce effortless, well-articulated sentences with

Table 13.3
Language Performance in Various Aphasias

Aphasia Type	Spontaneous Speech	Repetition	Paraphasia	Comprehension	Naming
Broca's	Non-fluent	Poor	Rare	Good	Fair, cues help
Wernicke's	Fluent	Poor	Semantic type	Poor	Poor, cues not helpful
Conduction	Fluent	Poor	Phonemic type	Good	Poor, because of paraphasias
Global	Non-fluent	Poor	Variable	Poor	Poor
Anomic	Fluent	Good	Never	Good	Poor
Transcortical motor	Non-fluent	Echolalia	Rare	Good	Poor
Transcortical sensory	Fluent	Echolalia	Common	Poor	Poor
Mixed transcortical	Non-fluent	Echolalia	Rare	Poor	Poor
Subcortical	Either	Good	Common	Variable	Variable

Note: All aphasics have aphasic writing.

normal grammatical skeletons, but they have neither hemiplegia nor a Broca's lesion. Their lesions are either temporal or parietal, yet their incorrect language output obviously constitutes an expressive aphasia. The speech is abnormal in being faster than usual and remarkably devoid of content despite being voluble (the similarity to politicians and press secretaries is striking). The speech has a normal rhythm and melody, but is filled with circumlocutions ("The thing you use to write with"), non-referential words ("thing," "they"), and errors of usage that are called *paraphasias*. Phonemic (or literal) paraphasias replace one sound with another, such as "takle" for "table." Semantic (or verbal) paraphasias substitute a real, but incorrect, word, such as "chair" for "table." Fluent paraphasic speech that makes no sense whatsoever is called *jargon aphasia*.

The speech of non-fluent aphasics is slow, labored, and poorly articulated. Small grammatical functors and endings are characteristically dropped, even when the patient attempts to repeat a correct sentence given by the examiner. Their speech is frankly

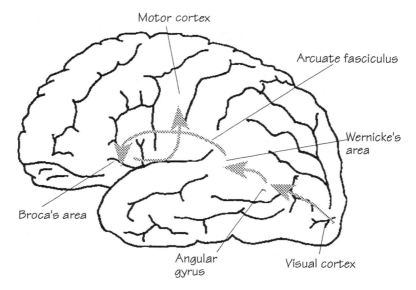

Motor cortex

Arcuate fasciculus

Wernicke's area

Broca's area

Angular gyrus

Visual cortex

Figure 13.1
The Wernicke model of language. Written language input is transformed into an auditory-based code that is subsequently accessible to either meaning or articulation. To speak a written word, its visual impression is transferred to Wernicke's area, where it is recoded into its corresponding auditory pattern. A representation of the word then is projected by the arcuate fasciculus to Broca's area, evoking the motor pattern for its articulation that is executed by the motor cortex. Similarly, a word that is heard is not understood until the auditory cortex projects it to Wernicke's area.

telegrammatic. Asked to describe the weather, a non-fluent aphasic may say only, "Sunny" and, if coaxed to produce a sentence, may effortfully reply, "Weather ... sunny." In striking contrast to this paltry verbal output is a retained musical capacity. Non-fluent aphasics may sing a melody correctly and even with artistic feeling. Language and music are separate communicative systems, though how we sing a song with words remains an issue of theoretical interest.

Wernicke provided a speculative analysis for the mechanism of aphasia (figure 13.1). He noted that Broca's area is contiguous to the cortical representation of the speech motor organs, and he surmised that it transformed language into motor patterns for articulation.

Similarly, because Wernicke's area lies adjacent to auditory cortex, Wernicke assumed that it participated in transforming the patterns of spoken language. He further assumed that these two areas must be connected, as indeed they are by the arcuate fasciculus. The general pattern of deficits is fairly straightforward.

Destruction of Broca's area leads to a non-fluent aphasia; damage extending to adjacent motor cortex often causes a hemiparesis that is greatest in the arm. In *Broca's aphasia*, comprehension is good but not normal, and repetition is poor. Poor confrontational naming is aided by either contextual or phonetic prompting. A moderate to severe ideomotor apraxia affecting the nonparetic left side is present. Imitation of the examiner's actions are better executed than are acts to command, whereas self-initiated actions can be entirely normal (as these are executed by non-pyramidal pathways as you by now know).

If any speech remains, the words "yes," "no," or expletives can be uttered in context and with considerable emotion, thus illustrating how patients are speechless but not wordless. Overlearned expressions such as, "Hello!" and "Good morning" not only may be retained but also may become compulsive utterances that are endlessly repeated (verbal stereotypy). Awareness of their own mistakes often leads patients to exasperation and, sometimes, despair.

Destruction of Wernicke's area stymies comprehension and the ability to repeat. Because the model assumed that written language is learned by reference to speech, a Wernicke's lesion should abolish comprehension of written language. In normal speaking, the auditory form of words was assumed to somehow be replayed via the arcuate fasciculus to Broca's area for articulation. Damage to Wernicke's area would therefore obviously impair language output.

At first, *Wernicke aphasics* appear strangely unaware of their deficit, then soon realize that they are talking in a vacuum, able to understand neither themselves nor others. Their verbal output is indeed fluent but so contaminated with semantic paraphasias as to be incomprehensible. Compared to Broca's aphasia, prompting rarely helps. (Strict fluency is not invariable: When hesitant, speech falters on the key descriptive noun or verb, an opposite feature from the telegrammatic but meaningful Broca's-type of output.) Wernicke's aphasics are deprived of all communication: They cannot understand what is said, read with comprehension, tell others what they want or write it down, name objects (even though they might repeat the name from dictation), or match words that they hear with those that they see.

Further details of Geschwind's formulation state that the comprehension of writing requires visual input to the speech regions, and that destruction of these projections should cause isolated impairment of reading comprehension. Second, language acquisition by the right hemisphere must depend on left-hemispheric projections via the corpus callosum. The Wernicke model was testable in that it predicted how certain lesions would produce symptoms that had not yet been described. These predictions turned out to be valid.

Conduction aphasia results from an interruption of the arcuate fasciculus; vascular anatomy usually places such an interruption deep in the parietal lobe just above the sylvian fissure. Patients comprehend spoken language normally, but cannot repeat the examiner's words. This impairment of repetition is most marked for short grammatical words ("the," "if," "is"), conditionals ("I *would* go if he *could* come"), and brief phrases ("This is it"). Conduction aphasics may be utterly incapable of repeating "He is here," while having no trouble rattling off "Presidential succession." (The underlying reason for this is unknown; an agrammatism is said to exist in this type of aphasia.) The hardest phrase to repeat is, "No ifs, ands, or buts," whereas they do best with numbers. Given a test phrase of "seventy-five percent," for example, they may effortlessly repeat "seventy-five" but falter on "percent." (By now, the reason this is so should be obvious: Numbers and language comprise different knowledge.)

Anomic aphasia (also called *amnestic aphasia*) is a fluent aphasia in which comprehension and repetition are preserved. When the aphasia is due to a stroke, the responsible lesion is in the vicinity of the angular gyrus, though localization of anomia often is impossible. One confound is that anomic aphasia often is a recovery stage in other types of aphasia or else a manifestation of diffuse brain dysfunction (e.g., Alzheimer's disease, metabolic encephalopathy). Furthermore, difficulty in naming objects is common in all varieties of aphasia. Therefore, the term *anomic aphasia* refers strictly to a fluent aphasia with essentially intact comprehension and repetition.

Global aphasia is non-fluent, and the loss of comprehension and repetition is severe. Responsible lesions destroy both Broca's and Wernicke's areas and leave the patient with a dense hemiplegia.

Isolation of one of the classic speech areas from the rest of the brain is a rare occurrence that is nonetheless mentioned in most texts because its clinical manifestations are readily explained by the Wernicke model. Though rare, the clinical manifestations are also of great theoretical concern. Prolonged hypotension, carbon monoxide poisoning, or other forms of anoxia typically destroy the border zones between adjoining territories perfused by the anterior, middle, and posterior cerebral arteries. Such lesions can isolate a functioning Broca's or Wernicke's area from the rest of the hemisphere, resulting in a *transcortical aphasia*.

In *transcortical motor aphasia* (isolation of the motor speech area), the patient cannot initiate propositional speech. In fact, the only verbal output usually is the parroting back of another's comments (echolalia). Auditory and reading comprehension are good. Except for the excellent ability to repeat, transcortical motor aphasia closely resembles Broca's aphasia.

In *transcortical sensory aphasia* (isolation of Wernicke's area), patients cannot comprehend spoken or written words. Speech is fluent with marked paraphasias, empty circumlocutions, and intact repetition that can be echolalic. What is striking in these patients, and even misleadingly suggestive of psychiatric disease, is the total irrelevance of their comments to what is asked or said by the examiner. Because obvious physical signs are lacking, and because speech output is a string of real words bearing no relation to the topic of conversation, this disorder usually is mistaken for psychosis by emergency room personnel. Causative lesions are posterior-inferior near the parietal-occipital junction. Over time, a neologistic jargon develops that gradually resolves through diminishing paraphasias. Comprehension of spoken language sometimes improves.

It is understandable that individuals who rapidly spew out abnormal speech might be considered confused or even psychotic. The differential diagnosis is not confusing at all, however. The "word salad" of schizophrenia occurs exclusively in chronic psychotics who have a history of repeated or lifelong institutionalization. The onset of either odd speech (normal but irrelevant) or frankly abnormal speech in an adult with no psychiatric history and no hemiparesis is a fluent aphasia until determined otherwise.

Mixed transcortical aphasia was previously called *isolation of the speech area*. Such patients have a fluent aphasia with severe loss of comprehension, but are able to repeat even lengthy phrases with ease. Indeed, they are speechless until spoken to, at which point echolalia and their remarkable compulsion to complete sentences become plain to everyone. The responsible lesion circumscribes but leaves intact the classic speech regions and their interconnections.

In a well-studied case produced by carbon monoxide poisoning (Geschwind et al., 1968), the patient never uttered a spontaneous propositional phrase, but could repeat lengthy sentences perfectly. She did this with perfect articulation and prosody, even surpassing repetition by completing spoken phrases. If the examiner said, "Roses are red," for example, she would respond, "violets are blue, sugar is sweet, and so are you." She could also learn new verbal material in the form of songs that did not exist before her illness. She could sing to a recording. When this was turned off, she would continue to sing the words and music correctly to the end, despite the lack of a model. At autopsy, the classic speech area was indeed isolated from the rest of the brain by surrounding cortical and white matter lesions. Her Wernicke and Broca areas, the connections between them, and her auditory inflow and motor outflow projections were all unscathed.

Non-Perisylvian Language Disorders

It should be evident from what we have covered in previous chapters that language can be disturbed by cerebral disorders that lie outside the perisylvian fissure of the language-dominant hemisphere. The subcortical aphasias, frontal aphasias, transcortical border-zone aphasias, and the aphasias of diffuse structural or metabolic disturbances all lie outside the traditional Wernicke model described above.

More fundamentally, occipital lesions prevent lexical input, whereas lesions of the supplementary motor cortex and orbital portions of the frontal lobe impair all motor activities, including speech. If fluent aphasics feature an increased speed and volubility of output, then non-fluent aphasics, whose lesions tend to be more anteriorly placed, show the opposite trend in their decreased spontaneous speech, limited response during interrogation, and a disinclination to speak at all.

Frontal types of aphasias are distinct from *akinetic mutism*, however, which is an akinesia typically produced by ruptured aneurysms of the anterior communicating artery or infarction of the anterior cerebral artery. Lesions in the posterior orbital portions of the frontal lobes couple reduced impulse (abulia) with indifference. When extreme abulia reaches the point of mutism and immobility, the state is called *akinetic mutism*. Patients are awake but unresponsive and, if they speak at all, they do so in barely audible monosyllables.

Following the advent of CT and other imaging technology, we recognized that aphasia sometimes was produced by a subcortical lesion. Subcortical aphasias are said to possess clinical features sufficiently distinct as to warrant a separate classification, though some researchers are unable to see any distinction other than the transience of severely disturbed language.

Thalamic lesions, for example, produce an aphasia that begins as mutism and evolves into paraphasic, hypophonic speech. Speech comprehension, naming, and repetition are unimpaired. Similar clinical pictures are said to be caused by lesions in the putamen, caudate, and pallidum, although some disagreement exists regarding whether aphasia can be produced by thalamic pathology alone (Benson, 1993).

Revisions to the Wernicke Model

It is easy to picture Broca's area because it is defined anatomically: It is the posterior third of the inferior frontal gyrus. Wernicke's area, on the other hand, is defined by its function: It is the area where a lesion impairs the comprehension of language. Because of this, it is impossible to draw a satisfactory picture of Wernicke's area. The simple question, "Where is it?" has distressed everyone who has asked it, including Wernicke himself (Bogen & Bogen, 1975).

There is no sharp boundary on one side of which a lesion causes aphasia and on the other side of which it does not. The ideal solution that is compatible with clinical data would be a topographic probability distribution showing the likelihood of impaired comprehension from a lesion at a given locus. Historically, our thinking has long been constricted by notions of a stable locus that would be identical in all brains. (Our concepts are additionally influenced by the word *area*. The word *zone* would be better than *area*, which is two-dimensional and implies that depth is not important. Lesions are deep, but the cortex is only 1 to 2 mm thick. This leads us to distinctions between neuronal groups and fiber projections, then cookie-cutter lesions versus ones that undermine the fiber projections, and so on.)

Electrical Stimulation Mapping

Beginning in the late 1970s, electrical stimulation studies directed by the American neurosurgeon George Ojemann gradually disclosed the need to revise the classic model of language organization that was based on strict neuroanatomy. (Others have reached the same conclusion, but I focus on Ojemann to keep us from going too far afield in this broad body of literature.) These studies confirmed that language was indeed discretely localized in any given individual, but that its exact location varied widely among individuals.

These results are important not only for those undergoing cortical resection in the language hemisphere, but also because they show how language cannot be reliably localized solely on anatomic grounds using tools such as scans or angiograms. The theoretical implications are broad. The variability of any given individual's functional language map really forces us to treat Broca's and Wernicke's areas less as concrete entities whose boundaries are sacrosanct and more as conceptual entities whose physical bases we are only now beginning to understand.

The use of electrical stimulation mapping during neurosurgery under local anesthesia was first devised by Penfield (Penfield & Roberts, 1959). The application of an electric current to the cortical surface is a complicated matter because it exerts both excitatory and inhibitory forces on neuronal groups and *en passage* fibers, both locally and at a distance (Yeomans, 1990; Devinsky et al., 1993). Penfield observed that a current applied to some cortical sites blocked the act of naming, whereas stimulating these sites in the quiet patient had no observable effect. Many sites that, when stimulated, evoked naming errors resided outside of the classically-defined language zones.

Ojemann used electrical stimulation mapping to show that the topographic extent of language cortex in a given individual bears little resemblance to classic maps (Ojemann et al., 1989). In a single individual, the potential language zone may occupy a broad expanse of the left lateral cortex, much larger than the language-possible stretch that was mapped by Penfield. Within this zone, discrete language sites are variably committed and yield graded effects in that, given a uniform current level, some areas always produce naming errors, others do only sometimes, and still other sites never produce errors. The transition from a place giving consistent naming errors to a site giving none can occur within millimeters over the continuous surface of a gyrus. Five tasks that seem to be selectively disruptable in a space just 5 mm across are naming, reading grammatical words (close procedure), phoneme identification (stop consonants), oral praxis (matching face gestures to a picture), and short-term verbal memory (Whitaker, 1979).

As figure 13.2 indicates, Ojemann showed that language, as measured by naming, is highly localized in a handful of "mosaics" that reach only 1 to 2 sq cm in size. One mosaic usually is in the frontal lobe, with additional units placed in either the temporal or parietal lobe. The total area of mosaics related to language is only one-fourth as large as the traditional Broca-Wernicke regions. In bilingual patients, the essential areas for the language in which they are least competent are larger than those for the language in which they have the most facility (Ojemann & Whitaker, 1978), suggesting that committed areas might involute with increasing facility in a given language. Some confirmation of this possibility comes from the observation that patients with lower verbal IQs have larger total language areas.

This type of mapping study shows that neither the location nor absence of a language function at a given cortical site can be reliably predicted by conventional anatomy. Because the study population is abnormal by virtue of the patients' need for craniotomies, it is reasonable to ask whether their cortex might not have reorganized relative to their lesions, especially those lesions acquired early in life. The results are the same, however, whether individ-

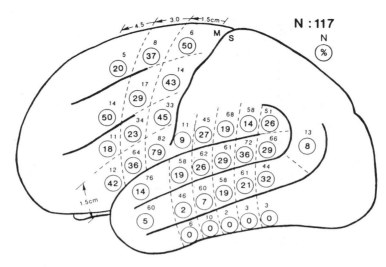

Figure 13.2
Variability of language location as identified by naming in 117 patients. Language sites are identified far beyond the traditional boundaries of Broca's and Wernicke's areas, and the presence of naming sites in the traditional areas is equally variable. "The detailed functional anatomy of our brains may be as individualized as the detailed anatomy of our faces" (Ojemann & Whitaker, 1978). From Ojemann et al. (1989), with permission.

uals damaged their brains as children or as adults. Neither is linguistic experience a variable, as similar results are obtained in those with the least language experience (a four-year-old boy) and those with the most (eighty-year-olds).

The variable location of language is marked in all regions related to language except the most posterior portion of the inferior frontal gyrus. Even there, however, enough variation exists so that, in a given individual, Broca's area sometimes does not even participate in language. (Parenthetically, small lesions confined to the classic Broca's area most often cause stuttering or oral apraxia rather than a frank Broca's aphasia [Mohr et al., 1978].) Such variability probably explains the historic difficulty in pinning down the *exact* location of Wernicke's area. As Bogen amusingly demonstrates, the classic Wernicke's language area is an artifact of combining the locations, in temporal and parietal cortex, of sites that are essential for language in different patients (Bogen & Bogen, 1975).

We have not been able to show that a cortical language area corresponds to any particular cytoarchitectonic area, although this idea has appealed to those who pondered whether language may really be a skill unique to humans. However, individual variability in cytoarchitecture in general has hardly been explored in either humans (Galaburda et al., 1978) or animals (Merzenich et al., 1987).

Psychological Investigations

We turn now to a different issue that also requires some revision of the classic language model. The neurological approach, as summarized by Geschwind (1965b, 1979), saw language as a linear procedure in which visual (lexical) input is transformed into an auditory-based code that then is accessed by either meaning (semantics) or articulation. Subsequent psychological investigations led to a language model in which modality-specific codes exist for words that are perceived either by vision or hearing. These modality-specific codes form part of a multiplex system in that they are said to have parallel access to shared output (articulation) and meaning (semantics).

The use of PET to explore what processes might be involved in the reading of single words reveals the participation of at least two distinct sets of cortical areas (Petersen et al., 1988). An occipital set appears to be specifically engaged in decoding visual patterns into words, whereas a frontal set seems to use those patterns for accessing stored semantic knowledge about them. This striking observation implicates very early visual processes in reading (visual perception had previously been neglected by experimental psychologists).

PET studies confirm that the auditory and visual awareness of words each has its own cortical representation and that each modality can independently access the supramodal entities of articulation and semantic knowledge. The existence of multiple parallel routes between localized modality-specific phonological, articulatory, and semantic coding areas is inconsistent with the earlier neurologic model. In that model, access to semantics is through phonology, whereas access to articulation is through semantics. That is, it proposes that a visual word must first be phonologically transformed in the angular gyrus and establish semantic associations in Wernicke's area before it can be recoded for articulation.

PET probes show no activation near Wernicke's area or in the angular gyrus during visual reading, and protocols that require semantic knowledge of single words activate frontal rather than posterior temporal regions. It therefore seems that lexical-based activity in occipital cortex can access articulation without first undergoing phonological recoding in the posterior temporal cortex. Sensory-specific information appears to have independent access to both semantic and articulation codes. Figure 13.3 shows a schematic of this proposed parallel network.

Further experiments clarified that the bilateral extrastriate occipital activations were in fact unique to words (Petersen et al., 1990). The visual presentation of words as well as pseudowords that obey English spelling rules activate regions of the left medial extrastriate cortex. (*Pseudowords* are word-like letter strings such as "polt" or "tweal.") The failure of nonsense letter strings or letter-like shapes to activate the same site suggests that the recognition of visual word forms is based on learned distinctions between words and non-words. Some spatial grouping is performed on words and word-like letter strings that identify their visual input as a single gestalt.

Rules of spelling and orthography are language-specific. The existence of a lesion in the left extrastriate cortex, which distinguishes between letter strings that either do or do not conform to English spelling rules, indicates that orthographic knowledge specific to English is accessed early in the flow of visual processing. (The existence of such a site may be relevant to priming. See p. 326 and Tulving & Schachter [1990].)

The left medial extrastriate cortex is activated by visual presentations of words and pseudowords, but not by the auditory presentation of words. (Recall that left occipital-temporal lesions produce alexia.) Furthermore, left frontal activation related to semantic processing occurs during the presentation of words but not pseudowords. Hence, separate brain regions are activated by stimulus sets that can be processed in different ways—as visual features, orthographically, or semantically.

The lesson from stimulation mapping—namely, that the processes underlying spoken language are not consistently localized

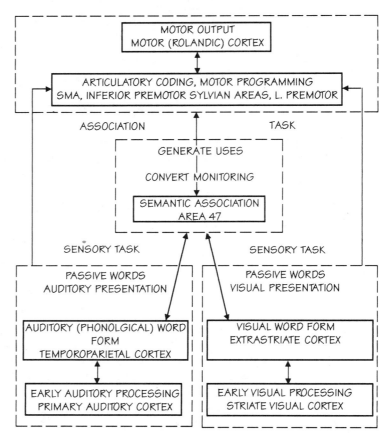

Figure 13.3
One possible configuration of cortical sites related to some apects of lexical processing, based on differential activation during PET. From Petersen
et al. (1988), with permission.

in the same cortical area in different people—contrasts with the results of PET probes during reading. Those investigators argue that, ontogenetically speaking, speech is relatively late compared to the development of the visual perception used in reading. The semantic skill accessed in reading may also have been present much earlier for use in object identification. One then can speculate that the processes employed in reading are more fixed than those used in other aspects of language and that early life experience can perhaps "initialize" an alternative set of language-processing sites in the brain.

In summary, language processing is not as tightly constrained by anatomical connections as the classic neurologic model originally proposed. We continue to reformulate the distributed system for language and ask both how genes hard-wire its constituents and how those parts are modified by experience.

FURTHER CONSIDERATIONS

Traditional Codicils

For historical reasons only, any number of topics usually are discussed in conjunction with language, even though contemporary research has shown them to be cognitive systems distinct from language. For this reason, I will do no more than enumerate a few here.

Amusia

Amusia, already mentioned briefly in chapter 6, is such topic. Double dissociations support the existence of two independent cognitive musical systems. One is consistent with conventional left lateralization models of language involving temporal sequence and analytical processing and the other with right lateralization models of implicit music cognition (Polk & Kertesz, 1993). Useful references for the interested reader are Sloboda (1987) and Ratner (1983).

Acalculia

Acalculia is another historical codicil to language. There are clearly sets of rules for such operations as addition, subtraction, and so forth that somewhat resemble language rules yet are most certainly independent of it. Acalculia was recognized in the latter part of the nineteenth century as resulting from a left-hemisphere lesion, but it was not recognized as an entity independent of any language deficit until the early twentieth century. Readers wishing to pursue the neuropsychology of acalculia should consult the special issue of *Brain and Cognition* edited by Helen Kahn (1991).

Contemporary interest in calculation is as a process that might shed light on both mental representation of numerical manipulation and the specific brain locations related to deficits in calculation. With the recent interest on the structural aspect of calculation, arithmetic may have been a better choice than language for promoting modular theories of the brain (see Fodor, 1983).

At present, evidence indicates that regardless of the functional modularity of calculation ability, there is neither a localized region nor a specific hemisphere that uniquely underlies the disorder.

Articulation

Disorders of phonation and articulation usually are discussed in the context of aphasia. *Phonation* is the production of vocal sounds and depends on the larynx and nasopharynx. Neurological lesions causing *dysphonia* are of the lower motor neuron type. Articulation mostly relies on the pharynx, palate, tongue, and lips. *Dysarthria* is produced by lower motor neuron lesions that paralyze one of these structures, by upper motor neuron spasticity or rigidity, or by cerebellar ataxia.

Motor lesions affecting speech output cover all levels of the neuraxis. For example, motor cortex lesions are seen in non-fluent aphasia, extrapyramidal lesions of the central nuclei are involved in Parkinson's disease and Huntington's chorea, striatal or pontine lesions are seen in pseudobulbar palsy, and medullary nuclei are present in motor neuron disease.

A rarely observed disorder of speech output that has been described both with and without aphasia is the *foreign accent syndrome*. Patients with dysarthric, ataxic, or apraxic speech sound funny because the properties of their native language are distorted. In contrast, the speech of those with foreign accent syndrome retains the normal attributes of their native language but has an unnatural intrinsic prosody. We noted earlier that right-hemisphere lesions can disturb affective prosody—namely, that which is either emotionally based or deliberately wrought. In a case of foreign accent syndrome accompanied by neither aphasia nor dysarthria, MRI disclosed a lesion in the middle fifth of the left precentral gyrus on its inter-sulcal posterolateral aspect (Takayama et al., 1993).

Agraphia

I mentioned that all aphasics have some degree of aphasic writing. This finding is more apparent, however, in patients with Broca's or Wernicke's aphasias, who display kindred types of aphasic errors. Writing is agrammatic in Broca's aphasia and overly fluent in the Wernicke type. Overfluency produces extra words and spelling errors related to duplication of letters and syllables. The problem in agraphia is a loss of writing skill that cuts across penmanship, spelling, semantics, and syntax.

In addition to *aphasic agraphia*, there are other kinds. *Spatial agraphia* involves an improper arrangement of written elements on the page (constructional apraxia usually is present). *Apraxic agraphia* is likewise not a disorder of language but an inability manually to shape letters and words. When severe, patients may not even know how to hold a pen properly or apply it to the paper.

You should examine writing for extra, incorrect, or missing words; misspellings; faulty sentence structure and other grammatical errors; speed; and quality of letter and word form, spatial configuration, slant, and the position and proportion of the margins. You can ask patients to copy nonsense or foreign words, as knowing what they mean is irrelevant to copying them.

Many in the population can talk but cannot read or write, illustrating both how spatial knowledge is a part of writing, and how writing is acquired in close association with reading during childhood development of language.

Thought and Language

What is the relationship among language, thought, and gesture? The traditions in philosophy that equate language with thought, or even with consciousness, are no longer easily defended. Earlier, sufficient examples were cited of knowledge that exists without language to make it clear that thought without language is not only possible (Weiskrantz, 1988) but may occur more often in mental life than most people concede. Only a portion of the neural process is accessible to language. Polar viewpoints on the relationship of language to thought are illustrated in Samuel Johnson's belief that "Words are but the signs of ideas," and Benjamin Whorf's assertion that, "Language is not simply a reporting device for an experience, but a defining framework for it."

The evidence for distinct modules of language subfunctions rests on the patterns of dissociations and associations between deficits that follow brain injury or experimental probes. Studies on thought and language range from cognition in severe aphasia to animal cognition, adult cognition compared to that of the infant, and metacognition (i.e., determination of whether introspection and the awareness of one's performance depends on language).

Whorf's hypothesis (1956) implies that individuals who speak different languages must differ in how they think. If so, then we can say further that speaking minds and those that never acquire grammar must differ immensely. To the real underlying question of how much of putative human uniqueness is indebted to language I have already suggested an answer: "Not everything." We can wonder how a protohuman mind before and after the accretion of language would be altered by the addition of speech, and approach such an issue by looking at children before and after they acquire language or at deaf children compared to speaking ones or by comparing children to primates, including primates that have been trained in symbolic manipulation that some label language. When we compare prelanguage children to apes, we find that the addition of language did not create the human advantage in cognition, but amplified one that already existed (Primack, 1988).

Perhaps less obvious than interludes of thought without language are those instances when language is eliminated from mental structure—namely, the opposite state of language without thought. Patients with spatial neglect, for example, also neglect half of their mental representations. Here, verbal representation alone does not fill the imaginal gap, and language cannot be an autonomous form of representation in the sense that it is not independent. Representation missing in the imagery model analogue is also missing in the verbal mode (Bisiach, 1988). When neglect extends to language performance one sees left-sided neglect in reading or spelling errors in the left half of words spelled both forward and backward (Baxter & Warrington, 1983).

Lastly, Vgotsky noted that the inner speech in a given train of thought would appear elliptical, asyntactical, and meaningless to an external observer because inner speech omits what is obvious to the speaker. However, what is omitted is most likely to be the most important aspect, the fundamental nonlinguistic component of thought.

Gesture

Everyone has observed that people gesture when they speak. Indeed, jokes circulate about how some ethnic groups cannot talk without using their hands. Gesture seems to flow naturally as part of language, but it is anything but superficial or secondary to the verbal discourse. The unity of language and gesture is deep, extending to the semantic and pragmatic levels of communication. Gestures of individuals who speak different languages follow identical principles. They do not merely form a part of what is said and what is meant, but shape thought itself in conveying ideas that language cannot always express. A meaningful gesture comprises its own gestalt. Whereas the progression of segments, sounds, and words in speech represents language's linear aspect, gesture conveys its "nonlinear, instantaneous, holistic and imagistic meanings" (McNeill, 1992).

Gestures occur only during speech. Speakers gesture, not listeners, and 90% of all gestures occur when the speaker actually is uttering something. The acts of speaking and gesturing are bound, synchronous, and semantically coëxpressive in presenting the same or closely related semantic meaning. At age four, gestures emerge in abundance. Gestures and speech develop together in children, and break down together in aphasia. There is no separate gestural language alongside spoken language. Although they follow general principles, gestures are not part of a fixed repertoire but represent thoughts in action that are free to reflect the idiosyncratic imagery of thought.

Gesture is different from signing, however. Given similar lesions, sign aphasia follows left-hemisphere lesions in a manner equal to verbal aphasias (Poizner et al., 1990). Spatial knowledge and language are particularly intertwined when language is communicated as a kinetic and spatial entity as it is in sign language. Interestingly, right-hemisphere lesions do not impair sign language despite profound alterations in visual-spatial capacity. This is a provocative observation that needs to be judged in light of Poizner's small sample size of six deaf patients.

Gestures differ from signs in being used referentially and in not being constructed from a restricted set of units that follow some principle of internal organization. For example, raising the arms to be picked up is a referential gesture. By contrast, syllabic babbling uses a reduced subset of possible phonetic sounds found in actual spoken languages, is organized in having well-formed consonant-vowel clusters, and is used without reference or apparent iconic meaning.

Language supposedly has a link to innate skills for articulation that are represented in Broca's area. Yet naturally occurring human signed languages are organized identically to spoken ones. They have a common phonology, morphology, syntax, and semantic structure (Klima & Bellugi, 1979).

A related issue is the "manual babbling" that occurs in deaf children who are exposed to sign languages from birth. Babbling in infants has normally been assumed to be a speech-based behavior that represents the developing capacity for spoken language. Similarities between manual and vocal modes of babbling, however, suggest that babbling per se is the product of an amodal, neurological language capacity in which the infant produces phonemic and syllabic units as a first step toward building a mature linguistic system.

Deaf infants demonstrate the same properties that are observed in hearing children's vocal babbling. They replicate units (movements instead of sounds), progress through stages on a similar time course, and begin their babbling by the age of ten months. Between the ages of twelve and fourteen months, hearing infants produce vocal jargon babbling, meaningless sequences that sound like sentences. At the same age, deaf infants likewise produce phonologically correct but nonexistent forms in the signed lexicon. These forms maintain the rhythm and duration of rudimentary signed sentences, just as hearing infants use stress and intonation in vocal jargon babbling.

Contrary to prevailing assumptions, the emergence of babbling does not appear to depend on speech. It is tied both to language's abstract structure and to an expressive capacity that can apparently process either signed or spoken signals. Despite radical differences in motor output, both vocal and manual babbling are similarly organized. Both contain singular units and combinations of units that are organized according to the phonetic and syllabic properties of human languages. Language is internally constrained with respect to the phonetic and syllabic units that it can realize but remains flexible in the face of environmental variations with respect to the way this capacity can be expressed.

Structure and Function

Is aphasia a single disorder or a collection of multiple syndromes? This question reflects two opposing schools of thought regarding aphasia, a quarrel that began in the past century and remains with us today. The holistic school argued that all aphasics have similar language problems that differ primarily in severity, whereas those who followed Wernicke's model state that no single brain region is critical for language, different regions contributing instead different language functions that are brought together by the connections among the regions. In the latter viewpoint, both language regions and their interconnections must be intact for normal language capacity to exist.

We have been unable to resolve this quarrel decisively because of the limits inherent in autopsy and structural imaging. I refer you back to the beginning chapters where I pointed out how structural brain damage says almost nothing about the functional consequences of a given injury. Recently, however, metabolic PET imaging has made it possible to explore whether common metabolic abnormalities are demonstrable in all aphasic patients. If so, this would favor a more holistic interpretation of aphasia.

An analysis of regional glucose metabolism in specific gyri and subcortical structures was carried out on forty-four aphasics who, as a group, were representative of the general distribution of aphasia

Table 13.4
Regional Hypometabolism in Aphasia

	Left	Right
Precentral gyrus	78	6
Postcentral gyrus	63	4
Lateral frontal	59	0
Middle frontal	59	0
Medial prefrontal	24	2
Superior parietal	38	—
Supramarginal	89	13
Superior temporal	87	4
Transverse superior temporal	87	4
Middle temporal	2	2
Inferior temporal	70	25
Lateral superior occipital	70	10
Lateral inferior occipital	38	9
Caudate, head	69	12
Caudate, body	31	13
Putamen	71	0
Thalamus	85	9

Regardless of severity and type, *all* aphasics have reduced glucose metabolism in either the left angular, supramarginal, or posterior-superior temporal gyri. In right hemisphere, the inferotemporal gyrus had the largest proportion of patients with hypometabolism (25%) although the ratio means between aphasics and controls in n.s. at $p < .05$. From Metter et al., 1990, with permission.

severity and type (Metter et al., 1990). Regardless of the type of aphasia, 97% of individuals had decreased metabolism in the left angular gyrus, 87% in the left supramarginal gyrus, and 85% in the left posterior-superior temporal (Wernicke's) area (table 13.4). Consistent with Ojemann's demonstration of variable language localization, all aphasics in the study, when taken together, had hypometabolism in their left temporal-parietal cortex (table 13.4).

As is so often the case in historical arguments, both sides turn out to be partially correct. Although the PET data demonstrate a high sensitivity for the left temporal-parietal region in aphasia, there are no data to argue for its specificity. The multiple behavioral differences observed among aphasics may depend on differential dysfunction and structural damage among the temporal-parietal cortex, and subcortical and frontal entities.

Another aspect relating to structure and function concerns the acquisition of multiple languages. Does the brain use the same area for learning a foreign language that it uses for its mother tongue, or does it initialize a new blob of brain? Instances of polyglot aphasia cannot address this question because these patients exhibit too much variability to devise rules that can predict the eventual language impairment or its restitution.

Earlier, we noted that the essential brain areas for the language in which bilingual patients are least competent are larger than those for the language in which they are most facile, suggesting that committed areas might involute with increasing facility in a given language (Ojemann & Whitaker, 1978). Electrical stimulation mapping in bilingual aphasics demonstrated that the center of their language zone is involved in both languages. Peripheral to it, however, sites in both frontal and parietal cortex participate in only one of their tongues. There is a tendency for those sites concerned with a given language to cluster together.

Alexia and Dyslexia

We discussed alexia with and without agraphia in chapter 9. Alexia with agraphia is based on a dominant parietal lesion, whereas alexia without agraphia is based on the combination of dominant occipital and splenial lesions. A so-called *third alexia* is described in aphasic individuals with frontal lesions.

Frontal alexics can understand some written material such as single words, nouns, or verbs. They usually can read aloud and comprehend verbs or substantive words. On the other hand, verbose sentences containing many prepositions and adjectives thwart their understanding. Their literal alexia is worse than their verbal alexia, meaning that they understand words better than they can understand portions of words. A severe agraphia is characteristic of frontal alexia, whereas the occipital alexia precludes agraphia, by definition.

Scientific fashion regarding alexia has changed from a neurologic model to a psycholinguistic approach that asks, for example, whether errors are related to the target word visually, semantically, or phonologically. The problem remains one of relating the psycholinguistic descriptions to those described neurologically.

The term *dyslexia* refers to a childhood developmental disorder, whereas *alexia* refers to an acquired reading impairment. Childhood dyslexia is many times more common than acquired alexia. Neurology customarily divides itself into adult and childhood branches because the pragmatic issues of patient care and the diseases encountered in each population are widely disparate. Despite this, adult neurology textbooks seem to discuss dyslexia rather often while neglecting other kinds of developmental disorders. Perhaps one reason for this quirk is that dyslexia serves as a good example for several points. I used it myself in discussing cerebral dominance, a process whereby the competition for synaptic targets sculpts each brain into a unique entity. The elevated frequency of personal and familial non-right-handedness in dyslexia and other developmental learning disorders has also attracted attention.

Though a common malady, dyslexia is more often mild than severely disruptive. Dyslexics have no other neurologic signs, and their disability can usually be overcome with persistence and good teaching. The trait is strongly familial, more frequently expressed in men, and probably autosomal dominant in its mode of inheritance. Dyslexics have a high incidence of frank left-handedness. Conversely, dyslexia is fifteen times more common in strong left-handers than in strong right-handers (Geschwind & Galaburda, 1987).

Is dyslexia a maturational delay of a normal process, a perceptual impairment (i.e., they can't read what they can't see), or a linguistic one, or possibly even an impairment in grasping the spatial configuration of words? The simple answer is that we are not sure. We are sure only that experts have disagreed on both the etiology and definition of dyslexia since the turn of the century when the condition was called *word blindness*. The notion that perception is impaired stemmed from observing dyslexics' frequent letter reversals. The comments in the preceding chapter regarding spatial knowledge in acquired alexia, coupled with the fact that dyslexics do poorly on constructional tasks, estimates of size and distance, and other tests of spatial knowledge, do suggest that study of configuration in dyslexia might be fruitful.

The so-called soft signs in dyslexia are numerous and are said to include faulty coördination, spatial reasoning, right-left confusion, temporal sequencing, color naming, and eye tracking. Numerous treatments have been offered, including eye-tracking exercises, colored spectacles, laterality and balance exercises, pointers and other mechanical devices, and even special diets, all of which suggest the true dismal state of our knowledge.

Dyslexia can be associated with other developmental disorders, attention deficit, and immune dysfunction. Evidence for neurologic dysfunction in dyslexia was circumstantial until cytoarchitectonic studies were performed. These suggested a fault in neuronal migration as well as significant lateral differences in which the left hemisphere is large (hemimegencephaly) and contains an excessive volume of subcortical white matter (Geschwind & Galaburda, 1987, pp. 58–66). The effects of androgen steroids on brain asymmetry and language cortex might well explain the greater risk for males to develop a variety of developmental disorders, including dyslexia. Other hormone-mediated, gender-specific, embryologic effects that respond to both genetic and environmental forces have implications for the heritability of language and learning impairments (Galaburda, 1993). It may be, though, that dyslexia will tell us more about brain development generally than it will tell us about language.

LANGUAGE MODELS AND MICROGENESIS

Though there have been numerous psychological theories of aphasia over its chaotic history, only one anatomic theory has ever been proposed—Wernicke's model. Electrical stimulation mapping and functional imaging are but two approaches that show this classical model and its modern revisions to be inadequate.

Many readers may think that there is nowhere to turn but to cognitive-type analyses for a better model of language, and perhaps even for a better model of "how the brain works" than biologically based theories can provide. There is, however, another reply to the inadequacy of the Wernicke model that is found in microgenesis

(Brown, 1988; Hanlon, 1991). Unfortunately, a satisfactory explication of microgenetic theory exceeds the space available here.

What I find interesting about microgenesis as a clinically based approach is that not only does it differ fundamentally from the Wernicke-type model but it also provides an escape from the computer metaphor that so heavily influences the methodology of cognitive science. It does this in part by focusing on positive symptoms rather than negative deficits. It also recommends itself by being consistent in all cognitive domains, from perception to thought to language to action. It even offers a self-consistent theory of time. Though I am not wholly satisfied with microgenesis, neither am I wholly satisfied with the results of cognitive science.

SUGGESTED READINGS

Crosson B. 1992 *Subcortical Functions in Language and Memory*. New York: Guilford Press

Galaburda AM, ed. 1993 *Dyslexia and Devlopment: Neurobiological Aspects of Extra-ordinary Brains*. Cambridge: Harvard University Press

Goodglass H. 1993 *Understanding Aphasia*. San Diego: Academic Press

McNeill D. 1992 *Hand and Mind: What Gestures Reveal About Thought*. Chicago: University of Chicago Press

Pinker S. 1994 *The Language Instinct: How Mind Creates Language*. New York: William Morrow

Sarno MT, ed. 1991 *Acquired Aphasia*, 2d ed. San Diego: Academic Press

References

Abraham HD. 1983 Visual phenomenology of the LSD flashback. *Archives of General Psychiatry* 40:884–889

Absher JR, Benson DF. 1993 Disconnection syndromes: An overview of Geschwind's contributions. *Neurology* 43:862–867

Adams JE, Rutkin BB. 1970 Visual responses to subcortical stimulation in the visual and limbic systems. Fourth Symposium of the International Society for Research in Stereoëncephalotomy. *Confina Neurologica* 32: 158–164

Adler N. 1972 *The Underground Stream. New Life Styles and the Antinomian Personality*. New York: Harper & Row

Agnati LF, Bjelke B, Fuxe K. 1992 Volume transmission in the brain. *American Scientist* 80(4):362–373

Ahern GL, Herring AM, Tackenberg J, et al. 1993 The association of multiple personality and temporolimbic epilepsy: Intracarotid amobarbital test observations. *Archives of Neurology* 50:1020–1025

Albert ML, Knoefel JE. 1994 *Clinical Neurology of Aging*, 2d ed. New York: Oxford University Press

Allman P. 1992 Drug treatment of emotionalism following brain damage. *Journal of the Royal Society of Medicine* 85:423–424

American Academy of Neurology AIDS Task Force. 1991 Nomenclature and research case definitions for neurologic manifestations of human immunodeficiency virus-type 1 (HIV-1) infection. *Neurology* 41:778–785

Anand BK, Dua J. 1955 Stimulation of the limbic system of brain in waking animals. *Science* 112:1139

Anderson SW, Damasio H, Tranel D. 1990 Neuropsychological impairments associated with lesions caused by tumor or stroke. *Archives of Neurology* 47:397–405

Andreasen NC, Arndt S, Swayze V, et al. 1994 Thalamic abnormalities in schizophrenia visualized through magnetic resonance image averaging. *Science* 266:294–298

Appollonio IM, Grafman J, Schwartz V, et al. 1993 Memory in patients with cerebellar degeneration. *Neurology* 43:1536–1544

Aronowitz BR, Hollander E, DeCaria C, et al. 1994 Neuropsychology of obsessive compulsive disorder: Preliminary findings. *Neuropsychiatry, Neuropsychology, and Behavioral Neurology* 7:81–86

Armstrong E. 1990 Evolution of the brain. In G Paxinos, ed, *The Human Nervous System*. San Diego: Academic Press

Armstrong E. 1991 The limbic system and culture: An allometric analysis of the neocortex and limbic nuclei. *Human Nature* 2:117

Aronson MK, Ooi WL, Morgenstern H, et al. 1990 Women, myocardial infarction, and dementia in the very old. *Neurology* 40:1102–1106

Arriagada PV, Growdon JH, Hedley-White T, Hyman BT. 1992 Neurofibrillary tangles but not senile plaques parallel duration and severity of Alzheimer's disease. *Neurology* 42:631–639

Baddeley A. 1992 Working memory. *Science* 255:556–559

Baker R. 1981 *Human Navigation and the Sixth Sense*. London: Hodder & Stoughton

Banks G, Short P, Martinez AJ, et al. 1989 The alien hand syndrome, clinical and postmortem findings. *Archives of Neurology* 46:456–459

Barinaga M. 1994 Learning by diffusion: Nitric oxide may spread memories. *Science* 263:466

Barrie JM, Freeman WJ. 1994 Perceptual topography: Spatio-temporal analysis of prepyriform, visual, auditory, and somesthetic EEGs in perception by trained rabbits. In FH Eeckman, ed, *Neural Systems: Analysis and Modeling*. Boston: Kluwer Academic Press

Barton S. 1994 Chaos, self-organization, and psychology. *American Psychologist* 49:5–14

Bassetti C, Bogousslavsky J, Regli F. 1993 Sensory syndromes in parietal stroke. *Neurology* 43:1942–1949

Baxter DM, Warrington EK. 1983 Neglect dysgraphia. *Journal of Neurology, Neurosurgery and Psychiatry* 46:1073–1078

Bayless GC, Rolls ET, Leonard CM. 1985 Selectivity between faces in the responses of a population of neurons in the cortex in the superior temporal sulcus of the monkey. *Brain Research* 342:91–102

Baynes K, Holtzman JD, Volpe BT. 1986 Components of visual attention: Alterations in response pattern to visual stimuli following parietal lobe infarction. *Brain* 109:99–114

Bear DM. 1983 Hemispheric specialization and the neurology of emotion. *Archives of Neurology* 40:195–202

Bear DM, Fedio P. 1977 Quantitative analysis of interictal behavior in temporal lobe epilepsy. *Archives of Neurology* 34:454–467

Beatty WW, 1989 Geographical knowledge throughout the life span. *Bulletin of the Psychonomic Society* 27:379–381

Beatty WW, Tröster AI. 1987 Gender differences in geographical knowledge. *Sex Roles* 16:565–590

Becker JB, Breedlove SM, Crews D. 1992 *Behavioral Neuroendocrinology.* Cambridge: MIT Press

Benbow CP. 1988 Sex differences in mathematical reasoning ability in intellectually talented preadolescents: Their nature, effects and possible causes. *Behavioral and Brain Sciences* 11:169–232

Benson BF. 1993 Aphasia. Benton AL. 1992a Clinical Neuropsychology: 1960–1990. *Journal of Clinical and Experimental Neuropsychology* 14: 407–417

Benton AL. 1992a Gerstmann's syndrome. *Archives of Neurology* 49:445–447

Benton A. 1992b Clinical neuropsychology: 1960–1990. *Journal of Clinical and Experimental Neuropsychology* 14:407–417

Benton AL. 1993 Visuoperceptual, visuospatial, and visuoconstructive disorders. In KM Heilman, E Valenstein, eds, *Clinical Neuropsychology,* 3d ed. New York: Oxford University Press

Benton AL, Levin AS, Van Allen MW. 1974 Geographical orientation in patients. *Neuropsychologia* 12:183–191

Berent S, Giordani B, Gilman S, et al. 1990 Neuropsychological changes in olivopontocerebellar atrophy. *Archives of Neurology* 47:997–1001

Bernard LC. 1990 Prospects for faking believable memory deficits on neuropsychological tests and the use of incentives in simulation research. *Journal of Clinical and Experimental Neuropsychology* 12:715–728

Berrios GE, Brook P. 1982 The Charles Bonnett syndrome and the problem of visual perceptual disorders in the elderly. *Age and Ageing* 11:17–23

Bisiach E. 1988 Language without thought. In Weiskrantz L, ed, *Thought without language,* pp 464–484. New York: Oxford University Press

Bogen JE. 1972. Neowiganism (concluding statements). In WL Smith, ed, *Drugs, Development and Cerebral Function.* Springfield: Charles C Thomas

Bogen JE. 1993 The callosal syndromes. In KM Heilman, E Valenstein, eds, *Clinical Neuropsychology,* 3d ed. New York: Oxford University Press

Bogen JE, Bogen GM. 1975 Wernicke's region–where is it? *Annals of the New York Academy of Science* 280:834–843

Boorstin DJ. 1983 *The Discoverers*. New York: Random House, pp 394–395.

Botez MI. 1993 Cerebellar cognition. *Neurology* 43:2153

Botez-Marquard T, Botez MI. 1992 Visual memory deficits after damage to the anterior commissure and right fornix. *Archives of Neurology* 49:321–324

Bowers H, Bowers JE. 1961 *Arithmetical Excursions*. New York: Dover Publications

Bózzola FC, Gorelick PB, Freels S. 1992 Personality changes in Alzheimer's disease. *Archives of Neurology* 49:297–300

Braun CMJ, Denault C, Cohen H, Rouleau I. 1994 Discrimination of facial identity and facial affect by temporal and frontal lobectomy patients. *Brain and Cognition* 24:198–212

Brindley CS, Lewin WS. 1968 The sensations produced by electrical stimulation of the visual cortex. *Journal of Physiology* 196:479–493

Brion S, Jedynak C-P. 1972 Trouble du transfert interhémisphérique à propos de trois observations de tumeurs du corps calleus: Le signe de la main étrangère. *Revue Neurologique* 126:257–266

Broca P. 1865 Sur la faculté du langage articulé. *Bulletin de la société d'Anthropologie* 6:337–393

Broca P. 1878 Anatomie comparée des circunvolutions cerebrales. Le grand lobe limbique et la scissure limbique dans la série des mammiféere. *Revue d'Anthropologie* 1:385–432

Brodal A. 1969 *Neurological Anatomy in Relation to Clinical Medicine*. New York: Oxford University Press

Brodmann K. 1909 *Vergleichende Lokalisationslehere der Großhirnrinde in ihren Prinzipien dargestellt auf Grund des Zellenbaues*. Leipzig: Barth

Brown JW. 1984 Hallucinations. In PJ Vinken, GW Bruyn, HL Klawans, eds, *Handbook of Clinical Neurology, vol. 45: Imagery and the Microstructure of Perception*. Amsterdam: Elsevier. pp 351–372

Brown JW. 1988 *The Life of the Mind*. Hillsdale, NJ: Lawrence Erlbaum & Associates

Brown RE. 1993 *An Introduction to Neuroëndocrinology*. New York: Cambridge University Press

Bruce V, Ellis AW, Perrett D. 1992 *Processing the Facial Image*. New York: Raven Press

Brust JCM, Behrens MM. 1977 "Release hallucinations" as the major symptom of posterior cerebral artery occlusion, a report of two cases. *Annals of Neurology* 2:432–436

Bruton CJ, Stevens JR, Frith CD. 1994 Epilepsy, psychosis, and schizophrenia: Clinical and neuropathologic correlations. *Neurology* 44:34–42

Bruyn GW. 1982 The seat of the soul. In FC Rose, WF Bynum, eds, *Historical Aspects of the Neurosciences: A Festschrift for Macdonald Critchley*. New York: Raven Press, pp 55–82

Buser P, Imbert M. 1992 *Audition* [RH Kay (transl)]. Cambridge: MIT Press

Butters N, Grant I, Haxby J, et al. 1990 Assessment of AIDS-related cognitive changes: Recommendations of the NIMH workshop on neuropsychological assessment approaches. *Journal of Clinical and Experimental Neuropsychology* 12:963–978

Byrne RW. 1982 *Geographical Knowledge and Orientation*. In AW Ellis, ed, *Normality and Pathology in Cognitive Functions*. London: Academic Press, pp 239–264

Cancelliere AEB, Kertesz A. 1990 Lesion localization in acquired deficits of emotional expression and comprehension. *Brain and Cognition* 13:133–147

Cascino GD, Luckstein RR, Sharbourough FW, Jack CR. 1993 Facial asymmetry, hippocampal pathology, and remote symptomatic seizures: A temporal lobe epileptic syndrome. *Neurology* 43:725–727

Caselli RJ. 1993 Ventrolateral and dorsomedial somatosensory association cortex damage produces distinct somesthetic syndromes in humans. *Neurology* 43:762–771

Caveness W, Gallup G. 1980 A survey of public attitudes toward epilepsy in 1979, with an indication of trends over the past thirty years. *Epilepsia* 21:509–518

Ceccaldi M, Milandre L. 1994 A transient fit of laughter as the inaugural symptom of capsular-thalamic infarction. *Neurology* 44:1762

Celesia GG, Bushnell D, Toleikis SC, Brigell MG. 1991 Cortical blindness and residual vision: Is the "second" visual system in humans capable of more than rudimentary visual perception? *Neurology* 41:862–869

Cherniak C. 1986 *Minimal Rationality*. Cambridge: MIT Press

Chomsky N. 1965 *Aspects of the Theory of Syntax*. Cambridge: MIT Press

Chomsky N. 1985 *Knowledge of Language: Its Nature, Origin, and Use*. New York: Praeger

Christman SD. 1994 The many sides of the two sides of the brain (review of "Hemispheric asymmetry: What's right and what's left?"). *Brain and Cognition* 26:91–98

Chugani HT, Shields WD, Shewmon DA, et al. 1990 Infantile spasms: I: PET identifies focal cortical dysgenesis in cryptogenic cases for surgical treatment. *Annals of Neurology* 27:406–413

Chui HC. 1989 Dementia: A review emphasizing clinicopathologic correlation and brain-behavior relationships. *Archives of Neurology* 46:806–814

Chui HC, Victoroff JI, Margolin D, et al. 1992 Criteria for the diagnosis of ischemic vascular dementia proposed by the state of California Alzheimer's disease diagnostic and treatment centers. *Neurology* 42:473–480

Cicchetti DV, Rourke BP, Sparrow SS, et al. 1991 Establishing the reliability and validity of neuropsychological disorders with low base rates: some recommended guidelines. *Journal of clinical and experimental neuropsychology* 13:328–338

Cicchetti DV, Volkmar F, Sparrow SS, et al. 1992 Assessing the reliability of clinical scales when the data have both nominal and ordinal features: Proposed guidelines for neuropsychological assessments. *Journal of Clinical and Experimental Neuropsychology* 14:673–686

Cobb S. 1960 Observations on the comparative anatomy of the avian brain. *Perspectives in Biology and Medicine* Spring:383–408

Cobb S. 1969 Adventures in Avian Neurology. In S Locke, ed, *Modern Neurology: Papers in Tribute to Derek Denny-Brown*. Boston: Little Brown, pp 1–13

Coffey CE, Wilkinson WE, Parashos, et al. 1992 Quantitative cerebral anatomy of the aging human brain. A cross-sectional study using magnetic resonance imaging. *Neurology* 42:527–536

Cohen H, Cohen D, eds. 1993 Tardive dyskinesia and cognitive dysfunction [special issue]. *Brain and Cognition* 23(1)

Cohen MM, Lessell S. 1984 Neuro-ophthalmology of aging. In ML Albert, ed, *Clinical Neurology of Ageing*. New York: Oxford University Press, pp 313–344

Cohen NJ, Eichenbaum H. 1993 *Memory, Amnesia, and the Hippocampal System*. Cambridge: MIT Press

Coker SB. 1991 The diagnosis of childhood neurodegenerative disorders presenting as dementia in adults. *Neurology* 41:794–798

Cole M. 1994 The foreign policy of the cerebellum. *Neurology* 44:2001–2005

Cooper SJ, Dourish CR, eds. 1990 *Neurobiology of Stereotyped Behavior*. New York: Oxford University Press

Cotman CW, Brinton RE, Galaburda A, et al. 1987 *The Neuro-Immune-Endocrine Connection*. New York: Raven Press

Courchesne E, Townsend J, Saitoh O. 1994 The brain in infantile autism: Posterior fossa structures are abnormal. *Neurology* 44:214–223

Cowell PE, Allen LS, Kertesz A, et al. 1994 Human corpus callosum: A stable mathematical model of regional neuroanatomy. *Brain and Cognition* 25:52–66

Crick F. 1984 Function of the thalamic reticular complex: The searchlight hypothesis. *Proceedings of the National Academy of Sciences of the United States of America.* 81:4586–4590

Critchley M. 1951 Types of visual perseveration: "Paliopsia" and "illusory visual spread." *Brain* 74:267–299

Critchley M. 1953 *The Parietal Lobes.* London: Arnold

Crosson B. 1992 *Subcortical Functions in Language and Memory.* New York: Guilford Press

Cummings JL. 1993 Frontal-subcortical circuits and human behavior. *Archives of Neurology* 50:873–880

Curtis BA, Jacobson S, Marcus EM. 1972 *An Introduction to the Neurosciences.* Philadelphia: WB Saunders

Cushing H. 1909 A note upon the faradic stimulation of the post central gyrus in conscious patients. *Brain* 32:44–53

Cytowic RE. 1976 Aphasia in Maurice Ravel. *Bulletin of the Los Angeles Neurological Society* 41:109–114

Cytowic RE. 1983 Taste—The unnecessary sense? *[letter] New England Journal of Medicine* 308(9):529–530

Cytowic RE. 1989 *Synesthesia: A Union of the Senses.* New York: Springer Verlag

Cytowic RE. 1990 *Nerve Block for Common Pain.* New York: Springer Verlag

Cytowic RE. 1993 *The Man Who Tasted Shapes: A Bizarre Medical Mystery Offers Revolutionary Insights into Emotions, Reasoning, and Consciousness.* New York: Jeremy P. Tarcher/Putnam

Cytowic RE. 1995 Synesthesia: Phenomenology and neuropsychology. A review of current knowledge. *Psyche* URL:ftp"//hcrl.open.ac.uk/pub/psyche/.... [Paper version Sept. 1995, MIT Press: Cambridge]

Cytowic RE, Stump DA, Larned DC. 1988 Closed Head Trauma: Somatic, Ophthalmic, and Cognitive Impairments in Nonhospitalized Patients. In HA Whitaker, ed, *Neuropsychological Studies of Nonfocal Brain Damage: Dementia and Trauma.* New York: Springer Verlag, pp 226–264

Daigneault S, Braün CMJ, Whitaker HA. 1992 An empirical test of two opposing theoretical models of prefrontal function. *Brain and Cognition* 19:48–71

Daly D. 1958 Ictal affect. *American Journal of Psychiatry* 115:97–108

Damasio AR, Damasio H, Van Hoesen GW. 1982 Prosopagnosia: Anatomic basis and behavioral mechanisms. *Neurology* 32:331–341

Damasio H, Damasio AR. 1989 *Lesion Analysis in Neuropsychology*. New York: Oxford University Press

Damasio H, Grabowski T, Frank R, et al. 1994 The return of Phineas Gage: Clues about the brain from the skull of a famous patient. *Science* 264: 1102–1105

D'Andrade RG. 1991 Cultural cognition. In MI Posner, ed, *Foundations of Cognitive Science* Cambridge: MIT Press, pp 795–830

Darwin C. 1872 *The Expression of the Emotions in Man and Animals.* Reprint, Chicago: University of Chicago Press, 1965

Dasheiff RM, Shelton J, Ryan C. 1993 Memory performance during the amytal test in patients with non-temporal lobe epilepsy. *Archives of Neurology* 50:701–705

Dawes RM, Faust D, Meehl PE. 1989 Clinical versus actuarial judgment. *Science* 243:1668–1674

Decarli C, Kaye JA, Horowitz B, Rappoport SI. 1990 Critical analysis of the use of computer-assisted transverse axial tomography to study human brain in aging and dementia of the Alzheimer type. *Neurology* 40:872–883

De Haan EHF, Young A, Newcombe F. 1987 Faces interfere with name classification in a prosopagnosic patient. *Cortex* 21:121–134

Delbrück M. 1986 *An Essay on Evolutionary Epistemology*. GS Stent, et al., eds. Oxford: Blackwell Scientific Publications

Dellatolas G, Annesi I, Jallon P, et al. 1990 An epidemiological reconsideration of the Geschwind-Galaburda theory of cerebral lateralization. *Archives of Neurology* 47:778–782

DeMeyer W. 1993 *Technique of the Neurologic Examination*, 4th ed. New York: McGraw Hill

Desimone R, Albright TD, Gross CD, Bryce C. 1984 Stimulus-selective responses of interior temporal neurons in the macaque. *Journal of Neuroscience* 4:2051–2062

de Sousa R. 1983 *The Rationality of Emotions* Cambridge: MIT Press

Devinsky O, Beric A, Dogali M, eds. 1993 *Electrical and Magnetic Stimulation of the Brain and Spinal Cord.* New York: Raven Press

Devinsky O, Feldman E, Burrowes K, Bromfield E. 1989a Autoscopic phenomena with seizures. *Archives of Neurology* 46:1080–1088

Devinsky O, Kelly K, Yacubian EMT, et al. 1994 Postictal behavior: A clinical and subdural electroencephalographic study. *Archives of Neurology* 51:254–259

Devinsky O, Putnam F, Grafman J, et al. 1989b Dissociative states and epilepsy. *Neurology* 39:835–840

Diamond IT, Neff WD. 1957 Ablation of temporal cortex and discrimination of auditory patterns. *Journal of Neurophysiology* 20:300–315

Dobelle WH, Mladejovsky MG. 1974 Phosphenes produced by electrical stimulation of human occipital cortex, and their application to the development of a prosthesis for the blind. *Journal of Physiology* 243:553–576

Dooneief G, Bello J, Todak G, et al. 1992 A prospective controlled study of magnetic resonance imaging of the brain in gay men and parenteral drug users with human immunodeficiency virus infection. *Archives of Neurology* 49:38–43

Doorenbos DI, Armin FH, Payment M, Clifton R. 1993 Stimulus-specific pathological laughter: A case report with discrete unilateral localization. *Neurology* 43:229–230

Downey JE. 1911 A case of colored gustation. *American Journal of Psychology* 22:528–539

Drevets WC, Raichle ME. 1995 Positron emission tomographic imaging studies of human emotional disorders. In MS Gazzaniga, ed, *The Cognitive Neurosciences*. Cambridge: MIT Press, pp 1153–1164

Drislane FW, Coleman AE, Schomer DL, Ives J, et al. 1994 Altered pulsatile secretion of lutenizing hormone in women with epilepsy. *Neurology* 44:306–310

Duckworth JC, Anderson WP. 1986 *MMPI Interpretation Manual for Counselors and Clinicians*, 3d ed. Muncie, IN: Accelerated Development Inc

Dyson F. 1971 Energy in the universe. In *Energy and Power*. San Francisco: WH Freeman

Eccles J. 1994 *How The Self Controls Its Brain*. New York: Springer Verlag

Efron R. 1990 *The Decline and Fall of Hemispheric Specialization*. Hillsdale, NJ: Lawrence Earlbaum and Associates

Engel J, ed. 1993 *Surgical Treatment of the Epilepsies*, 2d ed. New York: Raven Press

Engel J, Henry TR, Risinger MW, et al. 1990 Presurgical evaluation for partial epilepsy: Relative contributions of chronic depth-electrode recordings versus FDG-PET and scalp-sphenoidal ictal EEG. *Neurology* 40:1670–1677

Engel J, Shewmon DA. 1993 Overview: Who should be considered a candidate? IJ Engel, ed, *Surgical Treatment of the Epilepsies*, 2d ed. New York: Raven Press, pp 23–34

Esslinger PJ, Damasio H, Damasio AR, Butters N. 1993 Nonverbal amnesia and asymmetric cerebral lesions following encephalitis. *Brain and Cognition* 21:140–152

Fagan KJ, Lee SI. 1990 Prolonged confusion following convulsions due to generalized nonconvulsive status epilepticus. *Neurology* 40:1689–1694

Farah MJ. 1990 *Visual Agnosia: Disorders of Object Recognition and What They Tell Us About Normal Vision*. Cambridge: MIT Press

Farah MJ. 1994 Neuropsychological inference with an interactive brain: A critique of the "locality" assumption. *Behavioral and Brain Sciences* 17:43–104

Feinberg TE, Schindler RJ, Flanagan NG, Haber LD. 1992 Two alien hand syndromes. *Neurology* 42:19–24

Felton SY, Felton DL. 1991 Innervation of lymphoid tissue. In R Ader, DL Felton, N Cohen, eds, *Psychoneuroimmunology*, 2d ed. San Diego: Academic Press, pp 27–70

Flanagan O. 1992 *Consciousness Reconsidered*. Cambridge: MIT Press

Fisher CM. 1994 Hunger and the temporal lobe. *Neurology* 44:1577–1579

Fischer M, Ryan SB, Dobyns WB. 1992 Mechanisms of interhemispheric transfer and patterns of cognitive function in acallosal patients of normal intelligence. *Archives of Neurology* 49:271–277

Fodor JA. 1983 *The Modularity of Mind*. Cambridge: MIT Press

Forster FM. 1977 *Reflex Epilepsy, Behavioral Therapy, and Conditional Reflexes*. Springfield, IL: Charles C Thomas

Freeman W. 1990 Searching for signal and noise in the chaos of brain waves. In Krasner, ed, *The Ubiquity of Chaos*. Washington DC: American Association for the Advancement of Science, pp 47–55

Freeman WJ, Barrie JM. 1994 Chaotic oscillations and the genesis of meaning in cerebral cortex. In G Buzsaki, et al., eds, *Temporal Coding in the Brain*. Berlin: Springer Verlag, pp 13–37

Freeman WH, Skarda C. 1990 "Representations: Who needs them?" In JL McGaugh, NM Weinberger, G Lynch, eds. *Brain Organization and Memory: Cells, Systems, and Circuits*. New York: Oxford University Press, pp 375–380

Freud S. 1916 *Wit and its Relation to the Unconscious* [AA Brill, transl]. New York: Moffat, Yard & Co

Fritsch GT, Hitzig E. 1870 *Archiv für Anatomie und Psysiologie Leipzig*, pp 300–332

Fulham MJ, Brooks RA, Hallett M, DiChiro G. 1992 Cerebellar diaschisis revisited: Pontine hypometabolism and dentate sparing. *Neurology* 42:2267–2273

Fuster JM. 1995 *Memory in the Cerebral Cortex: An Empirical Approach to Neural Networks in the Human and Nonhuman Primate.* Cambridge: MIT Press

Fuxe K, Agnati LF, eds. 1991 *Volume Transmission in the Brain: Novel Mechanisms for Neural Transmission.* New York: Raven Press

Galaburda AM, ed. 1993 *Dyslexia and Development: Neurobiological Aspects of Extra-ordinary Brains.* Cambridge: Harvard University Press

Galaburda AM, Sanides F, Geschwind N. 1978 Human brain: Cytoarchitectonic left-right asymmetries in the temporal speech region. *Archives of Neurology* 35:812–817

Galaburda AM, Kemper TL. 1979 Cytoarchitectonic abnormalities in developmental dyslexia: A case study. *Annals of Neurology* 6:94–100

Galasko D, Kwo-on-Yuen PF, Klauber MR, Thai LJ. 1990 Neurological findings in Alzheimer's disease and normal ageing. *Archives of Neurology* 47:625–627

Galton F. 1907 *Inquiries into Human Faculty and Its Development.* London: JM Dent & Sons

Gardner H. 1983 *Frames of Mind: The Theory of Multiple Intelligences.* New York: Basic Books

Gasquoine PG. 1993 Alien hand sign. *Journal of Clinical and Experimental Neuropsychology* 15:653–667

Gatter KC, Winfield DA, Powel TPS. 1980 An electron microscopic study of the types and population of neurons in the cortex of the motor and visual areas of the cat and rat. *Brain* 103:245–258

Gazzaniga MS. 1989 Organization of the human brain. *Science* 245:947–952

Gazzaniga MS, Holtzman JD, Smylie CS. 1987 Speech without conscious awareness. *Neurology* 37:682–685

Gazzaniga MS, Kutas M, Van Petten C, Fendrich R. 1989 Human callosal function: MRI-verified neuropsychological functions. *Neurology* 39:942–946

Gearing M, Olson DA, Watts RL, Mirra SS. 1994 Progressive supranuclear palsy: Neurologic and clinical heterogeneity. *Neurology* 44:1015–1024

Gerard G, Weisberg LA. 1986 MRI periventricular lesions in adults. *Neurology* 36:990–1001

Gerstmann J. 1924 Fingeragnosie: Eine umschriebene Störung der Orientierung am eigenen Körper. *Weiner Klinische Wochenschrift* 37:1010–1012

Geschwind N. 1965a Disconnexion syndromes in animals and man. *Brain* 88:237–294, 585–644

Geschwind N. 1965b The organization of language in the brain. *Science* 170:940–944

Geschwind N. 1975 The borderland of Neurology and psychiatry: some common misconceptions. In DF Benson, D Blumer, eds, *Psychiatric Aspects of Neurological Disease*. New York: Grune & Stratton, pp 1–9

Geschwind N. 1979 Specializations of the human brain. *Scientific American* 241(3):180–201

Geschwind N., Galaburda AM. 1987 *Cerebral Lateralization: Biological Mechanisms, Associations, and Pathology*. Cambridge: MIT Press

Geschwind N, Kaplan E. 1962 A human cerebral disconnection syndrome: a preliminary report. *Neurology* 12:675–685

Geschwind N, Quadfasel FA, Segarra JM. 1968 Isolation of the speech area. *Neuropsychologia* 4:327–340

Gillberg C, Coleman M. 1993 *The Biology of the Autistic Syndromes* 2d ed. New York: Cambridge University Press

Gilovich T. 1991 *How We Know What Isn't So: The Fallibility of Human Reason in Everyday Life*. New York: Macmillan

Gladwin T. 1970 *East is a Big Bird*. Cambridge: Harvard University Press

Glickstein M. 1988 The discovery of the visual cortex. *Scientific American*, 118–127

Gloor P, Olivier A, Quesney LF, et al. 1982 The role of the limbic system in experiential phenomena of temporal lobe epilepsy. *Annals of Neurology* 12:129–144

Gold PE, Zornetzer SF. 1983 The mnemon and its juices: Neuromodulation of memory processes. *Behavior and Neural Biology* 38:151–189

Golgi C. 1873 Sulla struttura della sostanza grigia dell cervello. *Gazzetta Medica Lombarda* 33:244–246

Goon Y, Robinson S, Lavy S. 1973 Electroencephalographic changes in schizophrenic patients. *Israel Annals of Psychiatry* 11:99–107

Goossens LAZ, Anderman F, Anderman E, Remillard GM. 1990 Reflex seizures induced by calculation, card of board games, and spatial tasks: A review of 25 patients and delineation of the epileptic syndrome. *Neurology* 40:1171–1176

Gordon AG. 1994 Musical hallucinations. *Neurology* 44:986–987

Gordon HW. 1983 Cognitive asymmetry in dyslexic families. *Neuropsychologia* 18:645–656

Gorman DG, Cummings JL. 1992 Hypersexuality following septal injury. *Archives of Neurology* 49:308–310

Gorman DG, Unützer J. 1993 Brodmann's "missing" numbers. *Neurology* 43:226–227

Gowers WR. 1893 *A Manual of Diseases of the Nervous System*, vol. II, containing Part IV, "Diseases of the Brain and Cranial Nerves," and Part IV, "General and Functional Diseases of the Nervous System." London: J & A Churchill

Graffmann J, Levitan I, Massaquoi S, et al. 1992 Cognitive planning in patients with cerebellar atrophy. *Neurology* 42:1493–1496

Graf-Radford NR, Welsh K, Godersky J. 1987 Callosal apraxia. *Neurology* 37:100–105

Graham JR. 1993 *MMPI–2: Assessing Personality and Psychopathology.* New York: Oxford University Press

Gravenstein JS, Kalhan S, Balamoutsos NG. 1981 Of breath and spirits. *Journal of the American Medical Association* 246:1091–1092

Gray CM, Engel AK, Konig P, Singer W. 1990 Stimulus-dependent neuronal oscillations in cat visual cortex: Receptive field properties and feature dependence. *European Journal of Neuroscience* 2:607

Guberman A, Cantu-Reyna G, Stuss D, Broughton R. 1986 Nonconvulsive generalized status epilepticus: Clinical features, neuropsychological testing, and long-term follow-up. *Neurology* 36:1284–1291

Gur RC, Skolnick BE, Gur RE. 1994 Effects of emotional discrimination tasks on cerebral blood flow: Regional activation and its relation to performance. *Brain and Cognition* 25:271–286

Habib M, Gayraud D, Oliva A, et al. 1991 Effects of handedness and sex on the morphology of the corpus callosum: A study with brain magnetic resonance imaging. *Brain and Cognition* 16:41–61

Halgren E, Walter RD, Cherlow DG, Crandall PH. 1978 Mental phenomena evoked by stimulation of the human hippocampal formation and amygdala. *Brain* 101:83–117

Hallett M, Lebiedowska MK, Thomas SL, et al. 1993 Locomotion of autistic adults. *Archives of Neurology* 50:1304–1308

Halpern DF. 1991 *Sex Differences in Cognitive Abilities*, 2d ed. Hillsdale, NJ: Lawrence Earlbaum and Associates

Hanlon RE, ed. 1991 *Cognitive Microgenesis: A Neuropsychological Perspective*. New York: Springer Verlag

Harlow JM. 1868 Recovery from the passage of an iron bar through the head. *Massachusetts Medical Society Publication* 2:327–347 [See also the earlier Harlow JM. 1848 Passage of an iron rod through the head. *Boston Medical Surgery Journal* 39:389–393]

Hamilton M, ed. 1974 *Fish's Clinical Psychopathology*. Baltimore: Williams & Wilkins

Harrell LE, Duvall E, Folks DG, et al. 1991 The relationship of high-intensity signals on magnetic resonance images to cognitive and psychiatric state in Alzheimer's disease. *Archives of Neurology* 48:1136–1140

Hart JH, Lewis PJ, Lesser RP, et al. 1993 Anatomic correlates of memory from intracarotid amobarbital injections with technetium Tc 99m hexamethylpropyleneamine oxime SPECT. *Archives of Neurology* 50:745–750

Hartmann JA, Wolz WA, Roeltgen DP, Loverso FL. 1991 Denial of visual perception. *Brain and Cognition* 16:29–40

Harvey AS, Hopkins IJ, Bowe JM, et al. 1993 Frontal lobe epilepsy: Clinical seizure characteristics and localization with ictal ^{99m}Tc-HMPAO SPECT. *Neurology* 43:1966–1980

Haug H. 1984 Effect of secular acceleration on the human brain weight and its changes during ageing. *Gegenbaurs Morphologische Jahresblat* 130:481–500

Hausser-Hauw C, Bancaud J. 1987 Gustatory hallucinations in epileptic seizures: Electrophysiological, clinical and anatomical corelates. *Brain* 110:339–359

Haymaker W, Schiller F, eds. 1970 *The Founders of Neurology*, 2d ed. Springfield, IL: Charles C Thomas

Hearst E. 1991 Psychology and nothing. *American Scientist* 79:432–443

Heron W. 1957 The pathology of boredom. *Scientific American* 196:52–56

Hershey LA, Modic MT, Greenough PG, Jadde DF. 1987 Magnetic resonance imaging in vascular dementia. *Neurology* 37:29–36

Hess B, Mikhailov A. 1994 Self-organization in living cells. *Science* 264:223–225

Hinkin CH, van Gorp WG, Satz P, et al. 1992 Depressed mood and its relationship to neuropsychological test performance in HIV-1 seropositive individuals. *Journal of Clinical and Experimental Neuropsychology.* 14:289–297

Horowitz MJ. 1975 Hallucinations: An information processing approach. In RK Siegel, LJ West, eds, *Hallucinations: Behavior, Experience, and Theory*. New York: John Wiley & Sons, pp 163–196

Horsley V. 1886 Brain Surgery. *British Medical Journal* 2:670–675

Howieson DB, Holm LA, Kaye JA, et al. 1993 Neurologic function in the optimally healthy oldest old: Neuropsychological evaluation. *Neurology* 43:1882–1886

Hubel DH, Wiesel TN. 1972 Laminar and columnar distribution of geniculo-cortical fibers in the Macaque monkey. *Journal of Comparative Neurology* 158:267–294

Huber SJ, Cummings JL, eds. 1992 *Parkinson's Disease: Neurobehavioral Aspects*. New York: Oxford

Hulette CM, Earl NL, Crain BJ. 1992 Evaluation of cerebral biopsies for the diagnosis of dementia. *Archives of Neurology* 49:28–31

Huppert FA, Brayne C, O'Connor DW. 1994 *Dementia and Normal Ageing*. New York: Cambridge University Press

Husband AJ, ed. 1992 *Behavior and Immunity*. Boca Raton, FL: CRC Press

Huxley A. 1946 *Science, Liberty and Peace*. New York: Harper, pp 35–36

Hyman BT, van Hoesen GW, Damasio AR. 1990 Memory-related neural systems in Alzheimer's disease: An anatomic study. *Neurology* 40:1721–1730

ILAE. 1981 Commission on classification and terminology of the International League Against Epilepsy. Proposal for revised clinical and electroencephalographic classification of epileptic seizures. *Epilepsia* 30:389–399

Irle E, Peper M, Wowra B, Kunze S. 1994 Mood changes after surgery for tumors of the cerebral cortex. *Archives of Neurology* 51:164–174

Ironside R. 1956 Disorders of laughter due to brain lesions. *Brain* 79:589–609

Isaacson RL. 1982 *The Limbic System*, 2d ed. New York: Plenum Press

Jackson JH. 1870 *Selected Writings of John Hughlings Jackson*. Edited by J Taylor. Reprint, London: Staples Press, 1931

Jacobs BL. 1994 Serotonin, motor activity and depression-related disorders. *American Scientist* 82:456–463

Jacobs L, Karpick A, Bozian D, et al. 1981 Auditory-visual synesthesia: Sound induced photisms. *Archives of Neurology* 38:211–216

Jacome DE, Gumnit RJ. 1979 Audioalgesia and audiovisuoalgesic synesthesias: Epileptic manifestation. *Neurology* 29:1050–1053

James W. 1890 *The Principles of Psychology*. New York: Henry Holt & Co.

James W. 1902 *The Varieties of Religious Experience (being the Gifford lectures on natural religion at Edinburgh in 1901–1902)*. Reprint, New York: Vintage, 1990

Jeavons PM, Bishop A, Harding GFA. 1986 The prognosis of photosensitivity. *Epilepsia* 27:569–575

Jefferson JW, Marshall JR. 1981 *Neuropsychiatric Features of Medical Disorders*. New York: Plenum Press

Jelicic M, Bonke B, et al. 1992 Implicit memory for words presented during anæsthesia. *European Journal of Cognitive Psychology* 4:71–80

Johnson, R, Rorhbaugh JW, Ross JL. 1993 Altered brain development in Turner's syndrome: An event-related potential study. *Neurology* 43:801–808

Judd T, Gardner H, Geschwind N. 1983 Alexia without agraphia in a composer. *Brain* 106:435–457

Julesz B. 1981 Textons, the elements of texture perception, and their interactions. *Nature* (London) 290:91–97

Kahn HJ, ed. 1991 Cognitive and neuropsychological aspects of calculation disorders [special issue]. *Brain and Cognition* 17:97–308

Kandel ER. 1979 Psychotherapy and the single synapse: The impact of psychiatric thought on neurobiologic research. *New England Journal of Medicine* 301:1028–1037

Kawamura M, Hirayama K, Shinohara Y, et al. 1987 Alloæsthesia. *Brain* 10:225–236

Kenshalo DR, Isaac W. 1977 Informational and arousal properties of olfaction. *Physiology and Behavior* 18:1085–1087

Kieburtz KD, Epstein LG, Gelbard HA, Greenamyre T. 1991 Excitotoxicity and dopaminergic dysfunction in the acquired immunodeficiency syndrome dementia complex: Therapeutic implications. *Archives of Neurology* 48:1281–1284

Kihlstrom JF. 1987 The cognitive unconscious. *Science* 237:1445–1452

Kim JJ, Fanselow MS. 1992 Modality-specific retrograde amnesia of fear. *Science* 256:675–676

Kim S-G, Ugurbil K, Strick PL. 1994 Activation of a cerebellar output nucleus during cognitive processing. *Science* 265:949–951

Kish SJ, El-Awar M, Stuss D, et al. 1994 Neuropsychological test performance in patients with dominantly inherited spinocerebellar ataxia: Relationship to ataxia severity. *Neurology* 44:1738–1746

Klawans HL, ed. 1990 Emerging strategies in Parkinson's disease. *Neurology* 40[Suppl 3](10)

Klima ES, Bellugi U. 1979 *The Signs of Language*. Cambridge: Harvard University Press

Klüver H. 1937 "Psychic blindness" and other symptoms following bilateral temporal lobectomy in rhesus monkeys. *American Journal of Physiology* 119:352–353

Klüver H. 1966 Single reprint of the two earlier volumes, *Mescal* (1928) and *Mechanisms of Hallucination* (1942). Chicago: University of Chicago Press

Klüver H, Bucy PC. 1939 Preliminary analysis of functions of the temporal lobes in monkeys. *Archives of Neurology and Psychiatry* 42:979–1000

Kornhüber HH. 1974 Cerebral cortex, cerebellum and basal ganglia: An introduction to their motor function. In FO Schmitt, FG Worden, eds, *The Neurosciences Third Study Program*. Cambridge: MIT press, pp 267–280

Kornhüber HH, Deecke L. 1965 Hirnpotentialänderungen bei Wirlkürbewegungen und passiven Bewegungen des Menschen: Bereitschaftspotential und reafferente Potentiali. *Plfüger's Archiv für die Gesamte Psychiologie* 284:1–17

Kubovy M, Pomerantz JR, eds. 1981 *Perceptual Organization* Hillsdale, NJ: Lawrence Earlbaum and Associates

Lakoff G, Johnson M. 1980 *Metaphors We Live By*. Chicago: University of Chicago Press

Lance JW. 1986 Visual hallucinations and their possible pathophysiology. In JD Pettigrew, KJ Sanderson, WR Levick, eds. *Visual Neuroscience*. New York: Cambridge University Press, pp. 374–380

Lance JW. 1993 *Mechanisms and Management of Headache*, 5th ed. Boston: Butterworth-Heinemann

Lance JW, McLeod JG. 1981 *A Physiological Approach to Clinical Neurology* 3d ed. London: Butterworths

Land EH. 1977 The retinex theory of color vision. *Scientific American* 200:84–89

Landis T, Cummings JL, Benson DF, Palmer EP. 1986 Loss of topographic familiarity: An environmental agnosia. *Archives of Neurology* 43:132–136

Landis T, Graves R, Benson F, Hebben N. 1982 Visual recognition through kinæsthetic mediation. *Psychological Medicine* 12:515–531

Lanska DJ, Lanska MJ, Mendez MF. 1987 Brainstem auditory hallucinosis. *Neurology* 37:1685

Lashley KS. 1941 Patterns of cerebral integration indicated by scotomas of migraine. *Archives of Neurology and Psychiatry* 46:331–339

Laureno R. 1983 Central pontine myelinolysis following rapid correction of hyponatremia. *Annals of Neurology* 13:232–242

Lavine TZ. 1984 *From Socrates to Sartre: The Philosophic Quest.* New York: Bantam Books

Leão APP. 1944 Spreading depression of activity in cerebral cortex. *Journal of Neurophysiology* 7:359–390

Leary DE, ed. 1990 *Metaphors in the History of Psychology.* New York: Cambridge University Press

Ledoux JE, Wilson DH, Gazzaniga MS. 1979 Beyond Commissurotomy: Clues to Consciousness. In MS Gazzanniga, ed, *Handbook of Behavioral Neurobiology, vol 2: Neuropsychology.* New York: Plenum Press, pp 543–554

Lee SI, Phillips LH, Jane JA. 1991 Somato-somatic referred pain caused by suprasegmental spinal cord tumor. *Neurology* 41:928–930

Leiner HC, Leiner AL, Dow RS. 1991 The human cerebro-celebellar system: Its computing, cognitive, and language skills. *Behavioral Brain Research* 44:113–128

Lepore FE. 1990 Spontaneous visual phenomena with visual loss: 104 patients with lesions of retinal and neural afferent pathways. *Neurology* 40:444–447

Lessell S, Cohen MM. 1979 Phosphenes induced by sound. *Neurology* 29:1524–1527

LeVay S. 1993 *The Sexual Brain.* Cambridge: MIT Press

Levin HS. 1990 Cognitive rehabilitation: Unproved but promising. *Archives of Neurology* 47:223–224

Levin HS. 1994 A guide to clinical neuropsychological testing. *Archives of Neurology* 51:854–859

Levin HS, Eisenberg HM, Benton AL. 1991 *Frontal Lobe Function and Dysfunction.* New York: Oxford University Press

Levine DN. 1978 Prosopagnosia and visual object agnosia: A behavioral study. *Neuropsychologia* 5:341–365

Lezak MD. 1983 *Neuropsychological Assessment,* 2d ed. New York: Oxford University Press

Libet B. 1985 Unconscious cerebral initiative and the role of conscious will in voluntary action. *The Behavioral and Brain Sciences* 8:529–566

Lissauer H. 1890 Ein Fall von seelenblindheit nebst einem Beitrage zur Theorie derselben. *Archiv für Psychiatrie und Nervenkrankheiten* 21:222–270

Lopez JR, Adornato BT, Hoyt WF. 1993 "Entomopia": A remarkable case of cerebral polyopia. *Neurology* 43:2145–2146

Lorente de Nó R. 1943 Cerebral cortex: Architecture, intracortical connections, motor projections. In JF Fulton, ed, *Physiology of the Nervous System*, 2d ed. Oxford: Oxford University Press, pp 274–301

Lorenz K. 1965 *Über Tierisches und Menschliches Verhalten; Aus dem Werdegang der Verhaltenslehre* (Bd I, II). Munich: Peiper

Loring DW, Meador KJ, Lee GP, King DW. 1992 *Amobarbital Effects and Lateralized Brain Function. The Wada Test.* New York: Springer Verlag

Loring DW, Papanicolaou AC. 1987 Memory assessment in neuropsychology: Theoretical considerations and practical utility. *Journal of Clinical and Experimental Neuropsychology* 9:340–358

Luciano D, Devinsky O, Perrine K. 1993 Crying seizures. *Neurology* 43:2113–2117

Luria AR. 1959 Disorders of "simultaneous perception" in a case of bilateral occipitoparietal brain injury. *Brain* 83:437–449

MacIntyre A. 1988 *Whose Justice, Which Rationality?* Notre Dame, Indiana: University of Notre Dame Press

MacLean PD. 1949 Psychosomatic disease and the "visceral brain." Recent developments bearing on the Papez theory of emotion. *Psychosomatic Medicine* 11:338–353

MacLean PD. 1967 The brain in relation to empathy and medical education. *Journal of Nervous and Mental Diseases* 144:374–382

MacLean PD. 1978 Challenges of the Papez heritag. In K Livingston, O Hornkiewicz, eds, *Limbic Mechanisms*. New York: Plenum Press

MacLean PD. 1990 *The Triune Brain in Evolution: Role in Paleocerebral Functions.* New York: Plenum Press

Mair RG, McEntee WJ, Zattore RJ. 1985 Monoamine activity correlates with psychometric impairments in Korsakoff's disease. *Behavioral and Brain Research* 15:247–254

Malamut BL, Graf-Radford N. Chawluk J, et al. 1992 Memory in a case of bilateral thalamic infarction. *Neurology* 42:163–169

Manford M, Hart YM, Sander JWAS, Shorvon SD. 1992 The National General Practice Study of Epilepsy: The syndromic classification of the International league against epilepsy applied to epilepsy in a general population. *Archives of Neurology* 49:801–808

Mapou RL. 1988 Testing to detect brain damage: An alternative to what may no longer be useful. *Journal of Clinical and Experimental Neuropsychology* 10:271–278

Markowitsch HJ. 1993 Brodmann's numbers. *Neurology* 43:1863–1864

Martin WRW, Clark C, Ammann W, et al. 1992 Cortical glucose metabolism in Huntington's disease. *Neurology* 42:223–229

Mateer CA, Sohlberg MM. 1988 A Paradigm Shift in Memory rehabilitation. In HA Whitaker, ed, *Neuropsychological Studies of Nonfocal Brain Damage: Dementia and Trauma*. New York: Springer Verlag, pp 202–225

Mayo Clinic and Mayo Foundation. 1991 *Clinical Examinations in Neurology*, 6th ed. St Louis: Mosby Yearbook

McAdams S, Bigand E, eds. 1993 *Thinking in Sound: The Cognitive Psychology of Human Audition*. New York: Oxford University Press

McClelland JL, Rumelhart DE, Hinton GE. 1986 The appeal of parallel distributed processing. In DE Rumelhart, JL McClelland, eds, *Parallel Distributed Processing: Explorations in the Microstructure of Cognition*, vol 1. Cambridge: MIT Press, pp 3–44

McEntee WJ, Crook TH. 1990 Age-associated memory impairment: A role for catecholamines. *Neurology* 40:526–530

McGlone J, Gupta S, Humphrey D. et al. 1990 Screening for early dementia using memory complaints from patients and relatives. *Archives of Neurology* 47:1189–1193

McGlynn SM, Schacter DL. 1989 Unawareness of deficits in neuropsychological syndromes. *Journal of Clinical and Experimental Neuropsychology* 11:143–205

McLachlan RS, Chovaz CJ, Blume WT, Girvin JP. 1992 Temporal lobectomy for intractable epilepsy in patients over age 45 years. *Neurology* 42:662–665

McNeill D. 1992 *Hand and Mind: What Gestures Reveal About Thought* Chicago: University of Chicago Press

McWhirter DP, Sanders SA, Reinisch JM. 1990 *Homosexuality/Heterosexuality: Concepts of Sexual Orientation*. New York: Oxford University Press

Mendez MF, Grau R, Doss RC, Taylor JL. 1993 Schizophrenia in epilepsy: Seizure and psychosis variables. *Neurology* 43:1073–1077

Merzenich MM, Nelson RJ, Kaas JH, et al. 1987 Variability in hand surface representations in areas 3b and 1 in adult owl and squirrel monkeys. *Journal of Comparative Neurology* 258:281–296

Mesulam MM. 1981a A cortical network for directed attention and unilateral neglect. *Annals of Neurology* 10:309–325

Mesulam MM. 1981b Dissociative states with abnormal temporal lobe EEG: Multiple personality and the illusion of possession. *Archives of Neurology* 38:176–181

Mesulam MM. 1985a Patterns in behavioral neuroanatomy: Association areas, the limbic system, and hemispheric specialization. Mesulam MM. 1985b Attention, Confusional States, and Neglect. In M-Marsel Mesulam, ed, *Principles of Behavioral Neurology*. Philadelphia: FA Davis Company, pp 1–70, 125–168

Metter EJ, Hanson WR, Jackson CA, et al. 1990 Temporoparietal cortex in aphasia: Evidence from positron emission tomography. *Archives of Neurology* 47:1235–1238

Miller EN, Satz P, Visscher B. 1991 Computerized and conventional neuropsychological assessment of HIV-1-infected homosexual men. *Neurology* 41:1608–1616

Mirra SS, Heyman A, McKeel D, et al. 1991 The consortium to establish a registry for Alzheimer's disease (CERAD): II. Standardization of the neuropathologic assessment of Alzheimer's disease. *Neurology* 41:479–486

Mirsen TR, Lee DH, Wong CJ, et al. 1991 Clinical correlates of white-matter changes on magnetic resonance imaging scans of the brain. *Archives of Neurology* 48:1015–1021

Mittan, R. 1986 Fear of seizures. In *Psychopathology in Epilepsy: Social Dimensions*. New York: Oxford University Press, pp 90–121

Mohr LP, et al. 1978 *Neurology* 28:311–324

Moniz E (Antonio Caetanno deAbreu Freire). 1927 L'encèphalographe arterial son importance dans la localisation tumeres cèrèbrales. *Revue neurologique* 2:72–90

Moniz E (Antonio Caetanno deAbreu Freire). 1936 *Tentatives opératoires dans le traitment de certaines psychoses*. Paris: Masson

Moran F, Desimone R. 1985 Selective attention gates visual processing in the extrastriate cortex. *Science* 229:782–784

Mountcastle VN. 1957 Modality and topographic properties of single neurones of cat's somatic sensory cortex. *Journal of Neurophysiology* 20:408–434

Mountcastle VN. 1979 An organizing principle for cerebral function: The unit module and the distributed system. In FO Schmitt, FG Worden, eds, *The Neurosciences Fourth Study Program* Cambridge: MIT Press, pp 21–42

Murata S, Naritomi H, Sawada T. 1994 Musical auditory hallucinations caused by a brainstem lesion. *Neurology* 44:156–158

Nagel T. 1974 What is it like to be a bat? *Philosophical Review* 83. Reprinted in *Readings in Philosophy and Psychology*, vol 1, edited by N Block, Cambridge: Harvard University Press, 1980

Nagel T. 1986 *The View from Nowhere*. New York: Oxford University Press

Nauta WJH, Feirtag M. 1986 *Fundamental Neuroanatomy*. New York: WH Freeman

Niedenthal PM, Kitayama S. 1994 *The Heart's Eye: Emotional Influences in Perception and Attention*. San Diego: Academic Press

Nieuwenhuys R. 1985 *Chemoarchitecture of the Brain*. New York: Springer Verlag

Nieuwenhuys R, Voogd J. van Huijzen Chr. 1988 *The Human Central Nervous System: A Synopsis and Atlas*, 3d ed. New York: Springer Verlag

NIH Concensus Development Panel on Depression in Late Life. 1992 Diagnosis and treatment of depression in late life. *Journal of the American Medical Association* 268:1018–1024

NINDS-AIREN International Workshop. 1993 Vascular dementia: Diagnostic criteria for research studies. *Neurology* 43:250–260

Ojemann GA. 1974 Mental arithmetic during human thalamic stimulation. *Neuropsychologia* 12:1–10

Ojemann GA, Ojemann J, Lettich E, Berger M. 1989 Cortical language localization in left-dominant hemisphere. *Journal of Neurosurgery* 71:316–326

Ojemann GA, Whitaker HA. 1978 Language localization and variability. *Brain and Language* 6:239–260

O'Kusky J, Strauss E, Kosaka B, et al. 1988 The corpus callosum is larger with right-hemisphere cerebral speech dominance. *Annals of Neurology* 24:379–383

Oldfield RC. 1971 The assessment and analysis of handedness: The Edinburgh inventory. *Neuropsychologia* 9:97

Olszewski J. 1965 Subcortical arteriosclerotic encephalopathy: Review of the literature on the so-called Binswanger's disease and presentation of two cases. *World Neurology* 3:359–375

Ommaya AK. 1994 Emotion and the evolution of neural complexity. *Wescom 2* 1:23–28 (1992); *Wescom 3* 1:8–17 (1993)

Palca J. 1990 Insights from Broken brains. *Science* 248:812–814

Palmer S, Rock I. 1994 Rethinking perceptual organization: The role of uniform connectedness. *Psychonomic Bulletin and Review* 1:29–55

Palmini A, Gloor P. 1992 The localizing value of auras in partial seizures: A prospective and retrospective study. *Neurology* 42:801–808

Papez JW. 1937 A proposed mechanism of emotion. *Archives of Neurology and Psychiatry* 38:725–743

Peatfield RC, Rose FC. 1981 Migrainous visual symptoms in a woman without eyes. *Archives of Neurology* 38:466

Peiper A. 1951 Instinkt und angeborene scheme beim saugling. *Zeitschrift für Tierpsychologie* 8:449–456

Penfield W, Jasper H. 1954 *Epilepsy and the Functional Anatomy of the Human Brain*. Boston: Little, Brown

Penfield W, Roberts L. 1959 *Speech and Brain Mechanisms*. Princeton, NJ: Princeton University Press

Pepin EP, Auray-Pepin L. 1993 Selective dorsolateral frontal lobe dysfunction associated with diencephalic amnesia. *Neurology* 43:733–741

Peppard RF, Martin WRW, Carr GD, et al., 1992 Cerebral glucose metabolism in Parkinson's disease with and without dementia. *Archives of Neurology* 49:1262–1268

Perani D, Bressi S, Cappa SF, et al. 1993 Evidence of multiple memory systems in the human brain: An [^{18}F]FDG PET metabolic study. *Brain* 116:903–919

Persinger MA, Makarec K. 1992 The feeling of a presence and verbal meaningfulness in context of temporal lobe function: Factor analytic verification of the muses? *Brain and Cognition* 20:217–226

Petersen RC, Smith G, Kokmen E, et al. 1992 Memory function in normal aging. *Neurology* 42:396–401

Petersen SE, Fox PT, Posner MI, et al. 1988 Positron emission tomographic studies of the cortical anatomy of single-word processing. *Nature* 331:585–589

Petersen SE, Fox PT, Snyder AZ, Raichle ME. 1990 Activation of extrastriate and frontal cortical areas by visual words and word-like stimuli. *Science* 249:1041–1044

Petry A, Cummings JL, Hill MA, Shapira J. 1988 Personality alterations in dementia of the Alzheimer type. *Archives of Neurology* 45:1187–1190

Picard RW. 1995 Affective computing. *MIT Media Laboratory Perceptual Computing Section Technical Report* No. 321. Cambridge, MA. http://www.media.MIT.edu/~picard/

Pillon B, Dubois B, Ploska A, Agid Y. 1991 Severity and specificity of cognitive impairment in Alzheimer's, Huntington's, and Parkinson's diseases and progressive supranuclear palsy. *Neurology* 41:624–643

Pincus JH. 1993 Neurologist's role in understanding violence. *Archives of Neurology* 50:867–869

Piotrowski C, Lubin B. 1989 Assessment practices of division 38 practitioners. *Health Psychologist* 11:1–2

Poeck K. 1985 Pathological laughter and crying. In PJ Vinken, GW Bruyn, HL Klawans, eds, *Handbook of Clinical Neurology*. Amsterdam: Elsevier, pp 219–225

Poizner H, Klima ES, Bellugi U. 1990 *What the Hands Reveal About the Brain*. Cambridge: MIT Press

Polk M, Kertesz A. 1993 Music and language in degenerative disease of the brain. *Brain and Cognition* 22:98–117

Popper KR, Eccles JC. 1977 *The Self and its Brain*. Berlin: Springer Verlag

Primack D. 1988 Minds with and without language. In L Weiskrantz, ed, *Thought Without Language*. Oxford: Clarendon Press, pp 46–65

Progoff I. 1959 *Depth Psychology and Modern Man*. New York: Julian Press

Progoff I. 1994 *At a Journal Workshop*. New York: Putnam

Puglia JF, Brenner RP, Soso MJ. 1992 Relationship between prolonged and self-limited photoparoxysmal responses and seizure incidence: Study and review. *Journal of Clinical Neurophysiology* 9:137–144

Purves D. 1994 *Neural Activity and the Growth of the Brain*. New York: Cambridge University Press

Quin CE. 1994 The soul and the pneuma in the function of the nervous system after Galen. *Journal of the Royal Society of Medicine* 87:393–395

Racy A, Osborn MA, Vern BA, Molinari GF. 1980 Epileptic aphasia: First onset of a prolonged monosymptomatic status epilepticus in adults. *Archives of Neurology* 37:419–422

Ramón y Cajal S. 1901–1917 *Recuerdos de mi Vida* [Madrid]. Translated as *Recollections of My Life* by EH Craigie, J Cano, Cambridge: MIT Press, 1989

Ramón y Cajal S. 1933 Neuronismo o reticularismo? *Archives de Neurobiologica* 13 [Madrid]. Translated as *Neuron Theory or Reticular Theory? Objective Evidence of the Anatomical Unity of Nerve Cells* by Purkiss & Fox, Madrid: Consejo Sup. de. Invest. Cientificas, Instituto Ramón y Cajal, 1954

Ratner LG. 1983 *The Musical Experience*. New York: WH Freeman

Renault B, Signoret JL, Debruille L, et al. 1989 Brain potentials reveal covert facial recognition in prosopagnosia. *Neuropsychologia* 27:905–912

Reps P. 1994 *Zen Flesh, Zen Bones: A Collection of Zen and Pre-Zen Writings*. New York: Doubleday

Restak R. 1993 The neurological defense of violent crime: "Insanity defense" retooled. *Archives of Neurology* 50:869–871

Riddoch G. 1917 Dissociation of visual perception due to occipital injuries, with especial reference to appreciation of movement. *Brain* 40:15–57

Ritaccio AL, Hickling EJ, Ramani V. 1992 The role of dominant premotor cortex and grapheme to phoneme transformation in reading epilepsy: A neuroanatomic, neurophysiologic, and neuropsychological study. *Archives of Neurology* 49:933–939

Rizzo JF, Cronin-Golomb A, Growdon JH, et al. 1992 Retinocalcarine function in Alzheimer's disease: A clinical and electrophysiological study. *Archives of Neurology* 49:93–101

Rizzo M, Hurtig R. 1987 Looking but not seeing: Attention, perception, and eye movements in simultanagnosia. *Neurology* 37:1642–1648

Robertson IH, Marshall J, eds. 1993 *Unilateral Neglect: Clinical and Experimental Studies*. Hillsdale, NJ: Lawrence Earlbaum Associates

Rolak LA, Baram TZ. 1987 Charles Bonnett syndrome. *Journal of the American Medical Association* 257:2036

Roland RE. 1982 Cortical regulation of selective attention in man. A regional cerebral blood flow study. *Journal of Neurophysiology* 48:1059–1078

Rorty A, ed. 1980 *Explaining Emotions*. Berkeley: University of California Press

Rosenberg ML, Corbett JJ, Smith C, et al., 1993 Cerebrospinal fluid diversion procedures in pseudotumor cerebri. *Neurology* 43:1071–1072

Ross ED, Harner JH, de la Corte-Utamsing JH, Pardy PD. 1981 How the brain integrates affect and propositional language into a unified behavioral function. *Archives of Neurology* 38:745–748

Ruuskanen-Uoti H, Salmi T. 1994 Epileptic seizure induced by a product marketed as a "brainwave synchronizer." *Neurology* 44:180–181

Sackeim HA, Greenberg MS, Weiman AL, et al. 1982 Hemispheric asymmetry in the expression of positive and negative emotions: Neurologic evidence. *Archives of Neurology* 39:210–218

Sackein HA, Freeman, McElhiney M, et al. 1992 Effects of major depression on estimates of intelligence. *Journal of Clinical and Experimental Neuropsychology* 14:268–288

Sacks O. 1992 *Migraine: Understanding a Common Disorder*. Los Angeles: University of California Press, pp 51–98, 273–298

Sano F. 1918 James Henry Pullem, the genius of Earlswood. *Journal of Mental Science* 64:251–267

Sarnat HB, Netsky MG. 1981 *Evolution of the Nervous System*, 2d ed. New York: Oxford University Press

Saygi S, Katz A, Marks DA, Spencer SS. 1992 Frontal lobe partial seizures and psychogenic seizures: Comparison of clinical and ictal characteristics. *Neurology* 42:1274–1277

Sbordone RJ, Rudd M. 1986 Can psychologists recognize neurological disorders in their patients? *Journal of Clinical and Experimental Neuropsychology* 8:285–291

Schachter SC. 1988 Hormonal considerations in women with seizures. *Archives of Neurology.* 45:1267–1270

Schacter DL, Tulving E. 1994 *Memory Systems 1994*. Cambridge: MIT Press

Scheerer R. 1924 Die entoptische Sichtbarkeit der Blutbewegung im Auge und ihre klinische Bedeutung. *Klinische Monatsblatt der Augenheilkunde* 73:67–107

Schiffman SS. 1983 Taste and smell in disease (parts I and II). *New England Journal of Medicine* 308:1275–1279, 1337–1343

Schore AN. 1994 *Affect Regulation and the Origin of the Self: The Neurobiology of Emotional Development*. Hillsdale, NJ: Lawrence Earlbaum and Associates

Schmahmann JD. 1991 An emerging concept: The cerebellar contribution to higher function. *Archives of Neurology* 48:1178–1187

Schmidt R, Fazekas F, Offenbacher H, et al. 1991 Magnetic resonance imaging of white matter lesions and cognitive impairment in hypertensive individuals. *Archives of Neurology* 48:417–420

Scrambler G. 1987 *Sociological Aspects of Epilepsy*. In A Hopkins, ed, *Epilepsy*. New York: Demos, pp 497–510

Seilhean D, Duyckaerts C, Vazeux R, et al., 1993 HIV-1-associated cognitive/motor complex: Absence of neuronal loss in the cerebral neocortex. *Neurology* 43:1492–1499

Selnes OA, Jacobson L, Machado AM, et al. 1991 Normative data for a brief neuropsychological screening battery. Multicenter AIDS cohort study. *Perceptual and Motor Skills* 73:539–550

Selnes OA, Galai N, Bacellar H, et al., 1995 Cognitive performance after progression to AIDS: A longitudinal study from the Multicenter AIDS Cohort Study. *Neurology* 45:267–275

Sergent J. 1987 A new look at the human split brain. *Brain* 110:1375–1392

Sergent J. 1993 Music, the brain and Ravel. *Trends in Neuroscience* 16: 168–172

Sergent J, Zuck E, Terriah S, MacDonald B. 1992 Distributed neural network underlying musical sight-reading and keyboard performance. *Science* 257:106–109

Sherrington CD, Grünbaum AS. 1902 *British Medical Journal* 2:784

Siegel RK. 1977 Hallucinations. *Scientific American* 237:132–140

Siegel RK. 1978 Cocaine Hallucinations. *American Journal of Psychiatry* 135:309–314

Siegel RK, Jarvik ME. 1975 Drug-induced hallucinations in animals and man. In RK Siegel, LJ West, eds, *Hallucinations*. New York: John Wiley & Sons, pp 81–162

Silveri MC, Leggio MG, Molinari M. 1994 The cerebellum contributes to linguistic production: A case of agrammatic speech following a right cerebellar lesion. *Neurology* 44:2047–2050

Simon HA, Newell A. 1958 Heuristic problem solving: the next advance in operations research. *Operations Research* 6(Jan–Feb)

Sinoff SE, Rosenberg M. 1990 Permanent cerebral diplopia in a migraineur. *Neurology* 40:1138–1139

Skinner BF. 1974 *About Behaviorism*. New York: Alfred Knopf

Sloboda JA. 1987 *The Musical Mind: The Cognitive Psychology of Music*. New York: Oxford University Press

Smith BD, Meyers MB, Kline R. 1989 For better or worse: Left-handedness, pathology, and talent. *Journal of Clinical and Experimental Neuropsychology* 11:944–958

Smith GS, de Leon MJ, George AE, et al., 1992 Topography of cross-sectional and longitudinal glocuse metabolic deficits in Alzheimer's disease: Pathophysiologic implications. *Archives of Neurology* 49:1142–1150

Sohlberg MM, Mateer CA. 1989 Training use of compensatory memory books: A three stage behavioral approach. *Journal of Clinical and Experimental Neuropsychology* 11:871–891

Solomon RC. 1983 *The Passions: The Myth and Nature of Human Emotion*. Notre Dame, IN: Universitry of Notre Dame Press

Solomon RC. 1990 *A Passion for Justice: Emotion and the Origin of the Social Contract*. Reading, MA: Addison-Wesley

Sommer W. 1880 Erkrankung des Ammonshornes als ætologisches Moment der Epilepsie. *Archiv für Psychiatrie und Nervenkrankheiten* 10: 631–675

Sperling MR, O'Connor MJ, Saykin AJ, et al. 1992 A noninvasive protocol for anterior temporal lobectomy. *Neurology* 42:416–422

Sperry RW. 1961 Cerebral organization and behavior. *Science* 133:1749–1757

Spreen O, Strauss E. 1991 *A Compendium of Neuropsychological Tests: Administration, Norms, and Commentary.* New York: Oxford University Press

Squire LR. 1987 *Memory and The Brain.* New York: Oxford University Press

Squire LR, Weinberger NM, Lynch G, Mcgaugh JL, eds. 1992 *Memory: Organization and Locus of Change.* New York: Oxford University Press

Squire LR, Zola-Morgan S. 1991 The medial temporal lobe memory system. *Science* 253:1380–1386

Starkstein SE, Robinson RG. 1993 *Depression in Neurologic Disease.* Baltimore: Johns Hopkins University Press

Steiner JE. 1973 The gustofacial response: Observation on normal and anencephalic newborn infants. In *Symposium on Oral Sensation and Perception.* Bethesda: National Institutes of Health, pp 254–278

Steiner I, Shahin R, Melamed E. 1987 Acute "upside down" reversal of vision in transient vertebrobasilar ischemia. *Neurology* 37:1685–1686

Sternberg S. 1969 The discovery of processing stages: Extensions of Donders' method. *Acta Psychologia* 30:276–315

Stevens JR. 1992 Abnormal reinervation as a basis for schizophrenia: A hypothesis. *Archives of General Psychiatry* 49:238–243

Stoudemire A, Fogel BS. 1993 *Psychiatric Care of the Medical Patient.* New York: Oxford University Press

Strange PG. 1993 *Brain Biochemistry and Brain Disorders.* New York: Oxford University Press

Suarez de Mendoza F. 1890 *L'Audition Coloreé.* Paris: Octave Donin

Sumi SM, Bird TD, Nochlin D, Raskind MA. 1992 Familial presenile dementia with psychosis associated with cortical neurofibrillary tangles and degeneration of the amygdala. *Neurology* 42:120–127

Swayze VW, Andreasen NC, Ehrhardt JC, et al. 1990 Developmental abnormalaties of the corpus callosum in schizophrenia. *Archives of Neurology* 47:805–808

Szentágothai J. 1974 A structural overview. *Neurosciences Research Program Bulletin* 12:354–410

Szentágothai J, Arbib MA. 1975 The "module concept" in cerebral cortex architecture. *Brain Research* 95:475–496

Takayama Y, Sugishita M, Kido T, et al. 1993 A case of foreign accent syndrome without aphasia caused by a lesion of the left precentral gyrus. *Neurology* 43:1361–1363

Talbot JD, Marrett S, Evans AC, et al. 1991 Multiple representations of pain in human cerebral cortex. *Science* 251:1355–1358

Tatemichi TK. 1990 How acute brain failure becomes chronic: A view of the mechanisms of dementia related to stroke. *Neurology* 40:1652–1659

Teunisse S, Mayke MA, Derix MA, van Crevel H. 1991 Assessing the severity of dementia: Patient and caregiver. *Archives of Neurology* 48:274–277

Thomas P, Beaumanoir A, Genton P, et al. 1992 "De novo" absence status of late onset: Report of 11 cases. *Neurology* 42:104–110

Thompson E, Palacios A, Varela FJ. 1992 Ways of coloring: Comparative color vision for cognitive science. *Behavioral and Brain Sciences* 15:1–74

Tønnessen FE, Løkken A, Høien T, Lundberg I. 1993 Dyslexia, left-handedness, and immune disorders. *Archives of Neurology* 50:411–416

Tranel D, Damasio AR. 1985 Knowledge without awareness: An autonomic index of facial recognition by prosopagnosics. *Science* 228:1453–1454

Trimble MR. 1991 *The Psychoses of Epilepsy.* New York: Raven Press

Tuchman BW. 1984 *The March of Folly.* New York: Alfred Knopf

Tulving E, Schacter DL. 1990 Priming and human memory systems. *Science* 247:301–306

Van Dongen HR, Catsman-Berrevoets CE, van Mourik M. 1994 The syndrome of "cerebellar" mutism and subsequent dysarthria. *Neurology* 44: 2040–2046

Van Essen DC, Anderson CH, Felleman DJ. 1992 Information processing in the primate visual system: An integrated systems perspective. *Science* 255:419–423

Van Gorp WG, et al. 1991 Metacognition in HIV-1 seropositive asymptomatic individuals: self-ratings versus objective neuropsychological performance. *Journal of Clinical and Experimental Neuropsychology* 13:812–819

Valenstein ES. 1986 *Unkind Cuts: The Rise and Decline of Psychosurgery and Other Radical Treatments for Mental Illness.* New York: Basic Books

Vanneste J, Augustijn P, Dirven C, et al. 1992a Shunting normal-pressure hydrocephalus: Do the benefits outweigh the risks? *Neurology* 42:54–59

Vanneste J, Augustijn P, Davies GA, et al. 1992b Normal-pressure hydrocephalus: Is cisternography still useful in selecting patients for a shunt? *Archives of Neurology* 49:366–370

Verma A, Hirsch DJ, Glatt CE, et al. 1993 Carbon monoxide: A putative neural messenger. *Science* 259:381–384

Victor M, Adams RD. 1989 *The Wernicke-Korskoff Syndrome and Related Neurologic Disorders Due to Alcoholism and Malnutrition*, 2d ed. Philadelphia: FA Davis Company

Victoroff JI, Benson DF, Grafton ST, et al. 1994 Depression in complex partial seizures: Electroencephalography and cerebral metabolic correlates. *Archives of Neurology* 51:155–163

von Eckardt B. 1993 *What is Cognitive Psychology?* Cambridge: MIT Press

von der Malsburg C. 1981 Internal report 81–2. Göttingen, FRG: Department of Neurobiology, Max Planck Institute for Biophysical Chemistry

Waldvogel JA. 1990 The bird's eye view. *American Scientist* 78:342–353

Walsh C, Cepko CL. 1992 Widespread dispersion of neuronal clones across functional regions of the cerebral cortex. *Science* 255:434–440

Wasow T. 1991 Grammatical Theory. In MI Posner, ed, *Foundations of Cognitive Science*. Cambridge: MIT Press, pp 161–205

Weddell RA. 1994 Effects of subcortical lesion site on human emotional behavior. *Brain and Cognition* 25:161–193

Weinstein EA, Bender MD. 1943 Integrated facial patterns elicited by stimulation of the brain stem. *Archives of Neurology and Psychiatry* 50:34–42

Weinstein EA, Kahn RL, Slote WH. 1955 Withdrawal, inattention, and pain asymbolia. *Archives of Neurology and Psychitary* 74:235–248

Weinstein EA, Cole M, Mitchell MS. 1963 Agnosia, aphasia. *Trasactions of the American Neurological Association* 88:172–175

Weiser HG, Engel J, Williamson P, et al. 1993 Surgically remediable temporal lobe syndrome. In J Engel, ed, *Surgical Treatment of the Epilepsies*, 2d ed. New York: Raven Press, pp 49–63

Weiskrantz L. 1986 *Blindsight: A Case Study and Implications*. Oxford: Oxford University Press

Weiskrantz L, ed. 1988 *Thought Without Language*. Oxford: Clarendon Press

Weizenbaum J. 1976 *Computer Power and Human reason: From judgment to Calculation*. New York: WH Freeman

Welsch KMA. 1987 Migraine: A biobehavioral disorder. *Archives of Neurology* 44:323–327

Werbos PJ. 1992 The cytoskeleton: Why it may be crucial to human learning and neurocontrol. *Nanobiology* 1:75–96

Werbos PJ. 1994 The brain as a neurocontroller: New hypotheses and new experimental possibilities. In K Pribram, ed, *Origins: Brain and Self*. Hillsdale, NJ: Lawrence Earlbaum and Associates, pp 680–706

Wernicke K. 1874 *Der aphasische Symptomencomplex: Eine psychologische Studie auf anatomischer Basis* [Breslau]. Translated as *The Aphasia Symptom-Complex: A Psychological Study on an Anatomic Basis*, by Cohn & Weigert. In GH`Eggert, ed, *Wernicke's Works on Aphasia: A Sourcebook and Review*. The Hague: Mouton, 1977, pp 91–145

Whitaker HA. 1979 Electrical stimulation mapping of language cortex. In O Creutzfeld, H Scheich, C Schreiner, eds, *Experimental Brain Research Supplementum II: Hearing Mechanisms and Speech*. Berlin: Springer Verlag, pp 193–204

Whitaker HA, Cummings JL. 1994 *Brain and Cognition* 26(2):103–326 [special issue devoted to analysis of the Geschwind-Behan-Galaburda model of cerebral lateralization]

Whitaker HA, Ojemann GA. 1977 Graded localization of naming from electrical stimulation mapping of the left cerebral cortex. *Nature* 270:50–51

Whitaker HA, Habinger T, Ivers R. 1985 Acalculia from a lenticular-caudate infarction. *Neurology* 35:161

Whorf B. 1956 *Language, Thought, and Reality*. Cambridge: MIT Press

Wiesel TN. 1994 Genetics and Behavior [editorial]. *Science* 264:1647. [See also the remainder of volume 264 on the theme of genes and behavior]

Wigan AL. 1844 *A New View of Insanity: The Duality of the Mind, Proved by the Structure, Functions, and Diseases of the Brain and by the Phenomena of Mental Derangement, and Shown to be Essentail to Moral Responsibility*. London: Longmann, Brown, Green & Longmans. Reprinted with a foreword by JE Bogen, Los Angeles: Joseph Simon Publisher, 1985

Wilbush J. 1992 The Sherlock Holmes paradigm–detectives and diagnosis [discussion paper]. *Journal of the Royal Society of Medicine* 85:342–345

Wilkins AJ, Zifkin B, Anderman F, McGovern E. 1982 Seizures induced by thinking. *Annals of Neurology* 11:608–612

Williams JM. 1976 Synæsthetic adjectives: A possible law of semantic change. *Language* 52:461–478

Witelson SF. 1992 Cognitive neuroanatomy: A new era. *Neurology* 42: 709–713

Wolpert I. 1924 Die simultanagnosia: Storung der Gesamtauffassung. *Zeitschrift für die Gesamte Neurologie und Psychiatrie.* 93:397–415

Wolpert L. 1993 *The Unnatural Nature of Science.* Cambridge: Harvard University Press

Woolsey CN. 1952 *Biology of Mental Health and Disease.* New York: Hoeber, p 52

Yakovlev PI. 1948 Motility, behavior and the brain. Stereodynamic organization and neural co-ordinates of behavior. *Journal of Nervous and Mental Diseases* 107(4):313–335

Yakovlev PI. 1954 Paraplegia in flexion of cerebral origin. *Journal of Neuropathology and Experimental Neurology* 13:267–296

Yakovlev PI. 1970 The structural and functional "trinity" of the body, brain and behavior. In HT Wycis, ed, *Current Research in Neurosciences, Topical Problems in Psychiatry and Neurology*, Vol 10. New York: Karger, pp 197–208

Yeomans JS. 1990 *Principles of Brain Stimulation.* 1990 New York: Oxford University Press

Young RR, Delwaide PJ. 1992 *Principles and Practice of Restorative Neurology.* Stoneham, MA: Butterworth-Heinemann

Zeki S. 1993 *A Vision of the Brain.* Oxford: Blackwell Scientific Publications

Zihl J, von Cramon D, Mai N. 1983 Selective disturbance of movement vision after bilateral brain damage. *Brain* 106:313–340

Ziporyn T. 1992 *Nameless Diseases.* New Brunswick, NJ: Rutgers University Press

Zubenko GS, Moossy J. 1988 Major depression in primary dementia: Clinical and neuropathologic correlates. *Archives of Neurology* 45:1182–1186

Zubenko GS, Moossy J, Martinez AJ, et al. 1991 Neuropathologic and neurochemical correlates of psychosis in primary depression. *Archives of Neurology* 48:619–624

Zweig RM, Cardillo JE, Cohen M, et al., 1993 The locue ceruleus and dementia in Parkinson's disease. *Neurology* 43:986–991

Index